D1551057

DECISION ANALYSIS FOR HEALTHCARE MANAGERS

DECISION ANALYSIS FOR HEALTHCARE MANAGERS

Farrokh Alemi
David H. Gustafson

Health Administration Press, Chicago
AUPHA Press, Washington, DC

AUPHA
HAP

Your board, staff, or clients may also benefit from this book's insight. For more information on quantity discounts, contact the Health Administration Press Marketing Manager at (312) 424-9470.

11 10 09 08 07 5 4 3 2 1

Library of Congress Cataloging-in-Publication Data

Alemi, Farrokh.

Decision analysis for healthcare managers / Farrokh Alemi, David H. Gustafson.

p. cm.

Includes bibliographical references and index.

ISBN-13: 978-1-56793-256-0 (alk. paper)

ISBN-10: 1-56793-256-8 (alk. paper)

1. Health services administration—Decision making. 2. Hospitals—Quality control—Standards. I. Gustafson, David H. II. Title.

RA394.A44 2006

362.1068—dc22

2006041199

The paper used in this publication meets the minimum requirements of American National Standard for Information Sciences-Permanence of Paper for Printed Library Materials, ANSI Z39.48-1984.♾™

Acquisitions editor: Janet Davis; Project manager: Amanda Bove; Cover designer: Robert Rush

Health Administration Press
A division of the Foundation
of the American College of
Healthcare Executives
One North Franklin Street
Suite 1700
Chicago, IL 60606
(312) 424-2800

Association of University Programs
in Health Administration
2000 14th Street North
Suite 780
Arlington, VA 22201
(703) 894-0940

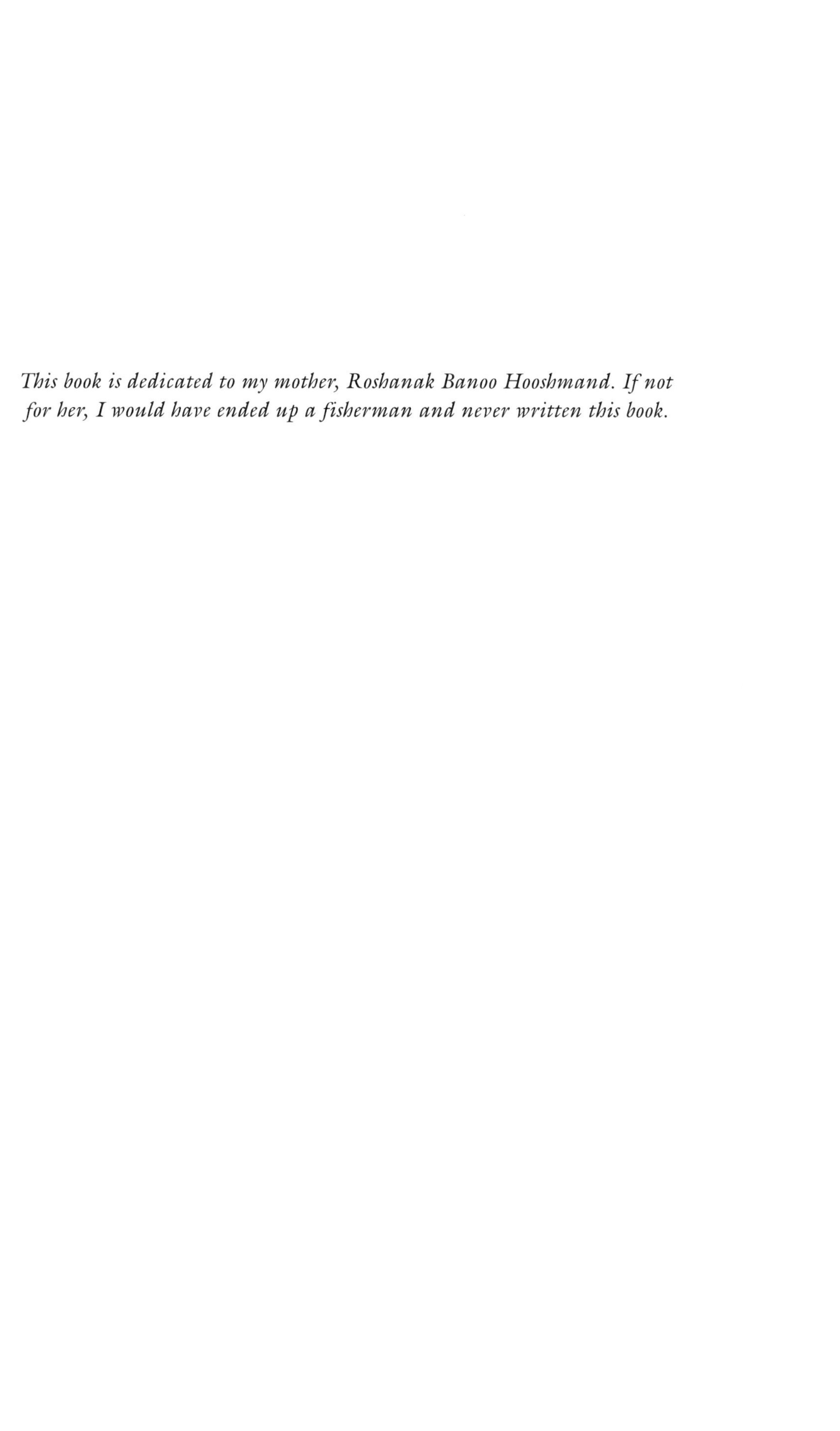

This book is dedicated to my mother, Roshanak Banoo Hooshmand. If not for her, I would have ended up a fisherman and never written this book.

CONTENTS

DETAILED CONTENTS

ACKNOWLEDGMENTS

Farrokh Alemi

I learned decision analysis from Dave Gustafson, who taught me to focus on insights and not mathematical rigor or numerical precision. It was a privilege to study with him, and now it is an even greater privilege to collaborate with him in writing this book. He remains a central influence in my career, and for that, I thank him.

I have worked with many program chairs and deans; P. J. Maddox stands out among them. She has an uncanny ability to challenge people and make them work harder than ever while supporting all they do. I am grateful to the environment she created at the Health System Management Program of George Mason University.

Jee Vang, one of my doctoral students, was a great help to me in explaining Bayesian networks. Jenny Sinkule, a psychology doctoral student and my research assistant, reviewed and improved the manuscript. Thanks to her efforts, I could focus on the bigger picture.

I should also thank the students in my decision analysis courses. When I first started teaching decision analysis, mostly to health administration and nursing students, the course was not well received. More than half of the students dropped the course; those who stuck with it, rated it one of the worst courses in their program. Their complaints were simple: the course content was not useful to them and it featured a lot of math they would never need or use. My students were and remain mostly professional women with little or no mathematical background; to them, all the talk of mathematical modeling seemed esoteric, impractical, and difficult.

I agreed with them and set out to change things. I knew the students were interested in improving quality of care, so I sought examples of modeling in improvement efforts. I tried to include examples of cost studies that would be relevant to their interests. I continuously changed the course content and made audio/visual presentations. Gradually, the course improved. Students stuck with it and evaluated it positively. It went from being rated one of the worst courses in the program to being rated as above average. The students acknowledged that math was their weakness but were excited about turning that weakness into one of their strengths. Word spread that graduates of the program could do things (such as using Bayesian networks) that graduates from other programs, sometimes even more rigorous MBA programs, could not do. For example, colleagues of a nursing student from our program were astonished when she conducted a root-cause analysis at her workplace. People became interested in the course, and faculty from other universities asked for permission to use some of the online material. The improvement efforts have continued and led to this book.

During the years that I wrote this book, I was supported with funded research projects from Health Resources and Services Administration, the National Institute of Drug Abuse (NIDA), the Substance Abuse and Mental Health Service Agency, the Robert Wood Johnson Foundation, and others. These research projects made a huge difference to my work and allowed me to explore areas I would not have had the time for otherwise. The risk assessment chapter grew directly out of one these funded research projects. I particularly want to thank Bill Cartwright, formerly of NIDA, who helped me a great deal with thinking through decision analytic approaches to cost studies. I also want to thank Mary Haack, a principal investigator in several of these grants, who remains my sounding board of what works in real situations.

Finally, I need to acknowledge my family—Mastee, Roshan, and Yara—who accepted, though never liked, how my worked spilled into my home life. There were times when we were on vacation and I needed to be on the Internet to fulfill a promise I had made to someone, somewhere, about something that seemed important at the time. When I committed to write this book, my workload greatly expanded. My family suffered from this expansion, but, in good humor, they supported me. Their support meant a lot to me, even when it was accompanied by eye rolls and expressions of incredulity that people actually do what I do.

PREFACE

Farrokh Alemi

Welcome to the world of decision analysis. This preface will introduce you to the purpose and organization of this book. This book describes how analytical tools can be used to help healthcare managers and policymakers make complex decisions. It provides numerous examples in healthcare settings, including benchmarking performance of clinicians, implementing projects, planning scenarios, allocating resources, analyzing the effect of HMO penetration, setting insurance rates, conducting root-cause analysis, and negotiating employment agreements.

More than 20 years ago, I wrote an article (Alemi 1986) arguing for the training of healthcare administrators in decision analysis. Despite widespread acceptance of the idea at the time, as demonstrated by published commentaries, decision analysis has not caught on with healthcare administrators as much as it has in other industries. Overall, the application of decision analysis in other industries is growing (Keefer, Kirkwood, and Corner 2004). MBA students are more likely to receive instruction in decision analysis; and when they go to work, they are more likely to use these tools. Goodwin and Wright (2004) give several descriptive examples of the use of decision analysis by managers:

- DuPont uses it to improve strategic decision making;
- Nuclear planners used decision analysis to select countermeasures to the Chernobyl disaster;
- ICI America uses it to select projects;
- Phillips Petroleum uses it to make oil exploration decisions;
- The U.S. military uses it to acquire new weapon systems;
- EXEL Logistics uses it to select a wide-area network; and
- ATM Ltd. uses it for scenario planning.

The list goes on. In contrast, there are only few applications to healthcare management reported in the literature. This would not be so ironic if it were not for the fact that there are numerous applications of decision analysis to clinical decision making and an increasing emphasis in healthcare on basing clinical decisions on evidence and data (Detsky et al. 1998). In this book we hope to change the situation in one of two ways. First, this book will highlight the applications of decision analysis to healthcare management. Healthcare managers can see for themselves how useful analysis can be in central problems they face. Second, this book covers decision analysis in enough depth so that readers can apply the tools to their own settings.

This book is ideally suited for students in healthcare administration programs. It may help these programs to develop courses in decision analysis. At the same time, the book will be useful for existing survey courses on quantitative analysis in terms of providing a more in-depth understanding of decision analysis so that students will feel confident in their abilities to apply these skills in their careers.

The book is also intended for clinicians who are interested in the application of decision analysis to improving quality of care. Often, practicing physicians, medical directors, nurse mangers, and clinical nurse leaders need to take a system perspective of patient care. This book provides them with analytical tools that can help them understand systems of care and evaluate the effect of these operations on patient outcomes. There are a number of books on clinical decision analysis, but this book includes applications to quality improvement that are not typically discussed in other clinical decision analysis books, including conducting a root-cause analysis, assessing severity of patients' illness, and benchmarking performance of clinicians. These are tools that can serve clinicians well if they want to improve healthcare settings.

Finally, this book may be useful in training healthcare policy analysts. Policy analysts have to provide accurate analysis under time pressures. Decision analysis is one tool that can help them provide relevant analysis in a timely fashion. The book contains a number of applications of decision analysis to policy decisions, including the design of health insurance programs and security analysis.

Organization of the Book

This book is organized into two broad sections. In the first section, various analytical tools (multi-attribute value models, Bayesian probability models, and decision trees) are introduced. In particular, the following chapters are included in the first part of the book:

1. **An Introduction to Decision Analysis.**
2. **Modeling Preferences.** This chapter demonstrates how to model a decision maker's values and preferences. It shows how to construct multi-attribute value and utility models—tools that are helpful in

evaluation tasks. In particular, it shows how to use multi-attribute value models in constructing severity indexes.

3. **Measuring Uncertainty.** This chapter introduces the concepts of probability and causal networks. It lays the groundwork for measuring uncertainty by a subjective assessment of probability. It also shows how to assess the concept of probabilistic independence—a concept central to model building.
4. **Modeling Uncertainty.** This chapter demonstrates how to assess the probability of uncertain, rare events based on several clues. This chapter introduces Bayes's odds form and shows how it can be used in forecasting future events. In particular, the chapter applies the Bayes's odds form to a market assessment for a new type of HMO.
5. **Decision Trees.** This chapter discusses how to combine utility and uncertainty in analyzing options available to healthcare managers. It includes analyzing the sensitivity of conclusions to errors in model parameters, and it shows how a decision tree can be used to analyze the effect of a new PPO on an employer.
6. **Modeling Group Decisions.** This chapter advises on how to obtain the preferences and uncertainties of a group of decision makers. This chapter describes the integrative group process.

In the second part of the book, the tools previously described are applied to various management decisions, including the following:

7. **Root-Cause Analysis.** This chapter applies Bayesian networks to root-cause modeling. The use of causal networks to conduct root-cause analysis of sentinel events is addressed.
8. **Cost-Effectiveness of Clinics.** This chapter demonstrates the use of decision trees for analyzing cost-effectiveness of clinical practices and cost of programs.
9. **Security-Risk Analysis.** This chapter applies Bayesian probability models to an assessment of privacy and security risks.
10. **Program Evaluation.** This chapter uses decision-analysis tools for program evaluation, using Bayesian probability models to analyze markets for new health services.
11. **Conflict Analysis.** This chapter shows the use of multi-attribute value modeling in analyzing conflict and conflict resolution. It also demonstrates how multi-attribute value models could be used to model conflict around a family-planning program. In addition, an example is given of a negotiation between an HMO manager and a physician.
12. **Benchmarking Clinicians.** This chapter addresses the use of decision analysis to construct measures of severity of illness of patients and to compare clinicians' performance across different patient populations.

13. **Rapid Analysis.** This chapter shows how subjective and objective data can be combined to conduct a rapid analysis of business and policy decisions.

Suggested Chapter Sequences

Some of the chapters in this book are interrelated and should be read in order. Chapter 6: Modeling Group Decisions should only be covered after the reader is familiar with modeling an individual's decision.

If you are modeling a decision maker's values, you may want to start with Chapter 2: Modeling Preferences and then read Chapter 10: Program Evaluation and Chapter 11: Conflict Analysis, both of which show the application of this tool.

Readers interested in learning about the use of probability models may want to start with Chapter 3: Measuring Uncertainty and then read Chapter 4: Modeling Uncertainty before reading Chapter 7: Root-Cause Analysis and Chapter 9: Security-Risk Analysis.

Healthcare administrators trying to understand and analyze complex decisions might want to look at decision trees. To do so, they need to read all of the chapters through Chapter 5: Decision Trees. Once they have read the fifth chapter, they should read Chapter 8: Cost-Effectiveness of Clinics and Chapter 12: Benchmarking Clinicians to see example applications.

Readers interested in conflict analysis may want to start with Chapter 2: Modeling Preferences and Chapter 6: Modeling Group Decisions before reading Chapter 11: Conflict Analysis.

This book was written to serve the needs of healthcare administration students. But other students can also benefit from a selection of chapters in this book. If this book is used as part of a course on risk analysis, for example, then readers should start with the Chapter 3: Measuring Uncertainty, Chapter 4: Modeling Uncertainty, and Chapter 6: Modeling Group Decisions before reading Chapter 9: Security-Risk Analysis.

In a course on policy analysis, this book might be used differently. The sequence of chapters that might be read are all chapters through Chapter 5: Decision Analysis, and then Chapter 8: Cost-Effectiveness of Clinics, Chapter 10: Program Evaluation, Chapter 11: Conflict Analysis, and Chapter 13: Rapid Analysis.

A course on quality improvement and patient safety may want to take an entirely different path through the book. These students would read all chapters through Chapter 5: Decision Trees, and then read Chapter 7: Root-Cause Analysis, Chapter 8: Cost-Effectiveness of Clinics, and Chapter 12: Benchmarking Clinicians.

Book Companion Web Site

This book has been based on an earlier book by Gustafson, Cats-Baril, and Alemi (1992). All of the chapters have gone through radical changes, and some are entirely new, but some, especially Chapter 6, Chapter 10, and Chapter 11, continue to be heavily influenced by the original book.

Writing a book is very time consuming; the first book took a decade to write, and this one took nearly three years. With such schedules, books can become out-of-date almost as soon as they are written. To remedy this problem, this book features a companion web site that should make the book significantly more useful. At this site, readers of this book can

- access software and online tools that aid decision analysis;
- listen to narrated lectures of key points;
- view students' examples of rapid-analysis exercises;
- follow animated examples of how to use computer programs to conduct an analysis;
- link to websites that provide additional information;
- download PowerPoint slides that highlight important concepts of each chapter; and
- see annotated bibliographies of additional readings.

Perhaps the most useful materials included on the web site are examples of decision analysis done by other students. Most chapters end with Rapid-Analysis Exercises. These are designed to both test the knowledge of the student as well as to give them confidence that they can do decision analysis without relying on consultants. Many students have said that what helps them the most in learning decision analysis is doing the Rapid-Analysis Exercises, and what helps them in doing these assignments is seeing the work of other students. This book's companion web site will feature such examples of students' work.

The idea is relatively simple: learn one, do one, and teach one. If you would like to include examples of how you have used the decision analytic tools you have learned to complete the Rapid-Analysis Exercises, please e-mail author Farrokh Alemi at falemi@gmu.edu so that your work can be posted on the companion web site.

When you learn decision analysis, you are admitted to a "club" of people who cherish the insights it provides. You will find that most decision analysts will be delighted to hear from you and will be intrigued with your approach to a problem. Most authors of books and articles on decision analysis would welcome your comments and queries. Use the resources on the web to network with your colleagues. Welcome to our midst!

Summary

We live in a fast-changing society where analysis is of paramount importance. Our hope is to help students solve pressing problems in our organizations and society. Good decisions based on a systematic consideration of all relevant factors and stakeholder opinions and values lead to good outcomes, both for those involved in the decision-making process and for the customers who are directly affected by the consequences and effects of such decisions.

References

Alemi, F. 1986. "Decision Analysis in Healthcare Administration Programs: An Experiment." *Journal of Health Administration Education* 4 (1): 45–61.

Detsky, A. S., G. Naglie, M. D. Krahn, D. Naimark, and D. A. Redelmeier. 1998. "Primer on Medical Decision Analysis: Part 1. Getting Started." *Medical Decision Making* 18 (2): 237–8.

Goodwin, P., and G. Wright. 2004. *Decision Analysis for Management Judgment, Third Edition*. Hoboken, NJ: John Wiley and Sons.

Gustafson, D. H., W. L. Cats-Baril, and F. Alemi. 1992. *Systems to Support Health Policy Analysis: Theory, Models, and Uses*. Chicago: Health Administration Press.

Keefer, D. L., C. W. Kirkwood, and J. L. Corner. 2004. "Perspective on Decision Analysis Applications, 1990–1991." *Decision Analysis* 1 (1): 4–22.

CHAPTER

1

INTRODUCTION TO DECISION ANALYSIS

Farrokh Alemi and David H. Gustafson

This chapter introduces the ideas behind decision analysis, the process of analysis, and its limitations. The discussion is directed toward decision analysts who help decision makers in healthcare institutions and healthcare policy analysts.

Any time a selection must be made among alternatives, a decision is being made, and it is the role of the analyst to assist in the decision-making process. When decisions are complicated and require careful consideration and systematic review of the available options, the analyst's role becomes paramount. An analyst needs to ask questions to understand who the decision makers are, what they value, and what complicates the decision. The analyst deconstructs complex decisions into component parts and then reconstitutes the final decision from those parts using a mathematical model. In the process, the analyst helps the decision maker think through the decision.

Some decisions are harder to make than others. For instance, some problems are poorly articulated. In other cases, the causes and effects of potential actions are uncertain. There may be confusion about what events could affect the decision. This book helps analysts learn how to clarify and simplify such problems without diminishing the usefulness or accuracy of the analysis. Decision analysis provides structure to the problems a manager faces, reduces uncertainty about potential future events, helps decision makers clarify their values and preferences, and reduces conflict among decision makers who may have different opinions about the utility of various options. This chapter outlines the steps involved in decision analysis, including exploring problems and clarifying goals, identifying decision makers, structuring problems, quantifying values and uncertainties, analyzing courses of action, and finally recommending the best course of action. This chapter provides a foundation for understanding the purpose and process of decision analysis. Later chapters will introduce more specific tools and skills that are meant to build upon this foundation.

This book has a companion web site that features narrated presentations, animated examples, PowerPoint slides, online tools, web links, additional readings, and examples of students' work. To access this chapter's learning tools, go to ache.org/DecisionAnalysis and select Chapter 1.

Who Is an Analyst?

This book is addressed to analysts who are trying to assist healthcare managers in making complex and difficult decisions. The definition of systems analysis[1] can be used to explain what an analyst is. An *analyst* studies the choices between alternative courses of action, typically by mathematical means, to reduce uncertainty and align the decision with the decision makers' goals.

This book assumes that the decision maker and the analyst are two different people. Of course, a decision maker might want to self-analyze his own decisions. In these circumstances, the tools described in the book can be used, but one person must play the roles of both the analyst and the decision maker. When managers want to think through their problems, they can use the tools in this book to analyze their own decisions without the need for an analyst.

Who Is a Decision Maker?

The *decision maker* receives the findings of the analysis and uses them to make the final decision. One of the first tasks of an analyst is to clarify who the decision makers are and what their timetable is. Many chapters in this book assume that a single decision maker is involved in the process, but sometimes more than one decision maker may be involved. Chapter 11 and Chapter 6 are intended for situations when multiple decision makers are involved.

Throughout the book, the assumption is that at least one decision maker is always available to the analyst. This is an oversimplification of the reality of organizations. Sometimes it is not clear who the decision maker is. Other times, an analysis starts with one decision maker who then leaves her position midway through the analysis; one person commissions the analysis and another person receives the findings. Sometimes an analyst is asked to conduct an analysis from a societal perspective, where it is difficult to clearly identify the decision makers. All of these variations make the process of analysis more difficult.

What Is a Decision?

This book is about using analytical models to find solutions to complex decisions. Before proceeding, various terms should be defined. Let's start with a definition of a decision. Most individuals go through their daily work without making any decisions. They react to events without taking the time to think about them. When the phone rings, they automatically answer it if they are available. In these situations, they are not deciding but just working. Sometimes, however, they need to make decisions. If they have to hire someone and there are many applicants, they need to make a decision. One situation is making a decision as opposed to following a routine. To make a *decision*[2] is to arrive at a final solution after consideration, ending dispute about what to do. A decision is made when a course of action is selected among alternatives. A decision has the following five components:

1. Multiple alternatives or options are available.
2. Each alternative leads to a series of consequences.
3. The decision maker is uncertain about what might happen.
4. The decision maker has different preferences about outcomes associated with various consequences.
5. A decision involves choosing among uncertain outcomes with different values.

What Is Decision Analysis?

Analysis[3] is defined as the separation of a whole into its component parts. *Decision analysis* is the process of separating a complex decision into its component parts and using a mathematical formula to reconstitute the whole decision from its parts. It is a method of helping decision makers choose the best alternative by thinking through the decision maker's preferences and values and by restructuring complex problems into simple ones. An analyst typically makes a mathematical model of the decision.

What Is a Model?

A *model* is an abstraction of the events and relationships influencing a decision. It usually involves a mathematical formula relating the various concepts together. The relationships in the model are usually quantified using numbers. A model tracks the relationship among various parts of a decision and helps the decision maker see the whole picture.

What Are Values?

A decision maker's *values* are his priorities. A decision involves multiple outcomes and, based on the decision maker's perspective, the relative worth of these outcomes would be different. Values show the relative desirability of the various courses of action in the eyes of the decision maker.

Values have two sides: cost and benefits. *Cost* is typically measured in dollars and may appear straightforward. However, true costs are complex measures that are difficult to quantify because certain costs, such as loss of goodwill, are nonmonetary and not easily tracked in budgets. Furthermore, monetary costs may be difficult to allocate to specific operations as overhead, and other shared costs may have to be divided in methods that seem arbitrary and imprecise.

Benefits need to be measured on the basis of various constituencies' preferences. Assuming that benefits and the values associated with them are unquantifiable can be a major pitfall. Benefits should not be subservient to cost, because values associated with benefits often drive the actual decision. By assuming that values cannot be quantified, the analysis may ignore concerns most likely to influence the decision maker.

An Example

A hypothetical situation faced by the head of the state agency responsible for evaluating nursing home quality can demonstrate the use of decision analysis. A nursing home has been overmedicating its residents in an effort to restrain them, and the administrator of the state agency must take action to improve care at the home. The possible actions include fining the home, prohibiting admissions, and teaching the home personnel how to appropriately use psychotropic drugs.

Any real-world decision has many different effects. For instance, the state could institute a training program to help the home improve its use of psychotropic drugs, but the state's action could have effects beyond changing this home's drug utilization practices. The nursing home could become more careful about other aspects of its care, such as how it plans care for its patients. Or the nursing home industry as a whole could become convinced that the state is enforcing stricter regulations on the administration of psychotropic drugs. Both of these effects are important dimensions that should be considered during the analysis and in any assessment performed afterward.

The problem becomes more complex because the agency administrators must consider which constituencies' values should be taken into account and what their values are regarding the proposed actions. For example, the administrator may want the state to portray a tougher image to the nursing home industry, but one constituent, the chairman of an important legislative committee, may object to this image. Therefore, the choice of action will depend on which constituencies' values are considered and how much importance each constituency is assigned.

Prototypes for Decision Analysis

Real decisions are complex. Analysis does not model a decision in all its complexity. Some aspects of the decision are ignored and not considered fundamental to the choice at hand. The goal is not to impress, and in the process overwhelm, the decision maker with the analyst's ability to capture all possibilities. Rather, the goal of analysis is to simplify the decision enough to meet the decision maker's needs. An important challenge, then, is to determine how to simplify an analysis without diminishing its usefulness and accuracy. When an analyst faces a decision with interrelated events, a tool called a decision tree might be useful (see Chapter 4).

Over the years, as analysts have applied various tools to simplify and model decisions, some prototypes have emerged. If an analyst can recognize that a decision is like one of the prototypes in her arsenal of solutions, then she can quickly address the problem. Each prototype leads to some simplification of the problem and a specific analytical solution. The existence of these prototypes helps in addressing the problem with known tools and methods. Following are five of these prototypes:

1. The unstructured problem
2. Uncertainty about future events
3. Unclear values
4. Potential conflict
5. The need to do it all

Prototype 1: The Unstructured Problem

Sometimes decision makers do not truly understand the problem they are addressing. This lack of understanding can manifest itself in disagreements about the proper course of action. The members of a decision-making team may prefer different reasonable actions based on their limited perspectives of the issue. In this prototype, the problem needs to be structured so the decision makers understand all of the various considerations involved in the decision. An analyst can promote better understanding of the decision by helping policy makers to explicitly identify the following:

- Individual assumptions about the problem and its causes
- Objectives being pursued by each decision maker
- Different perceptions and values of the constituencies
- Available options
- Events that influence the desirability of various outcomes
- Principal uncertainties about future outcomes

A good way to structure the problem is for the analyst to listen to the decision maker's description of various aspects of the problem. As Figure 1.1 shows, uncertainty and constituencies' values can cloud the decision; the analyst usually seeks to understand the nature of the problem by clarifying the values and uncertainties involved. When the problem is fully described, the analyst can provide an organized summary to the decision makers, helping them see the whole and its parts.

Prototype 2: Uncertainty About Future Events

Decision makers are sometimes not sure what will happen if an action is taken, and they may not be sure about the state of their environment. For example, what is the chance that initiating a fine will really change the way the nursing home uses psychotropic drugs? What is the chance that a hospital administrator opens a stroke unit and competitors do the same? In this prototype, the analyst needs to reduce the decision maker's uncertainty.

In the nursing home example, there were probably some clues about whether the nursing home's overmedication was caused by ignorance or greed. However, the clues are neither equally important nor measured on a common scale. The analyst helps to compress the clues to a single scale for comparison. The analyst can use the various clues to clarify the reason for the use of psychotropic drugs and thus help the decision maker choose between a punitive course of action or an educational course of action.

Some clues suggest that the target event (e.g., eliminating the overmedication of nursing home patients) might occur, and other clues suggest the opposite. The analyst must distill the implications of these contradictory clues into a single forecast. Deciding on the nature and relative importance of these clues is difficult, because people tend to assess complex uncertainties poorly unless they can divide them into manageable components. Decision analysis can help make this division by using probability models that combine components after their individual contributions have been determined. This book addresses such a probability model, the Bayes's theorem, in Chapter 4.

Prototype 3: Unclear Values

In some situations, the options and future outcomes are clearly identified, and uncertainty plays a minor role. However, the values influencing the

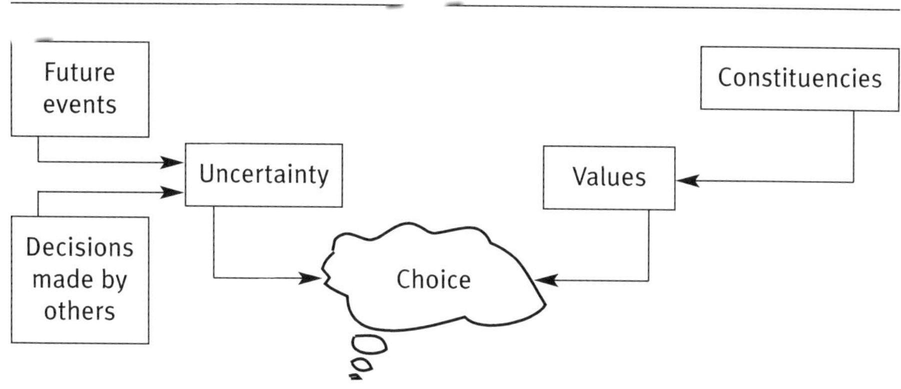

FIGURE 1.1 Decisions Are Difficult When Values and Uncertainty Are Unstructured

options and outcomes might be unclear. A value is the decision maker's judgment of the relative worth or importance of something. Even if there is a single decision maker, it is sometimes important to clarify his priorities and values.

The decision maker's actions will have many outcomes, some of which are positive and others negative. One option may be preferable on one dimension but unacceptable on another. The decision maker must trade off the gains in one dimension with losses in another.

In traditional attempts to debate options, advocates of one option focus on the dimensions that show it having a favorable outcome, while opponents attack it on dimensions on which it performs poorly. The decision maker listens to both sides but has to make up her own mind. Optimally, a decision analysis provides a mechanism to force consideration of all dimensions, a task that requires answers to the following questions:

- Which objectives are paramount?
- How can an option's performance on a wide range of measurement scales be collapsed into an overall measure of relative value?

For example, a common value problem is how to allocate limited resources to various individuals or options. The British National Health Service, which has a fixed budget, deals with this issue quite directly. Some money is allocated to hip replacement, some to community health services, and some to long-term institutional care for the elderly. Many people who request a service after the money has run out must wait until the next year. Similarly, a CEO has to trade off various projects in different departments and decide on the budget allocation for the unit. The decision analysis approach to these questions uses multi-attribute value (MAV) modeling, which is discussed in Chapter 2.

Prototype 4: Potential Conflict

In this prototype, an analyst needs to help decision makers better understand conflict by modeling the uncertainties and values that different constituencies see in the same decision. Common sense tells us that people with different values tend to choose different options, as shown in Figure 1.2. The principal challenges facing a decision-making team may be understanding how different constituencies view and value a problem and determining what trade-offs will lead to a win-win, instead of a win-lose, solution. Decision analysis addresses situations like this by developing an MAV model (addressed further in Chapter 2) for each constituency and by using these models to generate new options that are mutually beneficial (see Chapter 11).

Consider, for example, a contract between a health maintenance organization (HMO) and a clinician. The contract will have many components. The parties will need to make decisions on cost, benefits, professional independence, required practice patterns, and other such issues. The HMO representatives and the clinician have different values and preferred outcomes. An analyst can identify the issues and highlight the values and preferences of the parties. The conflict can then be understood, and steps can be taken to avoid escalation of conflict to a level that disrupts the negotiations.

Prototype 5: The Need to Do it All

Of course, a decision can have all of the elements of the last four prototypes. In these circumstances, the analyst must use a number of different tools and integrate them into a seamless analysis.

Figure 1.3 shows the multiple components of a decision that an analyst must consider when working in this prototype.

An example of this prototype is a decision about a merger between two hospitals. There are many decision makers, all of whom have different values and none of whom fully understand the nature of the problem. There are numerous actions leading to outcomes that are positive on some levels and negative on others. There are many uncertain consequences associated with the merger that could affect the different outcomes, and the outcomes do not have equal value. In this example, the decision analyst needs to address all of these issues before recommending a course of action.

Steps in Decision Analysis

Good analysis is about the process, not the end results. It is about the people, not the numbers. It uses numbers to track ideas, but the analysis is

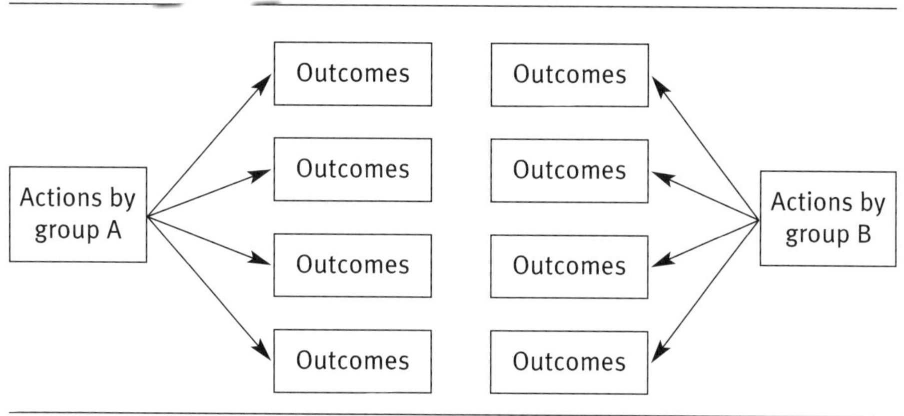

FIGURE 1.2 Decisions Are Difficult When Constituencies Prefer Different Outcomes

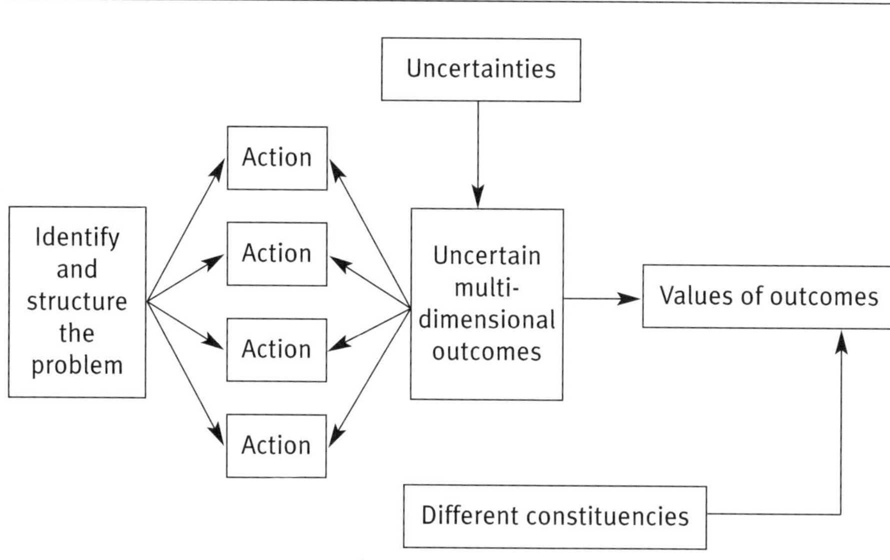

FIGURE 1.3 Components of a Decision

about the ideas and not the numbers. One way to analyze a decision is for the analyst to conduct an independent analysis and present the results to the decision maker in a brief paper. This method is usually not very helpful to the decision maker, however, because it emphasizes the findings as opposed to the process. Decision makers are more likely to accept an analysis in which they have actively participated.

The preferred method is to conduct decision analysis as a series of increasingly sophisticated interactions with the decision maker. At each interaction, the analyst listens and summarizes what the decision maker says. In each step, the problem is structured and an analytical model is created. Through these cycles, the decision maker is guided to his own conclusions, which the analysis documents.

Whether the analysis is done for one decision maker or for many, there are several distinct steps in decision analysis. A number of investigators have suggested steps in conducting decision analysis (Soto 2002; Philips et al. 2004; Weinstein et al. 2003). Soto (2002), working in the context of clinical decision analysis, recommends that all analyses should take the following 13 steps:

1. Clearly state the aim and the hypothesis of the model.
2. Provide the rationale of the modeling.
3. Describe the design and structure of the model.
4. Expound the analytical time horizon chosen.
5. Specify the perspective chosen and the target decision makers.
6. Describe the alternatives under evaluation.
7. State entirely the data sources used in the model.
8. Report outcomes and the probability that they occur.
9. Describe medical care utilization of each alternative.
10. Present the analyses performed and report the results.
11. Carry out sensitivity analysis.
12. Discuss the results and raise the conclusions of the study.
13. Declare a disclosure of relationships.

This book recommends the following eight steps in the process of decision analysis.

Step 1: Identify Decision Makers, Constituencies, Perspectives, and Time Frames

Who makes the decision is not always clear. Some decisions are made in groups, others by individuals. For some decisions, there is a definite deadline; for others, there is no clear time frame. Some decisions have already been made before the analyst comes on board; other decisions involve much uncertainty that the analyst needs to sort out. Sometimes the person who sponsors the analysis is preparing a report for a decision-making body that is not available to the analyst. Other times, the analyst is in direct contact with the decision maker. Decision makers may also differ in the perspective they want the analysis to take. Sometimes providers' costs and utilities are central; other times, patients' values drive the analysis. Sometimes societal perspective is adopted; other times, the problem is analyzed from the perspective of a company. Decision analysis can help in all of these situations, but in each of them the analyst should explicitly specify the decision makers, the perspective of the analysis, and the time frame for the decision.

It is also important to identify and understand the constituencies, whose ideas and values must be present in the model. A decision analyst can always assume that only one constituency exists and that disagreements arise primarily from misunderstandings of the problem rather than from different value systems among the various constituencies. But when several constituencies have different assumptions and values, the analyst must examine the problem from the perspective of each constituency.

A choice must also be made about who will provide input into the decision analysis. Who will specify the options, outcomes, and uncertainties? Who will estimate values and probabilities? Will outside experts be called in? Which constituencies will be involved? Will members of the decision-making team provide judgments independently, or will they work as a team to identify and explore differences of opinion? Obviously, all of these choices depend on the decision, and an analyst should simply ask questions and not supply answers.

Step 2: Explore the Problem and the Role of the Model

Problem exploration is the process of understanding why the decision maker wants to solve a problem. The analyst needs to understand what the resolution of the problem is intended to achieve. This understanding is crucial because it helps identify creative options for action and sets some criteria for evaluating the decision. The analyst also needs to clarify the purpose of the modeling effort. The purpose might be to

- keep track of ideas,
- have a mathematical formula that can replace the decision maker in repetitive decisions,
- clarify issues to the decision maker,
- help others understand why the decision maker chose a course of action,
- document the decision,
- help the decision maker arrive at self-insight,
- clarify values, or
- reduce uncertainty.

Let's return to the earlier example of the nursing home that was restraining its residents with excessive medication. The problem exploration might begin by understanding the problem statement: "Excessive use of drugs to restrain residents." Although this type of statement is often taken at face value, several questions could be asked: How should nursing home residents behave? What does "restraint" mean? Why must residents be restrained? Why are drugs used at all? When are drugs appropriate, and when are they not appropriate? What other alternatives does a nursing home have to deal with problem behavior?

The questions at this stage are directed at (1) helping to understand the objective of an organization, (2) defining frequently misunderstood terms, (3) clarifying the practices causing the problem, (4) understanding the reasons for the practice, and (5) separating desirable from undesirable aspects of the practice.

During this step, the decision analyst must determine which ends, or objectives, will be achieved by solving the problem. In the example, the decision analyst must determine whether the goal is primarily to

1. protect an individual patient without changing overall methods in the nursing home;
2. correct a problem facing several patients (in other words, change the home's general practices); or
3. correct a problem that appears to be industry-wide.

Once these questions have been answered, the decision analyst and decision maker will have a much better grasp on the problem. The selected objective will significantly affect both the type of actions considered and the particular action selected.

Step 3: Structure the Problem

Once the decision makers have been identified and the problem has been explored, the analyst needs to add conceptual detail by structuring the problem. The goals of structuring the problem are to clearly articulate the following:

- What the problem is about, why it exists, and whom it affects
- The assumptions and objectives of each affected constituency
- A creative set of options for the decision maker
- Outcomes to be sought or avoided
- The uncertainties that affect the choice of action

Structuring is the stage in which the specific set of decision options is identified. Although the generation of options is critical, it is often overlooked by decision makers, which is a pitfall that can easily promote conflict in cases where diametrically opposed options falsely appear to be the only possible alternatives. Often, creative solutions can be identified that better meet the needs of all constituencies. To generate better options, one must understand the purpose of analysis. The process of identifying new options relies heavily on reaching outside the organization for theoretical and practical experts, but the process should also encourage insiders to see the problem in new ways.

It is important to explicitly identify the objectives and assumptions of the decision makers. Objectives are important because they lead to the preference of one option over the other. If the decision-making team can understand what each constituency is trying to achieve, the team can analyze and understand its preferences more easily. The same argument holds for assumptions: Two people with similar objectives but different assumptions about how the world operates can examine the same evidence and reach widely divergent conclusions.

Take, for example, the issue of whether two hospitals should merge. Assume that both constituencies—those favoring and those opposing such merger—want the hospital to grow and prosper. One constituency believes the merger will help the hospital grow faster, and the other believes the merger will make the organization lose focus. One constituency believes the community will be served better by competition, and the other believes the community will benefit from collaboration between the institutions. In each case, the assumptions (and their relative importance) influence the choice of objectives and action, and that is why they should be identified and examined during problem structuring.

Problem structuring is a cyclical process—the structure may change once the decision makers have put more time into the analysis. The cyclical nature of the structuring process is desirable rather than something to be avoided. An analyst should be willing to go back and start all over with a new structure and a new set of options.

Step 4: Quantify the Values

The analyst should help the decision maker break complex outcomes into their components and weight the relative value of each component. The components can be measured on the same scale, called a value scale, and an equation can be constructed to permit the calculation of the overall value of an option.

Step 5: Quantify the Uncertainties

The analyst interacts with decision makers and experts to quantify uncertainties about future events. Returning to the previous example, if the nursing home inspectors were asked to estimate the chances that the home's chemical restraint practice resulted from ignorance or greed, they might agree that the chances were 90 percent ignorance and 10 percent greed. In some cases, additional data are needed to assess the probabilities. In other cases, too much data are available. In both cases, the probability assessment must be divided into manageable components. Bayes's theorem (see Chapter 4) provides one means for disaggregating complex uncertainties into their components.

Step 6: Analyze the Data and Recommend a Course of Action

Once values and uncertainties are quantified, the analyst uses the model of the decision to score the relative desirability of each possible action. This can be done in different ways, depending on what type of a model has been developed. One way is to examine the expected value of the outcomes. *Expected value* is the weighted average of the values associated with outcomes of each action. Values are weighted by the probability of occurrence for each outcome. Suppose, in the nursing home example, that the following two actions are selected by the decision maker for further analysis:

1. Teach staff the proper use of psychotropic drugs
2. Prohibit admissions to the home

The possible outcomes of the above actions are as follows:

1. Industry-wide change: Chemical restraint is corrected in the home, and the nursing home industry gets the message that the state intends tougher regulation of drugs.
2. Specific nursing home change: The specific nursing home changes, but the rest of industry does not get the message.
3. No change: The nursing home ignores the chosen action, and there is no impact on the industry.

Suppose the relative desirability of each outcome is as follows:

1. Industry-wide change has a value score of 100, which is the most desirable possible outcome.
2. Specific nursing home change has a value score of 25.
3. No change has a value score of zero, which is the worst possible outcome.

The probability that each action will lead to each outcome is shown in the six cells of the matrix in Figure 1.4.

The *expected value principle* says the desirability of each action is the sum of the values of each outcome of the action weighted by the probability of the outcome. If P_{ij} is the probability of action i leading to outcome j and V_j is the value associated with outcome j, then expected value is

$$\text{Expected value of action } i = \sum P_{ij} \times V_j.$$

In the case of the example, expected values are as follows:

$$\text{Expected value of consultation} = (0.05 \times 100) + (0.60 \times 25) + (0.35 \times 0) = 20,$$

FIGURE 1.4
Decision Matrix

		Possible Outcomes			
		Industry-wide Change Value = 100	Specific Nursing Home Change Value = 25	No Change Value = 0	Expected Value
Possible Actions	Teach staff the appropriate use of psychotropic drugs	5% chance of occurrence .05 × 100 = 5	60% chance of occurrence .60 × 25 = 15	35% chance of occurrence .35 × 0 = 0	20
	Prohibit admissions to the hospital	40% chance of occurrence .40 × 100 = 40	20% chance of occurrence .20 × 25 = 5	40% chance of occurrence .40 × 0 = 0	45

Expected value for stopping admission =
$(0.40 \times 100) + (0.20 \times 25) + (0.40 \times 0) = 45.$

As shown in Figure 1.4, the expected value for teaching staff about psychotropic drugs is 20, whereas the expected value for prohibiting admissions is 45. This analysis suggests that the most desirable action would be to prohibit admissions because its expected value is larger than teaching the staff. In this simple analysis, you see how a mathematical model is used, how uncertainty and values are quantified, and how the model is used to track ideas and make a picture of the whole for the decision maker.

Step 7: Conduct a Sensitivity Analysis

The analyst interacts with the decision maker to identify how various assumptions affect the conclusion. The previous analysis suggests that teaching staff is an inferior decision to prohibiting admissions. However, this should not be taken at face value because the value and probability estimates might not be accurate. Perhaps the estimates were guesses, or the estimates were average scores from a group, some of whose members had little faith in the estimates. In these cases, it would be valuable to know whether the choice would be affected by using a different set of estimates. Stated another way, it might make sense to use sensitivity analysis to determine how much an estimate would have to change to alter the expected value of the suggested action.

Usually, one estimate is changed until the expected value of the two choices become the same. Of course, several estimates can also be modified at once, especially using computers. Sensitivity analysis can be vital not only to examining the impact of errors in estimation but also to determining which variables need the most attention.

At each stage in the decision analysis process, it is possible and often essential to return to an earlier stage to

- add a new action or outcome,
- add new uncertainties,
- refine probability estimates, or
- refine estimates of values.

This cyclical approach offers a better understanding of the problem and fosters greater confidence in the analysis. Often, the decision recommended by the analysis is not the one implemented, but the analysis is helpful because it increases understanding of the issues. Phillips (1984) refers to this as the theory of requisite decisions: Once all parties agree that the problem representation is adequate for reaching the decision, the model is "requisite."

From this point of view, decision analysis is more an aid to problem solving than a mathematical technique. Considered in this light, decision analysis provides the decision maker with a process for thinking about her actions. It is a practical means for maintaining control of complex decision problems that involve risk, uncertainty, and multiple objectives (Phillips 1984; Goodwin and Wright 2004).

Step 8: Document and Report Findings

Even though the decision maker has been intimately involved in the analysis and is probably not surprised at its conclusions, the analysis should document and report the findings. An analysis has its own life cycle and may live well beyond the current decision. Individuals not involved in the decision-making process may question the rationale behind the decision. For such reasons, it is important to document all considerations that were put into the analysis. A clear documentation, one that uses multimedia to convey the issues, would also help create a consensus behind a decision.

Limitations of Decision Analysis

It is difficult to evaluate the effectiveness of decision analysis because often no information is available on what might have happened if decision makers had not followed the course of action recommended by the analysis.

One way to improve the accuracy of analysis is to make sure that the process of analysis is followed faithfully. Rouse and Owen (1998) suggest asking the following six questions about decision analysis to discern if it was done accurately:

1. Were all realistic strategies included?
2. Was the appropriate type of model employed?
3. Were all important outcomes considered?
4. Was an explicit and sensible process used to identify, select, and combine the evidence into probabilities?
5. Were values assigned to outcomes plausible, and were they obtained in a methodologically acceptable manner?
6. Was the potential impact of any uncertainty in the probability and value estimates thoroughly and systematically evaluated?

These authors also point out four serious limitations to decision analysis, which are important to keep in mind:

1. Decision analysis may oversimplify problems to the point that they do not reflect real concerns or accurately represent the perspective from which the analysis is being conducted.
2. Available data simply may be inadequate to support the analysis.
3. Value assessment, in particular assessment of quality of life, may be problematic. Measuring quality of life, while conceptually appealing and logical, has proven methodologically problematic and philosophically controversial.
4. Outcomes of decision analyses may not be amenable to traditional statistical analysis. Strictly, by the tenets of decision analysis, the preferred strategy or treatment is the one that yields the greatest value (or maximizes the occurrence of favorable outcomes), no matter how narrow the margin of improvement.

In the end, the value of decision analysis (with all of its limitations) is in the eye of the beholder. If the decision maker better understands and has new insights into a problem, or if the problem and suggested course of action can be documented and communicated to others more easily, then a decision maker may judge decision analysis, even an imperfect analysis, as useful.

Summary

This chapter introduces the concept of decision analysis and the role an analyst plays in assisting organizations make important choices amidst complicated situations. The analyst breaks the problem into manageable, understandable parts and ensures that important values and preferences are taken into consideration. This chapter introduces basic concepts, such as decision analysts, decision makers, and decisions. Key issues in decision analysis, such as how to simplify an analysis without diminishing its usefulness and accuracy, are also discussed. Several prototype methods for decision analysis are reviewed, including MAV modeling, Bayesian probability models, and decision trees. This chapter ends with a step-by-step guide to decision analysis and a discussion of the limitations of decision analysis.

Review What You Know

In the following questions, describe a nonclinical work-related decision. Describe who makes the decision, what actions are possible, what the resulting outcomes are, and how these outcomes are evaluated:

1. Who makes the decision?
2. What actions are possible (list at least two actions)?
3. What are the possible outcomes?
4. Besides cost, what other values enter these decision?
5. Whose values are considered relevant to the decision?
6. Why are the outcomes uncertain?

Audio/Visual Chapter Aids

To help you understand the concepts of decision analysis, visit this book's companion web site at ache.org/DecisionAnalysis, go to Chapter 1, and view the audio/visual chapter aids.

Notes

1. *Merriam-Webster's Collegiate Dictionary*, 11th ed., s.v. "Systems analysis."
2. *Merriam-Webster's Collegiate Dictionary*, 11th ed., s.v. "Decide."
3. *Merriam-Webster's Collegiate Dictionary*, 11th ed., s.v. "Analysis."

References

Goodwin, P., and G. Wright. 2004. *Decision Analysis for Management Judgment.* 3rd ed. Hoboken, NJ: John Wiley and Sons.

Philips, Z., L. Ginnelly, M. Sculpher, K. Claxton, S. Golder, R. Riemsma, N. Woolacoot, and J. Glanville. 2004. "Review of Guidelines for Good Practice in Decision-Analytic Modelling in Health Technology Assessment." *Health Technology Assessment* 8 (36): iii–iv, ix–xi, 1–158.

Phillips, L. D. 1984. "A Theory of Requisite Decision Models." *Acta Psychologica* 56: 29–48.

Rouse, D. J., and J. Owen. 1998. "Decision Analysis." *Clinical Obstetrics and Gynecology* 41 (2): 282–95.

Soto, J. 2002. "Health Economic Evaluations Using Decision Analytic Modeling. Principles and Practices: Utilization of a Checklist to Their Development and Appraisal." *International Journal of Technology Assessment in Healthcare* 18 (1): 94–111.

Weinstein, M. C, B. O'Brien, J. Hornberger, J. Jackson, M. Johannesson, C. McCabe, and B. R. Luce. 2003. "Principles of Good Practice for Decision Analytic Modeling in Health-Care Evaluation: Report of the ISPOR Task Force on Good Research Practices—Modeling Studies." *Value Health* 6 (1): 9–17.

CHAPTER

2

MODELING PREFERENCES

Farrokh Alemi and David H. Gustafson

This chapter introduces methods for modeling decision makers' values: multi-attribute value (MAV) and multi-attribute utility models. These models are useful in decisions where more than one thing is considered important.

In this chapter, a model is developed for one decision maker. (For more information on modeling a group decision, consult Chapter 6.) Altough the model-building effort focuses on the interaction between an analyst and a decision maker, the same process can be used for self-analysis: A decision maker can build a model of her own decisions without the help of an analyst.

Value models are based on Bernoulli's (1738) recognition that money's value does not always equal its amount. He postulated that increasing the amount of income has decreasing value to the wage earner. A comprehensive and rather mathematical introduction to constructing value models was written by Von Winterfeldt and Edwards (1986): This chapter ignores this mathematical foundation, however, to focus on behavioral instructions for making value models.

Value models quantify a person's priorities and preferences. Value models assign numbers to options so that higher numbers reflect more preferred options. These models assume that the decision maker must select from several options and that the selection should depend on grading the preferences for the options. These preferences are quantified by examining the various attributes (i.e., characteristics, dimensions, or features) of the options. For example, if a decision maker were choosing among different electronic health record (EHR) systems, the value of the different EHR systems could be scored by examining such attributes as compatibility with legacy systems, potential effect on practice patterns, and cost. First, the effect of each EHR system on each attribute would be scored—this is often called *single-attribute value function*. Second, scores would be weighted by the relative importance of each attribute. Third, the scores for all attributes would be aggregated, often by using a weighted sum. Fourth, the EHR with the highest weighted score would be chosen.

This book has a companion web site that features narrated presentations, animated examples, PowerPoint slides, online tools, web links, additional readings, and examples of students' work. To access this chapter's learning tools, go to ache.org/DecisionAnalysis and select Chapter 2.

If each option were described in terms of n attributes $A_1, A_2, \ldots, A_n$, then each option would be assigned a score on each attribute: $V(A_1)$, $V(A_2), \ldots, V(A_n)$. The overall value of an option is

$$\text{Value} = \text{Function}\ [V(A_1), V(A_2), \ldots, V(A_n)].$$

In other words, the overall value of an option is a function of the value of the option on each attribute.

Why Model Values?

Values (e.g., attitudes, preferences) play major roles in making management decisions. As mentioned in the first chapter, a *value* is a principle or quality that is intrinsically desirable. It refers to the relative worth, utility, or importance of something. In organizations, decision making is often very complex and a product of collective action. Frequently, decisions must be made concerning issues on which little data exist, forcing managers to make decisions on the basis of opinions rather than fact. Often, there is no correct resolution to a problem because all options are equally legitimate and values play major roles in the final choice.

Many everyday decisions involve value trade-offs. Often, a decision entails finding a way to balance a set of factors that are not all attainable at the same time. Thus, some factors must be given up in exchange for others. Decisions that can benefit from MAV modeling include the following:

- Purchasing software and equipment,
- Contracting with vendors,
- Adding a new clinic or program,
- Initiating float staffing,
- Hiring new staff or paying overtime,
- Balancing missions (e.g., providing service with revenue generating activities), and
- Pursuing quality improvement projects.

In all these decisions, the manager has to trade gains in one area against losses in other areas.

For example, initiating a quality improvement project in a stroke unit means you might not have resources to do the same in a trauma unit, or hiring a technically savvy person may mean you will have to put up with social ineptness. In business, difficult decisions usually involve giving up something to attain other benefits.

Most people acknowledge that a manager's decisions involve consideration of value trade-offs. This is not a revelation. What is unusual is that decision analysts model these values. Some may wonder why the analyst needs to model and quantify value trade-offs. The reasons for modeling decision maker's values include the following:

1. *To clarify and communicate decision makers' perspectives.* Modeling values helps managers communicate their positions by explicitly showing their priorities. These models clarify the basis of decisions so others can see the logic behind the decision and ideally agree with it. For example, Cline, Alemi, and Bosworth (1982) constructed a value model to determine the eligibility of nursing home residents for a higher level of reimbursement (i.e., the "super-skilled" level of nursing care). This model showed which attributes of an applicant affected eligibility and how much weight each attribute deserved. Because of this effort, the regulator, the industry, the care providers, and the patients became more aware of how eligibility decisions were made.
2. *To aid decision making in complex situations.* In complicated situations, decision makers face uncertain events as well as ill-expressed values. In these circumstances, modeling the values adds to the decision maker's understanding of the underlying problem. It helps the decision maker break the problem into its parts and manage the decision more effectively. In short, models help decision makers divide and conquer. Because of the modeling, decision makers may arrive at insight into their own values.
3. *To repeatedly consult the mathematical model instead of the decision maker.* Consider screening a large number of job applicants. If the analyst models the decision maker's values, then he could go through thousands of applicants and select a few that the manager needs to interview. Because the model reflects the manager's values, the analyst is reassured that he has not erroneously screened out applicants that the manager would have liked to interview.
4. *To quantify hard-to-measure concepts.* Concepts such as the severity of illness (Krahn et al. 2000), the medically underserved area (Fos and Zuniga 1999), or the quality of the remaining years of life (Chiou et al. 2005) are difficult concepts to define or measure. These hard-

to-measure concepts are similar to preferences because they are subjective and open to disagreement. Modeling describes these hard-to-measure concepts in terms of several objective attributes that are easier to measure.

Chatburn and Primiano (2001) used value models to examine large capital purchases, such as the decision to purchase a ventilator. Value models have also been used to evaluate drug therapy options (Eriksen and Keller 1993), to measure nurse practice patterns (Anthony et al. 2004), and to evaluate a benefit manager's preferences for smoking cessation programs (Spoth 1990).

Misleading Numbers

Though value models allow you to quantify subjective concepts, the resulting numbers are rough estimates that should not be mistaken for precise measurements. It is important that managers do not read more into the numbers than they mean. Analysts must stress that the numbers in value models are intended to offer a consistent method of tracking, comparing, and communicating rough, subjective concepts and not to claim a false sense of precision.

An important distinction is whether the model is to be used for rank ordering (ordinal scale) or for rating the worth of options (interval scale). Some value models produce numbers that are only useful for rank-ordering options. For example, some severity indexes indicate whether one patient is sicker than another, not how much sicker. In these circumstances, a patient with a severity score of four may not be twice as ill as a patient with a severity score of two. Averaging such ordinal scores is meaningless. In contrast, value models that score on an interval scale show how much more preferable one option is than another. For example, a severity index can be created to show how much more severe one patient's condition is than another's. A patient scoring four can be considered twice as ill as one scoring two. Further, averaging interval scores is meaningful.

Numbers can also be used as a means of classification, such as the nominal scale. Nominal scales produce numbers that are neither ordinal nor interval—for example, the numbers assigned to diseases in the international classification of diseases.

In modeling decision makers' values, single-attribute value functions must be interval scales. If single attributes are measured on an interval scale, these numbers can be added or multiplied to produce the overall score. If measured as an ordinal scale or a nominal scale, one cannot calculate the overall severity from the single-attribute values. In contrast, overall scores for options need only have an ordinal property. When choosing one option over another, most decision makers care about which option has the highest rating, not how much higher that rating is.

Keep in mind that the purpose of quantification is not to be precise in numerical assessment. The analyst quantifies values of various attributes so that the calculus of mathematics can be used to keep track of them and to produce an overall score that reflects the decision maker's preferences. Quantification allows the use of logic embedded in numbers in aggregation of values across attributes. In the end, model scores are a rough approximation of preferences. They are helpful not because they are precise but because they adequately track contributions of each attribute.

Examples of the Use of Value Models

There are many occasions in which value models can be used to model a decision. A common example is in hiring decisions. In choosing among candidates, the attributes shown in Table 2.1 might be used to screen applicants for subsequent interviews.

In Table 2.1, each attribute has an assigned weight. Each attribute level has an assigned value score. By common convention, attribute levels are set to range from zero to 100. Attribute levels are set so that only one level can be assigned to each applicant. Attribute weights are set so that all weights add up to one. The overall value of an applicant can be measured as the weighted sum of attribute-level scores. In this example, the model assigns to each applicant a score between zero and 100, where 100 is the most preferred applicant. Note that the way the decision maker has rated these attributes suggests that internal promotion is less important than appropriate educational degrees and computer experience. The model can be used to focus interviews on a handful of applicants.

Consider another example about organizing a health fair. Assume that a decision needs to be made about which of the following screenings should be included in the fair:

- Blood pressure
- Peak air flow
- Lack of exercise
- Smoking habits
- Knowledge of breast self-examination
- Depression
- Poor food habits
- Access to a primary care clinician
- Blood sugar levels

TABLE 2.1 A Model for Hiring Decisions

Attribute Weight	*Attribute*	*Attribute Level*	*Value of the Level*
.40	Applicant's education	No college degree	0
		Bachelor of Science or Bachelor of Arts	60
		Master of Science in healthcare field	70
		Master of Science in healthcare-related field	100
		Ph.D. or higher degree	90
.30	Computer skills	None	0
		Data entry	10
		Experience with a database or a worksheet program	80
		Experience with both databases and worksheet programs	100
.20	Internal promotion	No	0
		Yes	100
.10	People skills	Not a strength of the applicant	0
		Contributes to teams effectively	50
		Organizes and leads teams	100

The decision maker is concerned about cost but is willing to underwrite the cost of the fair if it leads to a significant number of referrals. Discussions with the decision maker led to the specification of the attributes shown in Table 2.2.

This simple model will score each screening based on three attributes: (1) the cost of providing the service, (2) the needs of the target group, and (3) whether the screening may generate a visit to the clinic. Once all screening options have been scored and the available funds considered, the top-scoring screening activities can be chosen and offered in the health fair.

A third example concerns constructing practice profiles. Practice profiles are helpful for hiring, firing, disciplining, and paying physicians (Vibbert 1992; McNeil, Pedersen, and Gatsonis 1992). A practice profile compares cost and outcomes of individual physicians to each other. Because patients differ in their severity of illness, it is important to adjust outcomes by the provider's mix of patients. Only then can one compare apples to apples. If there is a severity score, managers can examine patient outcomes to see if

TABLE 2.2
A Model for Health Fair Composition Decisions

Attribute Weight	Attribute	Attribute Level	Value of the Level
.45	Cost of providing the service	Interview cost	0
		Interview and nonintrusive test costs	60
		Interview and intrusive test costs	100
.35	Need in target group	Unknown	0
		Less than 1% are likely to be positive	10
		1% to 5% are likely to be positive	80
		More than 5% likely to be positive	100
.20	Generates a likely visit	No	0
		Yes	100

they are within expectations. Managers can compare two clinicians to see which one had better outcomes for patients with the same severity of illness. Armed with a severity index, managers can compare cost of care for different clinicians to see which one is more efficient. Value models can be used to create severity indexes—for example, a severity index for acquired immunodeficiency syndrome (AIDS).

After the diagnosis of human immunodeficiency virus (HIV) infection, patients often suffer a complex set of different diseases. The cost of treatment for each patient is heavily dependent on the course of their illness. For example, patients with skin cancer, Kaposi's sarcoma, have significantly lower first-year costs than patients with more serious infections (Freedberg et al. 1998). Thus, if a manager wants to compare two clinicians in their ability to care for AIDS patients, it is important to measure the severity of AIDS among their patients. Alemi and colleagues (1990) used a value model to create a severity index for AIDS. Even though much time has elapsed since the creation of this index, and care of AIDS patients has progressed, the method of developing the severity index is still relevant. The development of this index will be referred to at length throughout this chapter.

Steps in Modeling Values

Using the example of the AIDS severity index (Alemi et al. 1990), this section shows how to examine the need for a value model and how to create such a model.

Step 1: Determine if a Model Would Help

The first and most obvious question is whether constructing a value model will help resolve the problem faced by the manager. Defining the problem is the most significant step of the analysis, yet surprisingly little literature is available for guidance. To define a problem, the analyst must answer several related questions: Who is the decision maker? What are the objectives this person wishes to achieve? What role do subjective judgments play in these goals? Should a value model be used? How will it be used?

Who Is the Decision Maker?

In organizations, there are often many decision makers. No single person's viewpoint is sufficient, and the analyst needs a multidisciplinary consensus instead. Chapter 6 discusses how the values of a group of people can be modeled.

The core of the problem in the example was that AIDS patients need different amounts of resources depending on the severity of their illness. The federal administrators of the Medicaid program wanted to measure the severity of AIDS patients because the federal government paid for part of their care. The state administrators were likewise interested because state funds paid for another portion of their care. Individual hospital administrators were interested in analyzing a clinician's practice patterns and recruiting the most efficient. No single decision maker was involved. In short, the model focused on how a clinician makes severity judgments and thus brought together a group of physicians involved with care of and research on AIDS patients. For simplicity, the following discussion assumes that only one person is involved in the decision-making process.

What Are the Objectives?

Problem solving starts by recognizing a gap between the present situation and the desired future. Typically, at least one decision maker has noticed a difference between what is and what should be and begins to share this awareness with the relevant levels of the organization. Gradually, a motivation is created to change, informal social ties are established to promote the change, and an individual or group receives a mandate to find a solution.

Often, a perceived problem may not be the real issue. Occasionally, the decision maker has a solution in mind before fully understanding the problem, which shows the need for examining the decision maker's circumstances in greater depth. When solutions are proposed prematurely, it is important to sit back and gain a greater perspective on the problem. In these situations, it is the analyst's responsibility to redefine the problem to make it relevant to the real issues. An analyst can use tools that help the decision maker better define the problem. There are many ways to encourage creativity (Sutton 2001), including structured techniques such as brainstorming (Fields 1995) and less structured techniques such as analogies.

What Role Do Subjective Judgments Play?

After the problem has been defined, the analyst must examine the role subjective judgments will play in its resolution. One can do this by asking questions such as the following: What plans would change if the judgment were different? How are things being done now? If no one makes a judgment about the underlying concept, would it really matter, and who would complain? Would it be useful to tell how the judgment was made, or is it better to leave matters rather ambiguous? Must the decision maker choose among options, or should the decision maker let things unfold on their own? Is a subjective component critical to the judgment, or can it be based on objective standards?

In the severity index example, the administrators needed to budget for the coming years, and they knew judgments of severity would help them anticipate utilization rates and overall costs. Programs caring for low-severity patients would receive a smaller allocation than programs caring for high-severity patients. But no objective measures of severity were available, so clinicians' judgments concerning severity were used instead.

Should a Value Model Be Used?

Experts seem to intuitively know the prognosis of a patient and can easily recognize a very sick patient. Although in the AIDS example it was theoretically possible to have an expert panel review each case and estimate severity, it was clear from the outset that a model was needed because of the high cost of case-by-case review. Moreover, the large number of cases would require the use of several expert panels, each judging a subset of cases, and the panels might disagree. Further, judgments within a panel can be quite inconsistent over time. In contrast, the model provided a quick and consistent way of rating the severity of patients. It also explained the rationale behind the ratings, which allowed skeptics to examine the fairness of judgments, thus increasing the acceptance of those judgments.

How Will the Value Model Be Used?

In understanding what judgments must be made, it was crucial to attend to the limitations of circumstances in which these judgments are going to be made. The use of existing AIDS severity indexes was limited because they relied on physiological variables that were unavailable in many databases. Alemi and his colleagues (1990) were asked to predict prognoses from existing data. The only information widely available on AIDS patients was diagnoses, which were routinely collected after every encounter. Because these data did not include any known physiological predictors of survival (such as number of T4 cells), the manager needed an alternative way to predict survival. The severity index was created to serve as this alternative.

Step 2: Soliciting Attributes

After determining whether a model would be useful, the second step is to identify the attributes needed for making the judgment. For example, Alemi and his colleagues (1990) needed to understand and identify the patient attributes that should be used to predict AIDS severity. For the study, six experts known for clinical work with AIDS patients or for research on the survival of AIDS patients were assembled. Physicians came from several programs located in states with high rates of HIV/AIDS. The experts were interviewed to identify the attributes used in creating the severity index. When interviewing an expert to determine the attributes needed for a model, the analyst should keep introductions brief, use tangible examples, arrange the attributes in a hierarchy, take notes, and refrain from interrupting.

Keep Introductions Brief

Being as brief as possible, the analyst should introduce herself and explain the expert's role, the model's purpose, and how the model will be developed. An interview is going well if the analyst is listening and the expert is talking. If it takes five minutes just to describe the purpose of the interview, then something is amiss. Probably, the analyst does not understand the problem well, or possibly the expert is not familiar with the problem.

Be assertive in setting the interview's pace and agenda. Because the expert is likely to talk whenever the analyst pauses, the analyst should be judicious about pausing. For example, if one pauses after saying, "Our purpose is to construct a severity index to work with existing databases," the expert will likely use that opportunity for an in-depth discussion about the purpose. But if the analyst immediately follows the previous sentence with a question about the expert's experience in assessing severity, the expert is more likely to begin describing his background. The analyst sets the agenda and should pause in such a way as to make progress in the interview.

Use Tangible Examples

Concrete examples help the analyst understand which patient attributes should be used in the model and how they can be measured. Ask the expert to recall an actual situation and to contrast it with other occasions to discern the key discriminators. For example, the analyst might ask the expert to describe a severely ill patient in detail to ensure that the expert is referring to a particular patient rather than a hypothetical one. Then, the analyst asks for a description of a patient who was not severely ill and tries to elicit the key differences between the two patients; these differences are attributes the analyst can use to judge severity. The following is a sample dialog:

Analyst: Can you recall a specific patient with a very poor prognosis?
Expert: I work in a referral center, and we see a lot of severely ill patients. They seem to have many illnesses and are unable to recover completely, so they continue to worsen.

Analyst: Tell me about a recent patient who was severely ill.
Expert: A 28-year-old homosexual male patient deteriorated rapidly. He kept fighting recurrent influenza and died from gastrointestinal (GI) cancer. The real problem was that he couldn't tolerate AZT, so we couldn't help him much. Once a person has cancer, we can do little to maintain him.

Analyst: Tell me about a patient with a good prognosis—say, close to five years.
Expert: Well, let me think. A year ago, we had a 32-year-old male patient diagnosed with AIDS who has not had serious disease since—a few skin infections, but nothing serious. His spirit is up, he continues working, and we have every reason to expect he will survive four or five years.

Analyst: What key difference between the two patients made you realize that the first patient had a poorer prognosis than the second?
Expert: That's a difficult question. Patients are so different from each other that it's tough to point to one characteristic. But if you really push me, I would say two characteristics: the history of illness and the ability to tolerate AZT.

Analyst: What about the history is relevant?
Expert: If I must predict a prognosis, I want to know whether the patient has had serious illness in vital organs.

Analyst: Which organs?

Expert: Brain, heart, and lungs are more important than, say, skin.

In this dialog, the analyst started with tangible examples and used the terminology and words introduced by the expert to discuss concrete examples. There are two advantages to this process. First, it helps the expert recall the details without the analyst introducing unfamiliar words, such as "attributes." Second, soliciting attributes by contrasting patients helps single out those attributes that truly affect prognosis. Thus, it does not produce a wish list of information that is loosely tied to severity—an extravagance one cannot afford in model building.

After the analyst has identified some attributes, the analyst can ask directly for additional attributes that indicate prognosis. One might ask if there are other markers of prognosis, if the expert has used the word "marker." If necessary, the analyst might say, "In our terminology, we refer to the kinds of things you have mentioned as markers of prognosis. Are there other markers?" The following is an example dialog:

Analyst: Are there other markers for poor prognosis?
Expert: Comorbidities are important. Perhaps advanced age suggests poorer prognosis. Sex may matter.

Analyst: Does the age or sex really matter in predicting prognosis?
Expert: Sex does not matter, but age does. But there are many exceptions. You cannot predict the prognosis of a patient based on age alone.

Analyst: What are some other markers of poor prognosis?

As you can see in the dialog, the analyst might even express her own ideas without pushing them on the expert. In general, analysts are not there to express their own ideas; they are there to listen. However, they can ask questions to clarify things or even to mention things overlooked by the expert, as long as it does not change the nature of the relationship between the analyst and the expert.

The analyst should always use the expert's terminology, even if a reformulation might help. Thus, if the expert refers to "sex," the analyst should not substitute "gender." Such new terminology may confuse the conversation and create an environment where the analyst acts more like an expert, which can undermine the expert's confidence that she is being heard. It is reasonable, however, to ask for clarification—"sex" could refer to gender or to sex practices, and the intended meaning is important.

In general, less esoteric prompts are more likely to produce the best responses, so formulate a few prompts and use the prompts that feel most natural for the task. Avoid jargon, including the use of terminology from decision analysis (e.g., attribute, value function, aggregation rules).

Arrange the Attributes in a Hierarchy

An attribute hierarchy should move from broad to specific attributes (Keeney 1996). Some analysts suggest using a hierarchy to solicit and structure the attributes. For example, an expert may suggest that a patient's prognosis depends on medical history and demographics, such as age and sex. Medical history involves the nature of the illness, comorbidities, and tolerance of

AZT. The nature of illness breaks down into body systems involved (e.g., skin, nerves, blood). Within each body system, some diagnoses are minor and other diagnoses are more threatening. The expert then lists, within each system, a range of diseases. The hierarchical structure promotes completeness and simplifies tracking many attributes. A detailed example of arranging attributes in hierarchical structure is presented later in this chapter.

Take Notes and Refrain from Interrupting

The analyst should take notes and not interrupt. He should have paper and a pencil available, and write down the important points. Not only does this help the expert's recall, but it also helps the analyst review matters while the expert is still available. Experts tend to list a few attributes, then focus attention on one or two. The analyst should actively listen to these areas of focus. When the expert is finished, the analyst should review the notes for items that need elaboration. If certain points are vague, the analyst should ask for examples, which are an excellent means of clarification. For instance, after the expert has described attributes of vital organ involvement, the analyst may ask the expert to elaborate on something mentioned earlier, such as "acceptance of AZT." If the expert mentions other topics in the process, return to them after completing the discussion of AZT acceptance. This ensures that no loose ends are left when the interview is finished and reassures the expert that the analyst is indeed listening.

Other Approaches

Other, more statistical approaches to soliciting attributes are available, such as multidimensional scaling and factor analysis. However, the behavioral approach to soliciting attributes (i.e., the approach of asking the expert to specify the attributes) is preferred because it involves the expert more in the process and leads to greater acceptance of the model.

Step 3: Examine and Revise the Attributes

After soliciting a set of attributes, it is important to examine and, if necessary, revise them. Psychological research suggests that changing the framing of a question alters the response (Kahneman 2003). Consider the following two questions:

1. What are the markers for survival?
2. What are the markers for poor prognosis?

One question emphasizes survival, the other mortality. One would expect that patient attributes indicating survival would also indicate mortality, but researchers have found this to be untrue (see Chow, Haddad, Wong-Boren 1991; Nisbett and Ross 1980). Experts may identify entirely different attributes for survival and mortality. This research suggests that value-laden prompts tap different parts of the memory and can evoke recall of different pieces of information. Evidence about the impact of questions on recall and judgment is substantial. How questions are framed affects what answers are provided (Kim et al. 2005). Such studies suggest that analysts should ask their questions in two ways, once in positive terms and again in negative terms.

Several tests should be conducted to ensure that the solicitation process succeeded. The first test ensures that the listed attributes are exhaustive by using them to describe several hypothetical patients and asking the expert to rate their prognosis. If the expert needs additional information for a judgment, solicit new attributes until the expert has enough information to make the judgment.

A second test checks that the attributes are not redundant by examining whether knowledge of one attribute implies knowledge of another. For example, the expert may consider "inability to administer AZT" and "cancer of GI tract" redundant if no patient with GI cancer can accept AZT. In such cases, either the two attributes should be combined into one, or one must be dropped from the analysis.

A third test ensures that each attribute is important to the decision maker's judgment. The analyst can test this by asking the decision maker to judge two hypothetical situations: one with the attribute at its lowest level and another with the attribute at peak level. If the judgments are similar, the attribute may be ignored. For example, gender may be unimportant if male and female AIDS patients with the same history of illness have identical prognoses.

Fourth, a series of tests examines whether the attributes are related or are independent (Goodwin and Wright 2004; Keeney 1996).

In the AIDS severity study (Alemi et al. 1990), discussions with the expert and later revisions led to the following set of 18 patient attributes for judging the severity of AIDS:

1. Age
2. Race
3. Transmission mode
4. Defining diagnosis
5. Time since defining diagnosis
6. Diseases of nervous system
7. Disseminated diseases
8. GI diseases
9. Skin diseases
10. Lung diseases
11. Heart diseases
12. Recurrence of a disease
13. Functioning of the organs
14. Comorbidity
15. Psychiatric comorbidity
16. Nutritional status
17. Drug markers
18. Functional impairment

As the number of attributes in a model increases, the chances for preferential dependence also increases. The rule of thumb is that preferential dependencies are much more likely in value models with more than nine attributes.

Step 4: Set Attribute Levels

Once the attributes have been examined and revised, the possible levels of each attribute can be identified. The analyst starts by deciding if the attributes are discrete or continuous. Attributes such as age are continuous; attributes such as diseases of the nervous system are discrete. However, continuous attributes may be expressed in terms of a few discrete levels, so that age can be described in decades, not individual years. The four steps in identifying the levels of an attribute are to (1) define the range, (2) define the best and worst levels, (3) define some intermediate levels, and (4) fill in the other possible levels so that the listing of the levels is exhaustive and capable of covering all possible situations.

To define the range, the analyst must select a target population and ask the expert to describe the possible range of the attributes in it. Thus, for the AIDS severity index, the analyst asked the experts to focus on adult AIDS patients and, for each attribute, suggest the possible ranges. To assess the range of nervous system diseases, the analyst asked the following question:

> Analyst: In adult AIDS patients, what is a disease that suggests the most extensive involvement of the nervous system?

Next, the analyst asked the expert to specify the best and the worst possible levels of each attribute. In the AIDS severity index, one could easily identify the level with the best possible prognosis: the normal finding within each attribute—in common language, the healthy condition. The analyst accomplished the more difficult task of identifying the level with the worst possible prognosis by asking the expert the following question:

> Analyst: What would be the gravest disease of the central nervous system, in terms of prognosis?

A typical error in obtaining the best and the worst levels is failing to describe these levels in detail. For example, in assessing the value of nutritional status, it is not helpful to define the levels as simply the best nutritional status or the worst nutritional status. Nor does it help to define the worst level as "severely nutritionally deficient" because the adjective "severe" is not defined. Analysts should avoid using adjectives in describing levels, as experts perceive words like "severely" or "best" in different ways. The levels must be defined in terms of the underlying physical process measured in each attribute, and the descriptions must be connected to the nature of the attribute. Thus, a good level for the worst nutritional status might be "patients on total parenteral nutrition," and the best status might be "nutritional treatment not needed."

Next, the analyst should ask the expert to define intermediate levels. These levels are often defined by asking for a level between the best and worst levels. In the severity index example, this dialog might occur as follows:

Analyst: I understand that patients on total parenteral nutrition have the worst prognosis. Can you think of other relatively common conditions with a slightly better prognosis?
Expert: Well, a host of things can happen. Pick up any book on nutritional diseases, and you find all kinds of things.

Analyst: Right, but can you give me three or four examples?
Expert: Sure. The patient may be on antiemetics or nutritional supplements.

Analyst: Do these levels include a level with a moderately poor prognosis and one with a relatively good prognosis?
Expert: Not really. If you want a level indicative of moderately poor prognosis, then you should include whether the patient is receiving Lomotil or Imodium.

It is not always possible to solicit all possible levels of an attribute from the expert interviews. In these circumstances, the analyst can fill in the gaps afterward by reading the literature or interviewing other experts. The levels specified by the first expert are used as markers for placing the remaining levels, so that the levels range from best to worst. In the example, a clinician on the project team reviewed the expert's suggestions and filled in a long list of intermediate levels.

Step 5: Assign Values to Single Attributes

The analysis proceeds with the evaluation of single-attribute value function (i.e., a scoring procedure that assigns the relative value of each level in a single attribute). The procedure recommended here is called double-anchored estimation. In this method, the attribute levels are first ranked, or, if the attribute is continuous, the most and least preferred levels are specified and assigned scores of 0 and 100. Finally, the best and the worst levels are used as "anchors" for assessing the other levels.

For example, skin infections have the following levels:

- No skin disorder
- Kaposi's sarcoma

- Shingles
- Herpes complex
- *Candidiasis*
- Thrush

The following interaction typifies the questioning for the double-anchored estimation method:

Analyst: Which skin disorder has the worst prognosis?
Expert: None is really that serious.

Analyst: Yes, I understand that, but which is the most serious?
Expert: Patients with thrush perhaps have a worse prognosis than patients with other skin infections.

Analyst: Let's rate the severity of thrush at 100 and place the severity of no skin disorder at zero. How would you rate shingles?
Expert: Shingles is almost as serious as thrush.

Analyst: This tells me that you might rate the severity of shingles nearer 100 than zero. Where exactly would you rate it?
Expert: Maybe 90.

Analyst: Can you now rate the remaining levels?

Several psychologists have questioned whether experts are systematically biased in assessing value because using different anchors produces different value functions (Chapman and Johnson 1999). For example, in assessing the value of money, gains are judged differently than losses; furthermore, the value of money is judged according to the decision maker's current assets (Kahneman 2003). Because value may depend on the anchors used, it is important to use different anchors besides just the best or worst levels. Thus, if the value of skin infections is assessed by anchoring on shingles and no skin infections, then it is important to verify the ratings relative to other levels. Assume the expert rated skin infections as follows:

Attribute level	*Rating*
No skin disorder	0
Kaposi's sarcoma	10
Shingles	90
Herpes complex	95
Candidiasis	100
Thrush	100

The analyst might then ask the following:

Analyst: You have rated herpes complex halfway between shingles and *candidiasis.* Is this correct?
Expert: Not really. Prognosis of patients with herpes is closer to patients with *candidiasis.*

Analyst: How would you change the ratings?
Expert: Maybe we should rate herpes 98.

It is occasionally useful to change not only the anchors but also the assessment method. A later section describes several alternative methods of assessing single-attribute value functions. When a value is measured by two different methods, there would be inadvertent discrepancies; the analyst must ask the expert to resolve these differences.

By convention, the single-attribute value function must range from zero to 100. Sometimes, experts and decision makers refuse to assign the zero value. In these circumstances, their estimated values should be revised to range from zero to 100. The following formula shows how to obtain standardized value functions from estimates that do not range from zero to 100:

$$\text{Standardized value for level } X = 100 \times \frac{\text{Value assigned to level } X - \text{Value of least important level}}{\text{Value of most important level} - \text{Value of least important level}}.$$

For example, assume that the skin diseases attributes are rated as follows:

Attribute level	Rating
No skin disorder	10
Kaposi's sarcoma	20
Thrush	90

Then, the maximum value is 90 and the minimum value is 10, and standardized values can be assigned to each level using the formula above. For example, for Kaposi's sarcoma the value is

$$\text{Standardized value for Kaposi's sarcoma} = 100 \times \frac{20 - 10}{90 - 10} = 12.5.$$

Step 6: Choose an Aggregation Rule

In this step, the analysis proceeds when one finds a way to aggregate single-attribute functions into an overall score evaluated across all attributes.

Note that the scoring convention has produced a situation in which the value of each attribute is somewhere between zero and 100. Thus, the prognosis of patients with skin infection and the prognosis of patients with various GI diseases have the same range. Adding these scores will be misleading because skin infections are less serious than GI problems, so the analyst must find an aggregation rule that differentially weights the various attributes.

The most obvious rule is the ***additive value model.*** Assume that S represents the severity of AIDS. If a patient is described by a series of n attributes of $(A_1, A_2, \ldots, A_i, \ldots, A_n)$, then, using the additive rule, the overall severity is

$$S = \sum_i W_i \times V_i (A_j),$$

where

- $V_i (A_j)$ is the value of the *j*th level in the *i*th patient attribute,
- W_i is the weight associated with the *i*th attribute in predicting prognosis, and
- $\sum_i W_i = 1$.

Several other models are possible in addition to the additive model. The multiplicative model form is described in a later section of this chapter.

Step 7: Estimate Weights

The analyst can estimate the weights for an additive value model in a number of ways. It is often useful to mix several approaches. Some analysts estimate weights by assessing how many times one attribute is more important than the other (Edwards and Barron 1994; Salo and Hämäläinen 2001). The attributes are rank ordered, and the least important is assigned ten points. The expert is then asked to estimate the relative importance of the other attributes by estimating how many times the next attribute is more important. There is no upper limit to the number of points other attributes can be assigned. For example, in estimating the weights for the three attributes of skin infections, lung infections, and GI diseases, the analyst and the expert might have the following discussion:

Analyst: Which of the three attributes is most important?

Expert: Well, they are all important, but patients with either lung infections or GI diseases have worse prognoses than patients with skin infections.

Analyst: Do lung infections have a worse prognosis than GI diseases?

Expert: That's more difficult to answer. No, I would say that for all practical purposes, they have the same prognosis. Well, now that I think about it, perhaps patients with GI diseases have a slightly worse prognosis.

Having obtained the rank ordering of the attributes, the analyst can proceed to estimating the importance weights as follows:

Analyst: Let's say that we arbitrarily rate the importance of skin infection in determining prognosis at ten points. GI diseases are how many times more important than skin infections?

Expert: Quite a bit. Maybe three times.

Analyst: That is, if we assign 10 points to skin infections, we should assign 30 points to the importance of GI diseases?

Expert: Yes, that sounds right.

Analyst: How about lung infections? How many more times important are they than GI diseases?

Expert: I would say about the same.

Analyst: (Checking for consistency in the subjective judgments.) Would you consider lung infections three times more serious than skin infections?

Expert: Yes, I think that should be about right.

In the dialog above, the analyst first found the order of the attributes and then asked for the ratio of the weights of the attributes. Knowing the ratio of attributes allows the analyst to estimate the attribute weights. If the model has only three attributes, the weights for the attributes can be obtained by solving the following three equations:

$$\frac{W(\text{GI diseases})}{W(\text{skin infection})} = 3,$$

$$\frac{W(\text{lung diseases})}{W(\text{skin infection})} = 3,$$

$$W(\text{lung diseases}) + W(\text{skin infection}) + W(\text{GI diseases}) = 1.$$

One characteristic of this estimation method is that its emphasis on the ratio of the importance of the attributes leads to relatively extreme weighting compared to other approaches. Thus, some attributes may be judged critical, and others rather trivial. Other approaches, especially the direct magnitude process, may judge all attributes as almost equally important.

In choosing a method to estimate weights, the analyst should consider several trade-offs, such as ease of use and accuracy of estimates. The analyst can introduce errors by asking experts awkward and partially understood questions. It is best to estimate weights in several ways and use the resulting differences to help experts think more carefully about their real beliefs. In doing so, the analyst usually starts with a rank-order technique, then moves on to assess ratios, obtain a direct magnitude estimate, identify discrepancies, and finally ask the expert to resolve them.

One note of caution: Some scientists have questioned whether experts can describe how they weight attributes. Nisbett and Miyamoto (2005) argue that directly assessed weight may not reflect an expert's true beliefs. Other investigators find that directly assessing the relative importance of attributes is accurate (Naglie et al. 1997). In the end, what matters is not the weight of individual attributes but the accuracy of the entire model, which is discussed in the next section.

Step 8: Evaluate the Accuracy of the Model

Although researchers know the importance of carefully evaluating value models, analysts often lack the time and resources to do this. Because of the importance of having confidence in the models and being able to defend the analytical methodology, this section presents several ways of testing the adequacy of value models.

Most value models are devised to apply to a particular context, and they are not portable to other settings or uses. This is called *context dependence*. In general, it is viewed as a liability, but this is not always the case. For example, the AIDS severity index may be intended for evaluating practice patterns, and its use for evaluating prognosis of individual patients is inappropriate and possibly misleading.

The value model should require only available data for input. Relying on obscure data may increase the model's accuracy at the expense of practicality. Thus, the severity index should rely on reasonable sources of data, usually from existing databases. A physiologically based database, for instance, would predict prognosis of AIDS patients quite accurately. However, such an index would be useless if physiological information is generally unavailable and routine collection of this information would take considerable time and money. While the issue of data availability may seem obvious, it is a very common error in the development of value models. Experts used to working in organizations with superlative data systems may want data that are unavailable at average institutions, and they may produce a value model with limited usefulness. If there are no plans to compare scores across organizations, one can tailor indexes to each institution's capabilities and allow each institution to decide whether the cost of collecting new data is justified by the expected increase in accuracy. However, if scores will be used to compare institutions or allocate resources among institutions, then a single-value model based on data available to all organizations is needed.

The model should be simple to use. The index of medical underservice areas is a good example of the importance of simplicity (Health Services Research Group 1975). This index, developed to help the federal government set priorities for funding HMOs, community health centers, and health-facility development programs, originally had nine attributes; the director of the sponsoring federal agency rejected the index because of the number of variables. Because he wanted to be able to "calculate the score on the back of an envelope," the index was reduced to four attributes. The simplified version performed as well as one with a larger model; it was used for eight years to help set nationwide funding priorities. This example shows that simplicity does not always equal incompetence. Simplicity nearly always makes an index easy to understand and use.

When different people apply the value model to the same situation, they must arrive at the same scores; this is referred to as *interrater reliability*. In the example of the severity index (Alemi et al. 1990), different registered record abstractors who use the model to rate the severity of a patient should produce the same score. If a model relies on hard-to-observe patient attributes, the abstractors will disagree about the condition of patients. If reasonable people using a value model reach different conclusions, then one loses confidence in the model's usefulness as a systematic method of evaluation. Interrater reliability is tested by having different abstractors rate the severity of randomly selected patients.

The value model should also seem reasonable to experts—this is coined *face validity*. Thus, the severity index should seem reasonable to clinicians and managers. Otherwise, even if it accurate, one may experience problems with its acceptance. Clinicians who are unfamiliar with statistics will likely rely on their experience to judge the index, meaning that the variables, weights, and value scores must seem reasonable and practical to them. Face validity is tested by showing the model to a new set of experts and asking if they understand it and whether it is conceptually reasonable.

One way to establish the validity of a model is to show that it simulates the judgment of the experts; then, if the experts' acumen is believed, the model should be considered valid. In this approach, the expert is asked to score several (perhaps 100) hypothetical case profiles described only by attributes included in the model. If the model accurately predicts the expert's judgments, confidence in the model increases; but this measure has the drawback of producing optimistic results. After all, if the expert who developed the model cannot get the model to predict her judgments, who can? It is far better to ask a separate panel of experts to rate the patient profiles. In the AIDS severity project, the analyst collected the expert's estimate of survival time for 97 hypothetical patients and examined whether the value model could predict these ratings. The correlation between the additive model and the rating of survival was –0.53. (The negative correlation means that high severity scores indicate shorter survival; the magnitude of the correlation ranges between 1.0 and –1.0.) The correlation of –0.53 suggests low to moderate agreement between the model and the expert's intuitions; correlations closer to 1.0 or –1.0 imply greater agreement. A correlation of zero suggests no agreement. One can judge the adequacy of the correlations by comparing them with agreement among the experts themselves. The correlation between several pairs of experts rating the same 97 hypothetical patients was also in a similar range. The value model agreed with the average of the experts as much as the experts agreed with each other. Thus, the value model may be a reasonable approach to measuring severity of AIDS.

A model is considered valid if several different ways of measuring it lead to the same finding. This method of establishing validity is referred to as *construct validity*. For example, the AIDS severity model should be correlated with other measures of AIDS severity. If the analyst has access to other severity indexes, such as physiologically based indexes, the predictions of the different approaches can be compared using a sample of patients. One such study was done for the index described in this section. In a follow-up article about the severity index, Alemi and his colleagues (1999) reported that the index did not correlate well against physiological markers. If it had, confidence in the severity index would have been increased because physiological markers and the index were measuring the same thing. Given that the two did not have a high correlation, clearly they were measuring different aspects of severity, and the real question was which one was more accurate. As it turns out, the severity index presented in this chapter was more accurate in predicting survival than physiological markers.

In some situations, one can validate a value model by comparing the model's predictions against observable behavior. This method of establishing validity is referred to as *predictive validity*. If a model is used to measure a subjective concept, its accuracy can be evaluated by comparing predictions to an observed and objective standard, which is often called the *gold standard*, to emphasize its status as being beyond debate. In practice, gold standards are rarely available for judging the accuracy of subjective concepts (otherwise, one would not need the models in the first place). For example, the accuracy of a severity index can be examined by comparing it to observed outcomes of patients' care. When the severity index accurately predicts outcomes, there is evidence favoring the model. The model developed in this section was tested by comparing it to patients' survival rates. The medical histories of patients were analyzed using the model, and the ability of the severity score to predict patients' prognoses was examined. The index was more accurate than physiological markers in predicting patients' survival.

Other Methods for Assessing Single-Attribute Value Functions

Single-attribute value functions can be assessed in a number of different ways aside from the double-anchored method (Torrance et al. 1995). The *midvalue splitting technique* sets the best and worst levels of the attributes at 100 and zero. Then the decision maker finds a level of the attribute that psychologically seems halfway between the best and the worst levels. The value for this level is set to 50. Using the best, worst, and midvalue points, the decision maker continues finding points that psychologically seem halfway between any two points. After several points are identified, the values of other points are assessed by linear extrapolation from existing points. The following conversation illustrates how the midvalue splitting technique could be used to assess the value of age in assessing AIDS severity.

Analyst: What is the age with the best prognosis?
Expert: A 20-year-old has the best chance of survival.

Analyst: What is the age with the worst prognosis?
Expert: AIDS patients over 70 years old are more susceptible to opportunistic infections and have the worst prognosis. Of course, infants with AIDS have an even worse prognosis, but I understand we are focusing on adults.

Analyst: Which age has a prognosis half as bad as a 70-year-old?
Expert: I am going to say about 40, though I am not really sure.

Analyst: I understand. We do not need exact answers. Perhaps it may help to ask the question differently. Do you think an increase in age from 40 to 70 causes as much of a deterioration in prognosis as an increase from 20 to 40 years?

Expert: If you are asking roughly, yes.

Analyst: If 20 years is rated as zero and 70 years as 100, do you think it would be reasonable to rate 40 years as 50?

Expert: I suppose my previous answers imply that I should say yes.

Analyst: Yes, but this is not binding—you can revise your answers.

Expert: A rating of 50 for the age of 40 seems fine as a first approximation.

Analyst: Can you tell me what age would have a prognosis halfway between 20 and 40 years old?

Using the midvalue splitting technique, the analyst chooses a value score, and the expert specifies the particular attribute level that matches it. This is opposite to the double-anchored estimation, in which the analyst specifies an attribute level and asks for its value. The choice between the two methods should depend on whether the attribute is discrete or continuous. Often with discrete attributes, there are no levels to correspond to particular value scores, so analysts have no choice but to select the double-anchored method.

Another method for assessing a value function is to draw a curve in the following fashion: The levels of the attributes are sorted and set in the *x*-axis. The *y*-axis is the value associated with each attribute level. The best attribute level is assigned 100 and drawn on the curve. The worst attribute level is assigned zero. The expert is asked to draw a curve between these two points showing the value of remaining attribute levels. Once the graph is drawn, the analyst and the expert review its implications. For example, a graph can be constructed with age (20 to 70 years) on the *x*-axis and value (0 to 100) on the *y*-axis. Two points are marked on the graph (age 20 at zero value and age 70 at 100 value). The analyst asks the expert to draw a line between these two points showing the prognosis for intermediate ages.

Finally, an extremely easy method, which requires no numerical assessment at all, is to assume a linear value function over the attribute. This arbitrary assumption introduces some errors, but they will be small if an ordinal value scale is being constructed and if the single-attribute value function is monotonic (meaning that an increase in the attribute level will cause either no change or an increase in value).

For example, one cannot assume that increasing age will cause a proportionate decline in prognosis. In other words, the relationship between the variables is not monotonic: The prognosis for infants is especially poor, while 20-year-old patients have the best prognosis and 70-year-old patients have a poor outlook. Because increasing age does not consistently lead to increasing severity—and in fact it can also reduce severity—an assumption of linear value is misleading.

Other Methods for Estimating Weights

In the *direct magnitude estimate*, the expert is asked to rank order the attributes and then rate their importance by assigning each a number between zero and 100. Once the ratings are obtained, they are scaled to range between zero and one by dividing each weight by the sum of the ratings. Subjects rarely rate the importance of an attribute near zero, so the direct magnitude estimation has the characteristic of producing weights that are close together, but the process has the advantage of simplicity and comprehensibility.

Weights can also be estimated by having the expert distribute a fixed number of points, typically 100, among the attributes. The main advantage of this method is simplicity, as it is only slightly more difficult than the ranking method. But if there are a large number of attributes, experts will have difficulty assigning numbers that total 100.

One approach to estimating weights is to ask the expert to rate "corner" cases. A corner case is a description of a patient with one attribute at its most extreme level and the remainder at minimum levels. The expert's score for the corner case shows the weight of the attribute that was set at its maximum level. The process is continued until all possible corner cases have been rated, each indicating the weight for a different attribute. In multiplicative models (described later), the analyst can estimate other parameters by presenting corner cases with two or more attributes at peak levels. After the expert rates several cases, a set of parameters is estimated that optimizes the fit between model predictions and expert's ratings.

Another approach is to mix and match methods. Several empirical comparisons of assessment methods have shown that different weight-estimation methods lead to similar assessments. A study that compared seven methods for obtaining subjective weights, including 100-point distribution, ranking, and ratio methods, found no differences in their results (Jia, Fischer, and Dyer 1998; Cook and Stewart 1975). Such insensitivity to assessment procedures is encouraging because it shows that the estimates are not by-products of the method and thus are more likely to reflect the expert's true opinions. This allows the substitution of one method for another.

Other Aggregation Rules: Multiplicative MAV Models

The additive value model assumes that single-attribute value scores are weighted for importance and then added together. In essence, it calculates a weighted average of single-attribute value functions.

The *multiplicative model* is another common aggregation rule. In the AIDS severity study, discussions with physicians suggested that a high score in any single-attribute value function was sufficient ground for judging the patient severely ill. Using a multiplicative model, overall severity would be calculated as

$$S = \frac{-1 + \Pi_i \left[1 + k \times k_i \times U(A_i)\right]}{k},$$

where ki and k are constants chosen so that $k = -1 + \Pi_i\,(1 + k \times k_i)$.

In a multiplicative model when the constant k is close to -1, high scores in one category are sufficient to produce an overall severity score even if other categories are normal. This model better resembled the expert's intuitions. The additive MAV model would have led to less severe scores due to having numerous attributes at the normal level. To construct the multiplicative value model, the expert must estimate "n + 1" parameters: the n constants k_i; and one additional parameter, the constant k.

In the AIDS severity project, the analyst constructed a multiplicative value model. On 97 hypothetical patients, the severity ratings of the multiplicative and the additive models were compared to the expert's intuitive ratings. The multiplicative model was more accurate (correlation between additive model and experts' judgment was 0.53, while the correlation between multiplicative model and expert judgment was 0.60). The difference in the accuracy of the two models was statistically significant. Therefore, the multiplicative severity model was chosen.

Resulting Multiplicative Severity Index

Appendix 2.1 is an example of a multiplicative value model. Experts on HIV/AIDS were interviewed by Alemi and his colleagues (1990), and an index was built based on their judgments. This index is intended for assessing the severity of the course of AIDS based on diagnosis and without access to physiological markers. As such, it is best suited for analysis of data from regions of the world where physiological markers are not readily available or for analysis of data from large administrative databases where diagnoses are widely available. Kinzbrunner and Pratt (1994), as well as Alemi and his colleagues in a later article (1999), provide evaluations of this index. This index is in the public domain and can be used without royalty payments. Please note that advances in HIV/AIDS treatment may have changed the relative severity of various levels in the index.

In the multiplicative MAV model used in the Severity of the Course of AIDS index, the k value was set to –1 and all other parameters (single-attribute value functions and k_i constants) were estimated by querying a panel of experts. The scores presented in the index are the result of multiplying the single-attribute value function by its k_i coefficient. The index is scored by selecting a level within each attribute, finding the score associated with that level, multiplying all selected scores, and calculating the difference between one and the resulting multiplication.

Model Evaluation

In evaluating MAV models, it is sometimes necessary to compare model scores against experts' ratings of cases. For example, the analyst might want to see if a model makes a similar prediction on applicants for a job as a decision maker. Or the analyst might want to test if a model's score is similar to a clinician rating of severity of illness. This section describes how a model can be validated by comparing it to the expert or decision maker's judgments.

Models should be evaluated against objective data, but objective data do not always exist. In these circumstances, one can evaluate a model by comparing it against consensus among experts. A model is consider valid if it replicates the average rating of the experts and if there is consensus among experts about the ratings.

The steps in testing the ability of a model to predict an expert's rating are as follows:

1. Generate or identify cases that will be used to test the model.
2. Ask the experts to rate each case individually, discuss their differences, and rate the case again.
3. Compare the experts to each other and establish that there is consensus in ratings.
4. Compare the model scores against the averate of the experts' ratings. If there is more agreement between the model and the average of the experts than among the experts, consider the model effective in simulating the experts' consensus.

Generate Cases

The first step in comparing a model to experts' rating is to have access to a large number of cases. A *case* is defined as a collection of the levels of the attributes in the model. For each attribute, one level is chosen; a case is the combination of the chosen levels. For example, a case can be constructed for judging the severity of AIDS patients by selecting a particular level for each attribute in the severity index. There are two ways for constructing cases. The first is to rely on real cases, which are organized by using the model to abstract patients or situations. The second approach is to create a hypothetical case from a combination of attributes.

Relying on hypothetical rather than real cases is generally preferable for two reasons. First, the analyst does not often have time or resources to pull together a minimum of 30 real cases. Second, attributes in real cases are positively correlated, and any model in these circumstances, even models with incorrect attribute weights, will produce ratings similar to the experts. In generating hypothetical cases, a combination of attributes, called *orthogonal design*, is used to generate cases more likely to detect differences between the model and the expert. In an orthogonal design, the best and worst of each attribute are combined in such a manner that there is no correlation between the attributes.

The test of the accuracy of a model depends in part on what cases are used. If the cases are constructed in a way that all of the attributes point to the same judgment, the test will not be very sensitive, and any model, even models with improper attribute weights, will end up predicting the cases accurately. For example, if a hypothetical applicant is described to have all of the desired features, then both the model and the decision maker will not have a difficult time accurately rating the overall value associated with the applicant. A stricter test of the model occurs only when there are conflicting attributes, one suggesting one direction and the other the opposite. When cases are constructed to resemble real situations, attributes are often correlated and point to the same conclusions. In contrast, when orthogonal design is used, attributes have zero correlation, and it is more likely to find differences between the model score and expert's judgments.

The steps for constructing orthogonal cases, also called *scenario generation*, are as follows:

1. Select two extreme levels for each attribute (best and worst).
2. Start with two to the power of number of attribute cases. For example, if there are four attributes, you would need 16 cases.
3. Divide the cases in half and assign to each half the level of the first attribute.

4. Divide the cases into quartiles and assign to each quartile the level of the second attribute.
5. Continue this process until every alternate case is assigned the best and worst levels of the last attribute.
6. Review the cases to drop those that are not possible (e.g., pregnant males).
7. If there are too many cases, ask the expert or decision maker to review a randomly chosen sample of cases.
8. Summarize each case on a separate piece of paper so that the decision maker or expert can rate the case without being overwhelmed with information from other cases.

Table 2.3 shows an orthogonal design of cases for a three attribute model.

Rate Cases

The second step in comparing model scores to expert's judgments is to ask the expert or decision maker to review each case and rate it on a scale from zero to 100, where 100 is the best (defined in terms of the task at hand) and zero is the worst (again defined in terms of task at hand). If multiple experts are available, experts can discuss the cases in which they differ and rate again. This process is known as *estimate-talk-estimate* and is an efficient method of getting experts to come to agreement on their numerical ratings. In this fashion, a behavioral consensus and not just a mathematical average can emerge.

When asking an expert to rate a case, present each case on a separate page so that information from other cases will not interfere. Table 2.4 shows an orthogonal design for cases needed to judge severity of HIV/AIDS based on three attributes: skin disease, lung disease, and GI disease.

TABLE 2.3 Orthogonal Design for Three Attributes

Scenario/Case	*Attribute 1*	*Attribute 2*	*Attribute 3*
1	Best	Best	Best
2	Best	Best	Worst
3	Best	Worst	Best
4	Best	Worst	Worst
5	Worst	Best	Best
6	Worst	Best	Worst
7	Worst	Worst	Best
8	Worst	Worst	Worst

These cases are presented one at a time. Figure 2.1 shows an example case and the question asked of the expert.

Compare Experts

In step three, if there are multiple experts, their judgments are compared to each other by looking at pairwise correlations between the experts. Two experts are in excellent agreement if the correlation between their ratings are relatively high, at least more than 0.75. For correlations from 0.50 to 0.65, experts are in moderate agreement. For correlations lower than 0.5, the experts are in low agreement. If experts are in low agreement, it is important to explore the reason why. If there is one decision maker or one expert, this step is skipped.

TABLE 2.4
Orthogonal Design for Three Attributes in Judging Severity of AIDS

Scenario/ Case	*Skin Disease*	*Lung Disease*	*GI Disease*
1	No skin disorder	No lung disorder	No GI disease
2	No skin disorder	No lung disorder	GI cancer
3	No skin disorder	Kaposi's sarcoma	No GI disease
4	No skin disorder	Kaposi's sarcoma	GI cancer
5	Thrush	No lung disorder	No GI disease
6	Thrush	No lung disorder	GI cancer
7	Thrush	Kaposi's sarcoma	No GI disease
8	Thrush	Kaposi's sarcoma	GI cancer

FIGURE 2.1
An Example of a Scenario

Case number 4:
Rated by expert: XXXX
Patient has the following conditions:

Skin disorder:	None
Lung disorder:	Kaposi's sarcoma
GI disorder:	GI cancer

On a scale from 0 to 100, where 100 is the worst prognosis (i.e., a person with less than six months to live) and 0 is the best (i.e., a person with no disorders), where would you rate this case?

First rating before consultations: ______________
Second rating after consultations: ______________

Compare Model to Average of Experts

In step four, the average scores of experts (in cases where there are multiple experts) or the experts' ratings (in cases where there is a single expert) are compared to the model scores. For each case, an MAV model is used to score the case. The correlation between the model score and the expert's scores is used to establish the validity of the model. This correlation should be at least as high as agreement between the experts on the same cases.

Preferential Independence

Independence has many meanings. Following are various definitions for what it means to be independent:[1]

- Not subject to control by others
- Not affiliated with a larger controlling unit
- Not requiring or relying on something else
- Not looking to others for one's opinions or for guidance in conduct
- Not bound by or committed to a political party
- Not requiring or relying on others (for care or livelihood)
- Free from the necessity of working for a living
- Showing a desire for freedom
- Not determined by or capable of being deduced or derived from or expressed in terms of members (as axioms or equations) of the set under consideration
- Having the property that the joint probability (as of events or samples) or the joint probability density function (as of random variables) equals the product of the probabilities or probability density functions of separate occurrence
- Neither deducible from nor incompatible with another statement

To these definitions should be added yet another meaning known as *preferential independence.* Preferential independence can be defined as follows:

- One attribute is preferentially independent from another if changes in shared aspects of the attribute do not affect preferences in the other attribute.
- Two attributes are mutually preferentially independent from each other if each is preferentially independent of the other.

For example, the prognosis of patients with high cholesterol levels is always worse than the prognosis of patients with low cholesterol levels independent of shared levels of age. To test this, the expert should be asked which one of two patients has the worst prognosis:

Analyst: Let's look at two patients. Both of these patients are young. One has high cholesterol levels, and the other has low levels. Which one has the worst prognosis?

Expert: This is obvious—the person with high cholesterol levels.

Analyst: Yes, I agree it is relatively obvious, but I need to check for it. Let me now repeat the question, but this time both patients are frail elderly. Who has the worst prognosis, the one with high cholesterol or the one with low cholesterol?

Expert: If both are elderly, then my answer is the same: the one with high cholesterol.

Analyst: Great, this tells me in my terminology that cholesterol levels are preferentially independent of age.

Please note that in testing the preferential independence, the shared feature is changed but not the actual items that the client is comparing: the age for both patients is changed, but not the cholesterol levels.

Experts may say that two attributes are dependent (because they have other meanings in mind), but the attributes remain preferentially independent when the analyst checks. In many circumstances, preferential independence holds despite appearances to the contrary. However, there are occasional situations where preferential independence does not hold. Now take the previous example and add more facts in one of the attributes so that preferential independence does not hold:

Analyst: Let's look at two patients. Both of these patients are young. One has high cholesterol levels and low alcohol use. The other has high alcohol use and low cholesterol levels. Which one has worst prognosis?

Expert: Well, for a young person, alcohol abuse is a worse indicator than cholesterol levels.

Analyst: OK, now let's repeat the question, but this time both patients are frail elderly. The first patient has high cholesterol and low alcohol use. The second patient has low cholesterol and high alcohol use.

Expert: If both are elderly, I think the one with high cholesterol is at more risk. You see, for young people, I am more concerned with alcohol use; but for older people, I am more concerned with cholesterol levels.

Analyst: Great, this tells me that the combination of alcohol and cholesterol levels is not preferentially independent of age.

To assess preferential independence, a large number of comparisons need to be made, as any pair of attributes must be compared to any other attribute. Keeney and Raiffa (1976) show that if any two consecutive pairs are mutually preferentially independent from each other, then all possible pairs are mutually preferentially independent. This reduces the number of assessments necessary to only a comparison of consecutive pairs, as arranged by the analyst or the decision maker.

When preferential independence does not hold, the analyst should take this as a signal that the underlying attributes have not been fully explored. Perhaps a single attribute can be broken down into multiple attributes.

An additive or multiplicative MAV model assumes that any pair of attributes is mutually preferentially independent of a third attribute. When this assumption is not met, as in the above dialog, there is no mathematical formula that can combine single-attribute functions into an overall score that reflects the decision maker's preferences. In these circumstances, one has to build different models for each level of the attribute. For example, the analyst would need to build one model for young people, another for older people, and still another for frail elderly.

When the analyst identifies preferential independence, several different courses of actions could be followed. If the preferential dependence is not systematic or large, it could be ignored as a method of simplifying the model. On the other hand, if preferential independence is violated systematically for a few attributes, then a different model can be built for each value of the attributes. For example, in assessing risk of hospitalization, one model can be built for young people and a different model can be built for older people. Finally, one can search for a different formulation of attributes so that they are preferentially independent.

Multi-Attribute Utility Models

Utility models are value models that reflect the decision maker's risk preferences. Instead of assessing the decision maker's values directly, utility models reflect the decision maker's preferences among uncertain outcomes. Single-attribute utility functions are constructed by asking the decision maker to choose among a "sure return" and a "gamble." For example, to estimate return on investment, the decision maker should be asked to find a return that will make him indifferent to a gamble with a 50 percent chance of maximum return and a 50 percent chance of worst-possible return. The decision maker's sure return is assigned a utility of 50. This process is continued by posing gambles involving the midpoint and the best and worst points. For example, suppose you want to estimate the utility associated with returns ranging from zero to $1000. The decision maker is asked how much of a return she is willing to take for sure to give up a 50 percent chance of making $1,000 and a 50 percent chance of making $0.

If the decision maker gives a response that is less than midway (i.e., less than $500), then the decision maker is a risk seeker. The decision maker is assigning a utility to the midway point that is higher than the expected value of returns. If the decision maker gives a response above the midway point, then the decision maker undervalues a gamble and prefers the sure return. He is risk averse. The utility he assigns to gambles is less than the expected value of the gamble; risk itself is something this decision maker is trying to avoid. If the decision maker responds with the midpoint, then she is considered to be risk neutral. A risk-neutral person is indifferent between a gamble for various returns and the expected monetary value of the gamble.

Suppose the decision maker has responded with a value of $400. Then, 50 utilities should be assigned to the return of $400. The midpoint of the scale is $500. The decision maker is a risk seeker because he assigns to the gamble a utility more than its expected value. Of course, one point does not establish risk preferences, and several points need to be estimated before one has a reasonable picture of the utility function. The analyst continues the interview to assess the utility of additional gambles. The analyst can ask for a gamble involving the midpoint and the best return. The question would be stated as follows: "How much do you need to get for sure to give up a 50 percent chance of making $400 and a 50 percent chance of making $0." Suppose the response is $175; the return is assigned a utility of 25. Similarly, the analyst can ask, "How much do you need to get for sure to give up a 50 percent chance of making $400 and a 50 percent chance of making $1,000." Suppose the response is $675; the response is assigned a utility of 75. After the utility of a few points has been estimated, it is possible to fit the points to a polynomial curve so that a utility score for all returns can be estimated. Figure 2.2 shows the resulting utility curve.

Sometimes you have to estimate a utility function over an attribute that is not continuous or that does not have a natural physical scale. In this approach, the worst and the best levels are fixed at zero and 100 utilities. The decision maker is asked to come up with a probability that would make her indifferent between a new level in the attribute and a gamble involving the worst and best possible levels in the attribute. For

FIGURE 2.2 A Risk-Seeking Utility Function

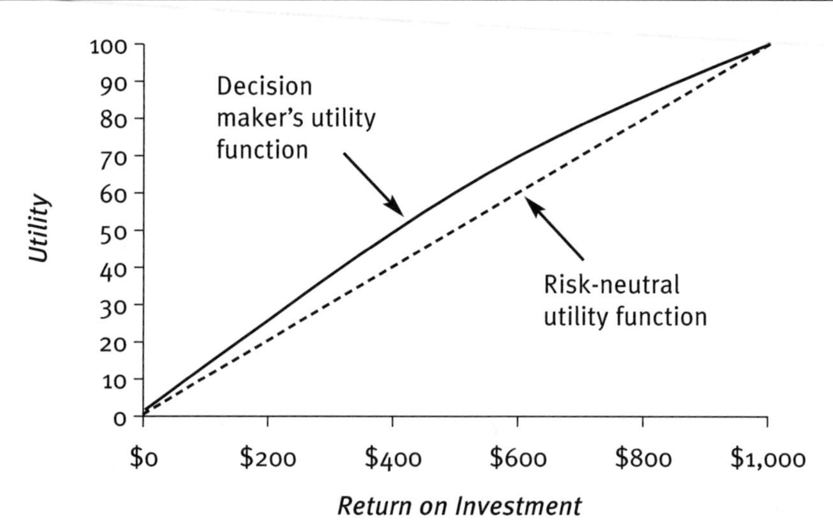

example, suppose you want to estimate the utility (or dis-utility) associated with the following six skin conditions (listed in increasing order of severity): (1) no skin disorder, (2) Kaposi's sarcoma, (3) shingles, (4) herpes complex, (5) *candidiasis,* and (6) thrush. The analyst then assigns the best possible level a utility of zero. The worst possible level, thrush, is assigned a utility of 100. The decision maker is asked to think if she prefers to have Kaposi's sarcoma or a 90 percent chance of thrush and a 10 percent chance of having no skin disorders. Regardless of the response, the decision maker is asked the same question again but with probabilities reversed: "Do you prefer to have Kaposi's sarcoma or a 10 percent chance of thrush and a 90 percent chance of having no skin disorders?" The analyst points out to the decision maker that the choice between the sure disease and the risky situation was reversed when the probabilities were changed.

Because the choice is reversed, there must exist a probability at which point the decision maker is indifferent between the sure thing and the gamble. The probabilities are changed until the point is found where the decision maker is indifferent between having Kaposi's sarcoma and the probability P of having thrush and probability $(1 - P)$ of having no skin disorders. The utility associated with Kaposi's sarcoma is 100 times the estimated probability, P. A utility function assessed in this fashion will reflect not only the values associated with different diseases but also the decision maker's risk-taking attitude. Some decision makers may consider a sure disease radically worse than a gamble involving a chance, even though remote, of having no diseases at all. These estimates thus reflect not only the decision makers' values but also their willingness to take risks. Value functions do not reflect risk attitudes; therefore, one would expect single-attribute value and utility functions to be different.

Hierarchical Modeling of Attributes[2]

It is sometimes helpful to introduce a hierarchical structure among the attributes, where broad categories are considered first and then, within these broad categories, weights are assigned to attributes. By convention, the weights for the broad categories add up to one, and the weight for the attributes within each category also add up to one. The final weight for an attribute is the product of the weight for its category and the weight of the attribute within the category. The following example shows the use of hierarchy in setting weights for attributes.

Chatburn and Primiano (2001) employed an additive, compensatory, multi-attribute utility model to assist the University Hospitals of Cleveland in their purchase of new ventilators for use in the hospitals' intensive care units. A decision-making model was useful in this instance because ventilators are expensive, complicated machines, and the administration and staff needed an efficient way to analyze the costs and benefits of the various purchase options.

The decision process began with an analysis of the hospitals' current ventilator situation. Many factors suggested that the purchase of new ventilators would be advantageous. First, all of the ventilators owned by the hospitals were between 12 and 16 years old, while the depreciable life span of a ventilator is only ten years. Thus, the age of the equipment put the hospitals at a greater risk to experience equipment failures. Because ventilators are used primarily for life support, the hospitals would be highly liable should this equipment fail. Second, the costs to maintain the older equipment were beginning to outweigh the initial capital investment. Third, the current fleet of ventilators varied in age and model. Some ventilators could be used only for adults, while others could only be used for infants or children, and different generations of machines ran under different operating systems. The result was that not all members of the staff were facile with every model of ventilator, yet it seemed impractical to invest in the type of extensive staff training that would be required to correct this problem. Therefore, the goals for the ventilator purchase were to advance patient care capabilities and increase staff competence, to reduce maintenance costs and staff training costs.

To begin the selection process, the consultants wanted to limit the analysis to only the most relevant choices: those machines that were designed for use in intensive care units with an ability to ventilate multiple types of patients. In addition, it was important to select a company with good customer support and the availability of software upgrades. Also, the analysis involved both a clinical and technical evaluation of each ventilator model, as well as cost analysis. Each possible ventilator was used in the hospital's units on a trial basis for 18 months so that staff could familiarize themselves with each model. The technical evaluation utilized previously published guidelines for ventilators as well as vendor-assisted simulations of various ventilator situations so that administrators and staff could compare the functionality of the different models. A checklist was used in this instance to evaluate each ventilator in three major areas: control scheme, operator interface, and alarms. Figure 2.3 depicts the attributes, their levels, and relative weights used in the final decision model.

Note that weights were first assessed across broad categories (cost, technical features, and customer service). Two of these broad categories were broken into additional attributes. Weights for broad categories were assessed; note that these weights add up to one. In addition, the weights for each attribute within the categories were also assessed; note that these weights also add up to one within the category. In the end, the model had eight attributes in total, and the weight for attributes was calculated as the product of the weight for the broad category and the weight of the attribute within that category.

Summary

In this chapter, a method is presented for modeling preferences. Often, decisions must be made through explicitly considering the priorities of decision makers. This chapter teaches the reader how to model decisions where qualitative priorities and preferences must be quantified so that an informed decision can be made. The chapter provides a rationale for modeling the values of decision makers and offers words of caution in interpreting quantitative estimates of qualitative values. The chapter concludes with examples of the use of value models, and it explains in detail the steps in modeling preferences.

The first step is determining if a model would be useful in making a particular decision. This includes identifying decision makers, objectives of the decision makers, what role subjective judgments play in the decision-making process, and if and how a value model should be employed.

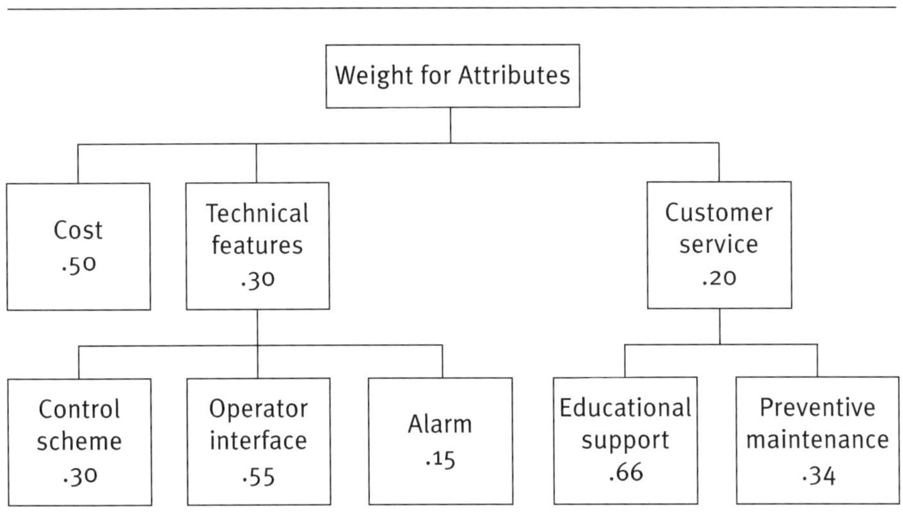

FIGURE 2.3 A Hierarchy for Assessing Attribute Weights

Next, the decision analyst must identify the attributes needed for making the judgment, and several suggestions are offered for completing this step. The third step entails narrowing the list of identified attributes to those that are the most useful. Once the attributes to be used in the decision have been finalized, the decision maker assigns values to the levels of each attribute. The next step entails the analyst determining how to aggregate single-attribute functions into an overall score evaluated across all attributes. These scores are then weighted based upon importance to the decision makers. The analyst finishes with an examination of the accuracy of the resulting decision model. The chapter concludes by providing several alternative methods for completing various steps in the process of modeling preferences.

Review What You Know

1. What are two methods for assessing a decision maker's preferences over a single attribute?
2. What are two methods for aggregating values assigned to different attributes into one overall score?
3. Make a numbered list of what to do and what not to do in selecting attributes.
4. Describe how attribute levels are solicited. In your answer, describe the process of soliciting attribute levels and not any specific list of attributes or attribute levels.

Rapid-Analysis Exercises

Construct a value function for a decision at work. Be sure to select a decision that does not involve predicting uncertain outcomes (see examples listed below). Select an expert who will help you construct the model and make an appointment to do so. Afterwards, prepare a report that answers the following questions:

1. What is the problem to be addressed? What judgment must be made, and how can the model of the judgment be useful? (Conduct research to report if similar studies have been done using MAV or utility models.)
2. Who is the decision maker?
3. What are the assumptions about the problem and its causes?
4. What objectives are being pursued by each constituency?
5. Do various constituencies have different perceptions and values?
6. What options are available?
7. What factors or attributes influence the desirability of various outcomes?
8. What values did the expert assign to each attribute and its levels?
9. How were single-attribute values aggregated to produce one overall score?
10. What is the evidence that the model is valid?
11. Is the model based on available data?
12. Did the expert consider the model simple to use?
13. Did the expert consider the model to be face valid?
14. Does the model correspond with other measures of the same concept (i.e., construct validity)?
15. Does the model simulate the experts' judgment on at least 15 cases?
16. Does the model predict any objective gold standard?

Audio/Visual Chapter Aids

To help you understand the concepts of modeling preferences, visit this book's companion web site at ache.org/DecisionAnalysis, go to Chapter 2, and view the audio/visual chapter aids.

Notes

1. *Merriam-Webster's Collegiate Dictionary*, 11th ed., s.v. "Independent."

2. This section is a summary prepared by Jennifer A. Sinkule based on Chatburn, R. L., F. P. Primiano, Jr. 2001. "Decision Analysis for Large Capital Purchases: How to Buy a Ventilator." *Respiratory Care* 46 (10): 1038–53.

References

Alemi, F., B. Turner, L. Markson, and T. Maccaron. 1990. "Severity of the Course of AIDS." *Interfaces* 21 (3): 105–6.

Alemi, F., L. Walker, J. Carey, and J. Leggett. 1999. "Validity of Three Measures of Severity of AIDS for Use in Health Services Research Studies." *Health Services Management Research* 12 (1): 45–50.

Anthony, M.K., P. F. Brennan, R. O'Brien, and N. Suwannaroop. 2004. "Measurement of Nursing Practice Models Using Multiattribute Utility Theory: Relationship to Patient and Organizational Outcomes." *Quality Management in Health Care* 13 (1): 40–52.

Bernoulli, D. 1738. "Spearman theoria novai de mensura sortus." *Comettariii Academiae Saentiarum Imperialses Petropolitica* 5:175–92. Translated by L. Somner. 1954. *Econometrica* 22:23–36.

Chapman, G. B, and E. J. Johnson. 1999. "Anchoring, Activation, and the Construction of Values." *Organizational Behavior and Human Decision Processes* 79 (2): 115–53.

Chatburn, R. L., and F. P. Primiano. 2001. "Decision Analysis for Large Capital Purchases: How to Buy a Ventilator." *Respiratory Care* 46 (10): 1038–53.

Chiou, C. F., M. R. Weaver, M. A. Bell, T. A. Lee, and J. W. Krieger. 2005. "Development of the Multi-Attribute Pediatric Asthma Health Outcome Measure (PAHOM)." *International Journal for Quality in Healthcare* 17 (1): 23–30.

Chow, C. W., K. M. Haddad, and A. Wong-Boren. 1991. "Improving Subjective Decision Making in Health Care Administration." *Hospital and Health Services Administration* 36 (2):191–210.

Cline, B., F. Alemi, and K. Bosworth 1982. "Intensive Skilled Nursing Care: A Multi-Attribute Utility Model for Level of Care Decision Making." *Journal of American Health Care Association* 8 (6): 82–87.

Cook, R. L., and T. R. Stewart. 1975. "A Comparison of Seven Methods for Obtaining Subjective Description of Judgmental Policy." *Organizational Behavior and Human Performance* 12:31–45.

Edwards, W., and F. H. Barron. 1994. "SMARTS and SMARTER: Improved Simple Methods for Multiattribute Utility Measurement." *Organizational Behavior and Human Decision Processes* 60: 306–25.

Eriksen, S., and L. R. Keller. 1993. "A Multiattribute-Utility-Function Approach to Weighing the Risks and Benefits of Pharmaceutical Agents." *Medical Decision Making* 13 (2): 118–25.

Fields, W. 1995. "Brainstorming: How to Generate Creative Ideas." *Nursing Quality Connection* 5 (3): 35.

Fos, P. J., and M. A. Zuniga. 1999. "Assessment of Primary Health Care Access Status: An Analytic Technique for Decision Making." *Health Care Management Science* 2 (4): 229–38.

Freedberg, K. A., J. A. Scharfstein, G. R. Seage, E. Losina, M. C. Weinstein, D. E. Craven, and A. D. Paltiel. 1998. "The Cost-Effectiveness of Preventing AIDS-Related Opportunistic Infections." *JAMA* 279 (2): 130–36.

Goodwin, P., and G. Wright. 2004. *Decision Analysis for Management Judgment.* 3rd ed. Hoboken, NJ: John Wiley and Sons.

Health Services Research Group, Center for Health Systems Research and Analysis, University of Wisconsin. 1975. "Development of the Index for Medical Under-service." *Health Services Research* 10 (2): 168–80.

Jia, J., G. W. Fischer, and J. S. Dyer. 1998. "Attribute Weighting Methods and Decision Quality in the Presence of Response Error: A Simulation Study." *Journal of Behavioral Decision Making* 11 (2): 85–105.

Kahneman, D. 2003. "A Perspective on Judgment and Choice: Mapping Bounded Rationality." *American Psychologist* 58 (9): 697–720.

Keeney, R. 1996. *Value-Focused Thinking: A Path to Creative Decisionmaking.* Cambridge, MA: Harvard University Press.

Keeney, R. L., and H. Raiffa. 1976. *Decisions and Multiple Objectives: Preferences and Value Tradeoffs.* New York: John Wiley and Sons.

Kim, S., D. Goldstein, L. Hasher, and R. T. Zacks. 2005. "Framing Effects in Younger and Older Adults." *Journals of Gerontology: Series B, Psychological Sciences and Social Sciences* 60 (4): P215–8.

Kinzbrunner, B., and M. M. Pratt. 1994. "Severity Index Scores Correlate with Survival of AIDS Patients." *American Journal of Hospice and Palliative Care* 11 (3): 4–9.

Krahn, M., P. Ritvo, J. Irvine, G. Tomlinson, A. Bezjak, J. Trachtenberg, and G. Naglie. 2000. "Construction of the Patient-Oriented Prostate Utility Scale (PORPUS): A Multiattribute Health State Classification System for Prostate Cancer." *Journal of Clinical Epidemiology* 53 (9): 920–30.

McNeil, B. J., S. H. Pedersen, and C. Gatsonis. 1992. "Current Issues in Profiles: Potentials and Limitations." In *Physician Payment Review Commission Conference on Profiling*, 46–70. Washington, DC: Physician Payment Review Commission.

Naglie, G., M. D. Krahn, D. Naimark, D. A. Redelmeier, and A. S. Detsky. 1997. "Primer on Medical Decision Analysis: Part 3—Estimating Probabilities and Utilities." *Medical Decision Making* 17 (2): 136–41.

Nisbett, R., and L. Ross. 1980. *Human Inferences.* Englewood Cliffs, NJ: Prentice-Hall.

Nisbett, R.E., and Y. Miyamoto. 2005. "The Influence of Culture: Holistic versus Analytic Perception." *Trends in Cognitive Sciences* 9 (10): 467–73.

Salo, A. A., and R. P. Hämäläinen. 2001. "Preference Ratios in Multi-Attribute Evaluation (PRIME)—Elicitation and Decision Procedures." *IEEE Transactions on Systems, Man, and Cybernetics* 31 (6): 533–45.

Spoth, R. 1991. "Multi-Attribute Analysis of Benefit Managers' Preferences for Smoking Cessation Programs." *Health Values* 14 (5): 3–15.

Sutton, R. I. 2001. "The Weird Rules of Creativity." *Harvard Business Review* 79 (8): 94–103, 161.

Torrance, G. W, W. Furlong, D. Feeny, and M. Boyle. 1995. "Multi-Attribute Preference Functions: Health Utilities Index." *Pharmacoeconomics* 7 (6): 503–20.

Vibbert, S. 1992. "Illinois Blues Target Doctors." *Medical Utilization Review*, April 2.

Von Winterfeldt, D., and W. Edwards. 1986. *Decision Analysis and Behavioral Research.* New York: Cambridge University Press.

Appendix 2.1: Severity of the Course of AIDS Index

Step 1: Choose the lowest score that applies to the patient's characteristics. If no exact match can be found, approximate the score by using the two markers most similar to the patient's characteristics.

Age

Less than 18 years, do not use this index

18 to 40 years, 1.0000
40 to 60 years, 0.9774
Over 60 years, 0.9436

Race

White, 1.0000
Black, 0.9525
Hispanic, 0.9525
Other, 1.0000

Defining AIDS diagnosis

Kaposi's sarcoma, 1.0000
Candida esophagitis, 0.8093
Pneumocystis carinii pneumonia, 0.8014
Toxoplasmosis, 0.7537
Cryptococcosis, 0.7338
Cytomegalovirus retinitis, 0.7259
Cryptosporidiosis, 0.7179
Dementia, 0.7140
Cytomegalovirus colitis, 0.6981
Lymphoma, 0.6981
Progressive multi-focal leukoencephalopathy, 0.6941

Mode of transmission

Blood transfusion for non-trauma, 0.9316
Drug abuse, 0.8792
Other, 1.0000

Skin disorders

No skin disorder, 1.0000
Kaposi's sarcoma, 1.0000
Shingles, 0.9036
Herpes simplex, 0.8735
Cutaneous candidiasis, 0.8555
Thrush, 0.8555

Heart disorders

No heart disorders, 1.0000
HIV cardiomyopathy, 0.7337

GI diseases

No GI disease, 1.0000
Isosporidiasis, 0.8091
Candida esophagitis, 0.8058
Salmonella infectum, 0.7905
Tuberculosis, 0.7897
Nonspecific diarrhea, 0.7803
GI cancer, 0.7060
Herpes esophagitis, 0.7536
Mycobacterium avium-intracellulare, 0.7494
Cryptosporidiosis, 0.7369
Kaposi's sarcoma, 0.7324
Cytomegalovirus colitis, 0.7086

Time since AIDS diagnosis

Less than 3 months, 1.0000
More than 3 months, 0.9841
More than 6 months, 0.9682
More than 9 months, 0.9563
More than 12 months, 0.9404
More than 15 months, 0.9245
More than 18 months, 0.9086
More than 21 months, 0.8927
More than 24 months, 0.8768
More than 36 months, 0.8172
More than 48 months, 0.7537
More than 60 months, 0.6941

Lung disorders

No lung disorders, 1.0000
Pneumonia, unspecified, 0.9208
Bacterial pneumonia, 0.8960
Tuberculosis, 0.8911
Mild *Pneumocystis carinii* pneumonia, 0.8664
Cryptococcosis, 0.8161
Herpes simplex, 0.8115
Histoplasmosis, 0.8135
Pneumocystis carinii pneumonia with respiratory failure, 0.8100
Mycobacterium avium-intracellulare, 0.8020
Kaposi's sarcoma, 0.7772

Nervous system diseases

No nervous system involvement, 1.0000
Neurosyphilis, 0.9975
Tubercular meningitis, 0.7776
Cryptoccoccal meningitis, 0.7616
Seizure, 0.7611
Myelopathy, 0.7511
Cytomegalovirus retinitis, 0.7454
Norcardiosis, 0.7454
Meningitis encephalitis unspecified, 0.7368
Histoplasmosis, 0.7264
Progressive multifocal leukoencephalopathy, 0.7213
Encephalopathy/HIV dementia, 0.7213
Coccidioidomycosis, 0.7189
Lymphoma, 0.7139

Disseminated disease

No disseminated illness, 1.0000
Idiopathic thrombocytopenic pupura, 0.9237
Kaposi's sarcoma, 0.9067
Non-*Salmonella* sepsis, 0.8163
Salmonella sepsis, 0.8043
Other drug-induced anemia, 0.7918
Varicella zoster virus, 0.7912
Tuberculosis, 0.7910
Norcardiosis, 0.7842
Non-tubercular mycobacterial disease, 0.7705
Transfusion, 0.7611
Toxoplasmosis, 0.7591
AZT drug-induced anemia, 0.7576
Cryptococcosis, 0.7555
Histoplasmosis, 0.7405
Hodgkin's disease, 0.7340
Coccidio-idomycosis, 0.7310
Cytomegalovirus, 0.7239
Non-Hodgkin's lymphoma, 0.7164
Thrombotic thrombocytopenia, 0.7139

Recurring acute illness

No, 1.0000
Yes, 0.8357

Functional impairment

No marker, 1.0000
Boarding home care, 0.7933
Hospice care, 0.7416
Home health care, 0.7655
Nursing home care, 0.7535

Psychiatric comorbidity

None, 1.0000
Psychiatric problem in psychiatric hospital, 0.8872
Psychiatric problem in medical setting, 0.8268
Severe depression, 0.8268

Drug markers

None, 1.0000
Lack of prophylaxis, 0.8756
Starting AZT on 1 gram, 0.7954
Starting and stopping of AZT, 0.7963
Dropping AZT by 1 gram, 0.7673
Incomplete treatment in herpes simplex virus, varicella-zoster virus, Mycobacterium avium-intracellulare, or Cytomegalovirus retinitis, 0.7593
Prescribed oral narcotics, 0.7512
Prescribed parenteral narcotics, 0.7192
Incomplete treatment of *Pneumocystis carinii* pneumonia, 0.7111
Incomplete treatment in toxoplasmosis, 0.7031
Incomplete treatment in cryptococcal infection, 0.6951

Organ involvement

None, 1.0000

Organ	*Failure*	*Insufficiency*	*Dysfunction*
Cerebral	0.7000	0.7240	0.7480
Liver	0.7040	0.7600	0.8720
Heart	0.7080	0.7320	0.7560
Lung	0.7120	0.7520	0.8000
Renal	0.7280	0.7920	0.8840
Adrenal	0.7640	0.8240	0.7960

Comorbidity

None, 1.0000
Hypertension, 1.0000
Alcoholism, 0.8406
Influenza, 0.9203
Legionella, 0.9402

Nutritional status

No markers, 1.0000
Antiemetic, 0.9282
Nutritional supplement, 0.7687
Payment for nutritionist, 0.7607
Lomotil®/Imodium®, 0.7447
Total parenteral nutrition, 0.7248

Step two: Multiply all selected scores and enter here:
Step three: Subtract 1 from above entry and enter here:
Step four: Divide by −0.99 and enter here:

CHAPTER

3

MEASURING UNCERTAINTY

Farrokh Alemi

This chapter describes how probability can quantify the degree of uncertainty one feels about future events. It answers the following questions:

- What is probability?
- What is the difference between objective and subjective sources of data for probabilities?
- What is Bayes's theorem?
- What are independence and conditional independence?
- How does one verify independence?

Measuring uncertainty is important because it allows one to make trade-offs among uncertain events, and to act in uncertain environments. Decision makers may not be sure about a business outcome, but if they know the chances are good, they may risk it and reap the benefits.

Probability

When it is certain that an event will occur, it has a probability of 1. When it is certain that an event will not occur, it has a probability of 0. When there is uncertainty that an event will occur, it has a probability of 0.5—or, a 50/50 chance of occurrence. All other values between 0 and 1 measure the uncertainty about the occurrence of an event.

The best way to think of probability is as the ratio of all ways an event may occur divided by all possible outcomes. In short, *probability* is the prevalence of the target event among the possible events. For example, the probability of a small business failing is the number of small businesses that fail divided by the total number of small businesses. Or, the probability of an iatrogenic infection in the last month in a hospital is the number of patients who last month had an iatrogenic infection in the hospital divided by the number of patients in the hospital during last month. The basic probability formula is

This book has a companion web site that features narrated presentations, animated examples, PowerPoint slides, online tools, web links, additional readings, and examples of students' work. To access this chapter's learning tools, go to ache.org/DecisionAnalysis and select Chapter 3.

$$P(A) = \frac{\text{Number of occurences of event } A}{\text{Total number of possible events}}.$$

Figure 3.1 shows a visual representation of probability. The rectangle represents the number of possible events, and the circle represents all ways in which event A might occur; the ratio of the circle to the rectangle is the probability of A.

Probability of Multiple Events

The rules of probability allow you to calculate the probability of multiple events. For example, the probability of either A or B occurring is calculated by first summing all the possible ways in which event A will occur and all the ways in which event B will occur, minus all the possible ways in which both event A and B will occur together (this is subtracted to avoid double counting). This sum is divided by all possible outcomes. This concept is shown in the Venn diagram in Figure 3.2. This concept is represented in mathematical terms as

$$P(A \text{ or } B) = P(A) + P(B) - P(A \text{ and } B).$$

The definition of probability gives you a simple calculus for combining the uncertainty of two events. You can now ask questions such as "What is the probability that frail elderly (age > 75 years old) or infant patients will join our HMO?" According to the previous formula, this can be calculated as

$$P(\text{Frail elderly or Infant}) = P(\text{Frail elderly}) + P(\text{Infant}) - P(\text{Frail elderly and Infant}).$$

Because the chance of being both a frail elderly person and an infant is 0 (i.e., the two events are mutually exclusive), the formula can be rewritten as

$$P(\text{Frail elderly or Infant}) = P(\text{Frail elderly}) + P(\text{Infant}).$$

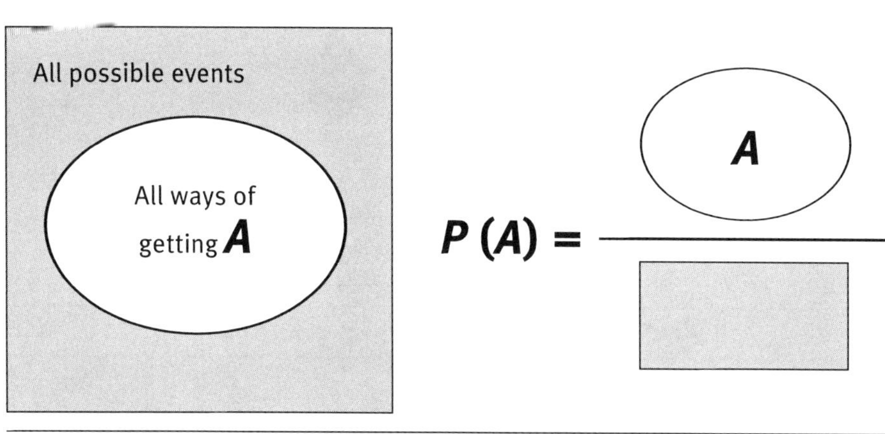

FIGURE 3.1 A Visual Representation of Probability

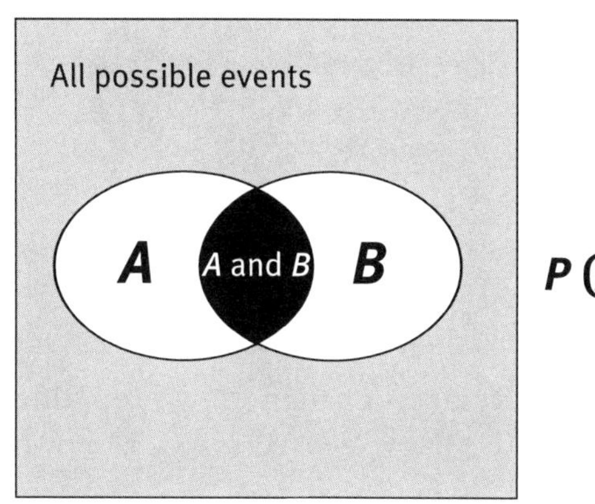

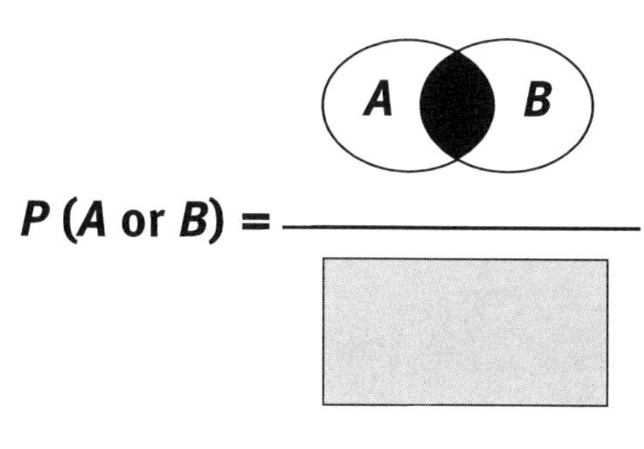

FIGURE 3.2 Visual Representation of Probability *A* or *B*

This definition of probability can also be used to measure the probability of two events co-occurring (probability of event *A* and event *B*). Note that the overlap between *A* and *B* is shaded in Figure 3.2; this area represents all the ways *A* and *B* might occur together. Figure 3.3 shows how the probability of *A* and *B* occurring together is calculated by dividing this shaded area by all possible outcomes.

Conditional, Joint, and Marginal Probabilities

The definition of probability also helps in the calculation of the probability of an event conditioned on the occurrence of other events. In mathematical terms, *conditional probability* is shown as $P(A|B)$ and read as probability of *A* given *B*. When an event occurs, the remaining list of possible outcomes is reduced. There is no longer the need to track events that

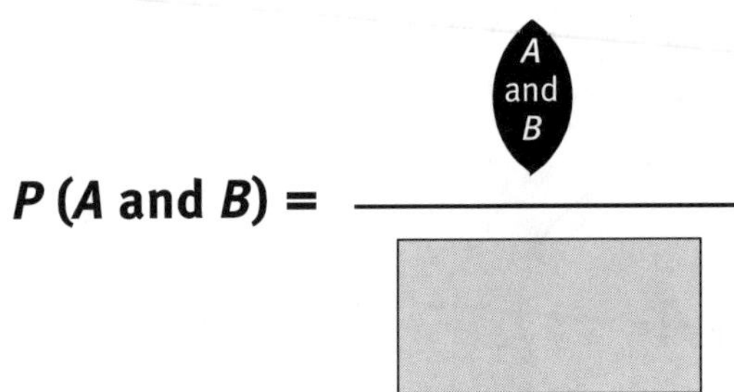

FIGURE 3.3 A Visual Representation of Joint Probability *A* or *B*

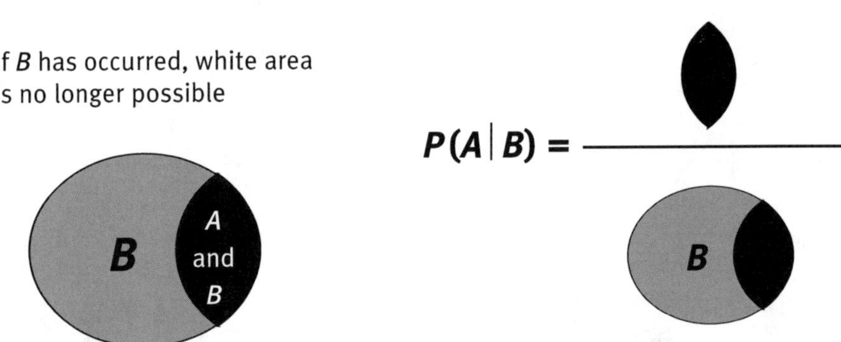

FIGURE 3.4 Probability of *A* Given *B* Is Calculated by Reducing the Possibilities

are not possible. You can calculate conditional probabilities by restricting the possibilities to only those events that you know have occurred, as shown in Figure 3.4. This is shown mathematically as

$$P(A \mid B) = \frac{P(A \text{ and } B)}{P(B)}.$$

For example, you can now calculate the probability that a frail elderly patient who has already joined the HMO will be hospitalized. Instead of looking at the hospitalization rate among all frail elderly patients, you need to restrict the possibilities to only the frail elderly patients who have joined the HMO. Then, the probability is calculated as the ratio of the number of hospitalizations among frail elderly patients in the HMO to the number of frail elderly patients in the HMO:

$$P(\text{Hospitalized} \mid \text{Joined HMO}) = \frac{P(\text{Hospitalized and Joined HMO})}{P(\text{Joined HMO})}.$$

Analysts need to make sure that decision makers distinguish between joint probability, or the probability of A and B occurring together, and conditional probability, or the probability of B occurring after A has occurred. Joint probabilities, shown as $P(A \text{ and } B)$, are symmetrical and not time based. In contrast, conditional probabilities, shown as $P(A|B)$, are asymmetrical and do rely on the passage of time. For example, the probability of a frail elderly person being hospitalized is different from the probability of finding a frail elderly person among people who have been hospitalized.

For an example calculation of conditional probabilities from joint probabilities, assume that an analysis has produced the joint probabilities in Table 3.1 for the patient being either in substance abuse treatment or in probation.

Table 3.1 provides joint and marginal probabilities by dividing the observed frequency of days by the total number of days examined. *Marginal probability* refers to the probability of one event; in Table 3.1, these are provided in the row and column labeled "Total." For example, the marginal probability of a probation day, regardless of whether it is also a treatment day, is 0.56. *Joint probability* refers to the probability of two events occurring at same time; in Table 3.1, these are provided in the remaining rows and columns. For example, the joint probability of having both a probation day and a treatment day is 0.51. This probability is calculated by dividing the number of days in which both probation and treatment occur by the total number of days examined.

If an analyst wishes to calculate a conditional probability, the total universe of possible days must be reduced to the days that meet the condition. This is a very important concept to keep in mind:

> Conditional probability is a reduction in the universe of possibilities.

Suppose the analyst wants to calculate the conditional probability of being in treatment given that the patient is already in probation. In this case, the universe is reduced to all days in which the patient has been in probation. In this reduced universe, the total number of days of treatment

TABLE 3.1 Joint Probability of Treatment and Probation

	Probation Day	*Not a Probation Day*	*Total*
Treatment Day	0.51	0.39	0.90
Not a Treatment Day	0.05	0.05	0.10
Total	0.56	0.44	1.00

becomes the number of days of having both treatment and probation. Therefore, the conditional probability of treatment given probation is

$$P(\text{Treatment} \mid \text{Probation}) = \frac{\text{Number of days in both treatment and probation}}{\text{Number of days in probation}}.$$

Because Table 3.1 provides the joint and marginal probabilities, the previous formula can be described in terms of joint and marginal probabilities:

$$P(\text{Treatment} \mid \text{Probation}) = \frac{P(\text{Treatment and Probation})}{P(\text{Probation})} = \frac{0.51}{0.56} = 0.93.$$

The point of this example is that conditional probabilities can be easily calculated by reducing the universe of possibilities to only those situations that meet the condition. You can calculate conditional probabilities from marginal and joint probabilities by keeping in mind how the condition has reduced the universe of possibility.

Conditional probabilities are a very useful concept. They allow you to think through an uncertain sequence of events. If each event can be conditioned on its predecessor, a chain of events can be examined. Then, if one component of the chain changes, you can calculate the effect of the change throughout the chain. In this sense, conditional probabilities show how a series of clues might forecast a future event. For example, in predicting who will join the HMO, the patient's demographics (age, gender, income level) can be used to infer the probability of joining. In this case, the probability of joining the HMO is the target event. The clues are the patient's age, gender, and income level. The objective is to predict the probability of joining the HMO given the patient's demographics—in other words, $P(\text{Join HMO} \mid \text{Age, gender, income level})$.

The calculus of probability is an easy way to track the overall uncertainty of several events. The calculus is appropriate if the following simple assumptions are met:

1. The probability of an event is a positive number between 0 and 1.
2. One event certainly will happen, so the sum of the probabilities of all events is 1.
3. The probability of any two mutually exclusive events occurring equals the sum of the probability of each occurring.

Most decision makers are willing to accept these three assumptions, often referred to by mathematicians as *probability axioms.*

If a set of numbers assigned to uncertain events meet these three principles, then it is a probability function and the numbers assigned in this fashion must follow the algebra of probabilities.

Sources of Data

There are two ways to measure the probability of an event:

1. One can observe the objective frequency of the event. For example, you can see how many out of 100 people who were approached about joining an HMO expressed intent to do so.
2. The alternative is to rely on subjective opinions of an expert. In these circumstances, ask an expert to estimate the strength of her belief that the event of interest might happen. For example, you might ask a venture capitalist who is familiar with new businesses the following question: On a scale from 0 to 100, where 100 is for sure, how strongly do you feel that the average employee will join an HMO?

Both approaches measure the degree of uncertainty about the success of the HMO, but there is a major difference between them: One approach is objective while the other is based on opinion. Objective frequencies are based on observations of the history of the event, while a measurement of strength of belief is based on an individual's opinion, even about events that have no history (e.g., What is the chance that there will be a terrorist attack in our hospital?).

Subjective Probability

More than half a century ago, Savage (1954) and de Finetti (1937) argued that the rules of probabilities can work with uncertainties expressed as strength of opinion. Savage termed the strength of a decision maker's convictions "subjective probability" and used the calculus of probability to analyze these convictions. Subjective probability remains a popular method for analyzing experts' judgments and opinions (Jeffrey 2004). Reviews of the field show that under certain circumstances, experts and nonexperts can reliably assess subjective probabilities that correspond to objective reality (Wallsten and Budescu 1983). Subjective probability can be measured along two different concepts: (1) intensity of feelings and (2) hypothetical frequency. Subjective probability based on intensity of feelings can be measured by asking the experts to rate their certainty on a scale of 0 percent to 100 percent. Subjective probability based on hypothetical frequency can be measured by asking the expert to estimate how many times the target event will occur out of 100 possible situations.

Suppose an analyst wants to measure the probability that an employee will join the HMO. Using the first method, an analyst would ask an expert on the local healthcare market about the intensity of his feelings:

> Analyst: Do you think employees will join the plan? On a scale from 0 to 100, with 100 being certain, how strongly do you feel you are right?

When measuring according to hypothetical frequencies, the expert would be asked to imagine what she expects the frequency would be, even though the event has not occurred repeatedly:

> Analyst: Out of 100 employees, how many do you think will join the plan?

Subjective Probability as a Probability Function

If both the subjective and the objective methods produce a probability for the event, then the calculus of probabilities can be used to make new inferences from these data. It makes no difference whether the frequency is objectively observed through historical precedents or subjectively described by an expert; the resulting number should follow the rules of probability.

Even though subjective probabilities measured as intensity of feelings are not actually probability functions, they should be treated as such. Returning to the formal definition of a probability measure, a probability function is defined by the following characteristics:

1. The probability of an event is a positive number between 0 and 1.
2. One event certainly will happen, so the sum of the probabilities of all events is 1.
3. The probability of any two mutually exclusive events occurring equals the sum of the probability of each occurring.

These assumptions are at the root of all mathematical work in probability, so any beliefs expressed as probability must follow them. Furthermore, if these three assumptions are met, then the numbers produced in this fashion will follow all rules of probabilities. Are these three assumptions met when the data are subjective? The first assumption is always true, because you can assign numbers to beliefs so they are always positive.

But the second and third assumptions are not always true, and people do hold beliefs that violate them. However, analysts can take steps to ensure that these two assumptions are also met. For example, when the estimates of all possibilities (e.g., probability of success and failure) do not total 1, the analyst can revise the estimates to do so. When the estimated probabilities of two mutually exclusive events do not equal the sum of their separate probabilities, the analyst can ask whether they should and adjust them as necessary.

Decision makers, left to their own devices, may not follow the calculus of probability. Experts' opinions also may not follow the rules of probability, but if experts agree with the aforementioned three principles, then such opinions should follow the rules of probability.

Probabilities and beliefs are not identical constructs; rather, probabilities provide a context in which beliefs can be studied. That is, if beliefs are expressed as probabilities, then the rules of probability provide a systematic and orderly method of examining the implications of these beliefs.

Bayes's Theorem

From the definition of conditional probability, one can derive the *Bayes's theorem*, an optimal model for revising existing opinion (sometimes called prior opinion) in light of new evidence or clues. The theorem states

$$\frac{P(H|C_1, \ldots, C_n)}{P(N|C_1, \ldots, C_n)} = \frac{P(C_1, \ldots, C_n|H)}{P(C_1, \ldots, C_n|N)} \times \frac{P(H)}{P(N)},$$

where

- $P(\ )$ designates the probability of the event within the parentheses;
- H marks a target event or hypothesis occurring;
- N designates the same event not occurring;
- $C_1, \ldots, C_n$ mark the clues 1 through n;
- $P(H|C_1, \ldots, C_n)$ is the probability of hypothesis H occurring given clues 1 through n;
- $P(N|C_1, \ldots, C_n)$ is the probability of hypothesis H not occurring given clues 1 through n;
- $P(C_1, \ldots, C_n|H)$ is the prevalence of the clues among the situations where hypothesis H has occurred and is referred to as the likelihood of the various clues given H has occurred; and
- $P(C_1, \ldots, C_n|N)$ is the prevalence of the clues among situation where hypothesis H has not occurred. This term is also referred to as the likelihood of the various clues given H has not occurred.

In other words, Bayes's theorem states that

Posterior odds after review of clues =
Likelihood ratio associated with the clues × Prior odds.

The difference between the left and right terms is the knowledge of clues. Thus, the theorem shows how opinions should change after examining clues 1 through *n*. Because Bayes's theorem prescribes how opinions should be revised to reflect new data, it is a tool for consistent and systematic processing of opinions.

Bayes's theorem claims that prior odds of an event are multiplied by the likelihood ratio associated with various clues to obtain the posterior odds for the event. At first glance, it might seem strange to multiply rather than add. You might question why other probabilities besides prior odds and likelihood ratios are not included. The following section makes the logical case for Bayes's theorem.

Rationale for Bayes's Theorem

Bayes's theorem sets a norm for decision makers regarding how they should revise their opinions. But who says this norm is reasonable? In this section, Bayes's theorem is shown to be logical and based on simple assumptions that most people agree with. Therefore, to remain logically consistent, everyone should accept Bayes's theorem as a norm.

Bayes's theorem was first proven mathematically by Thomas Bayes, an English mathematician, although he never submitted his paper for publication. Using Bayes's notes, Price presented a proof of Bayes's theorem (Bayes 1963). The following presentation of Bayes's argument differs from the original and is based on the work of de Finetti (1937). Suppose you want to predict the probability of joining an HMO based on whether the individual is frail elderly. You could establish four groups:

1. A group of size a joins the HMO and is frail elderly.
2. A group of size b joins the HMO and is not frail elderly.
3. A group of size c does not join the HMO and is frail elderly.
4. A group of size d does not join the HMO and is not frail elderly.

Suppose the HMO is offered to $a + b + c + d$ Medicare beneficiaries (see Table 3.2). The probability of an event is defined as the number of ways the event occurs divided by the total possibilities. Thus, since the total number of beneficiaries is $a + b + c + d$, the probability of any of them joining the HMO is the number of people who join divided by the total number of beneficiaries:

$$P(\text{Joining}) = \frac{a + b}{a + b + c + d}.$$

TABLE 3.2 Partitioning Groups Among Frail Elderly Who Will Join the HMO

	Frail Elderly	*Not Frail Elderly*	*Total*
Joins the HMO	*a*	*b*	*a* + *b*
Does not join the HMO	*c*	*d*	*c* + *d*
Total	*a* + *c*	*b* + *d*	*a* + *b* + *c* + *d*

Similarly, the chance of finding a frail elderly, P (Frail elderly), is the total number of frail elderly, $a + c$, divided by the total number of beneficiaries:

$$P(\text{Frail elderly}) = \frac{a + b}{a + b + c + d} .$$

Now consider a special situation in which one focuses only on those beneficiaries who are frail elderly. Given that the focus is on this subset, the total number of possibilities is now reduced from the total number of beneficiaries to the number who are frail elderly (i.e., $a + c$). If you focus only on the frail elderly, the probability of one of these beneficiaries joining is

$$P(\text{Joining} \mid \text{Frail elderly}) = \frac{a}{a + c} .$$

Similarly, the likelihood that you will find frail elderly among joiners is given by reducing the total possibilities to only those beneficiaries who join the HMO and then by counting how many were frail elderly:

$$P(\text{Frail elderly} \mid \text{Joining}) = \frac{a}{a + c} .$$

From the above four formulas, you can see that

$$P(\text{Joining} \mid \text{Frail elderly}) = P(\text{Frail elderly} \mid \text{Joining}) \times \frac{P(\text{Joining})}{P(\text{Frail elderly})} .$$

Repeating the procedure for not joining the HMO, you find that

$$(\text{Not joining} \mid \text{Frail elderly}) = P(\text{Frail elderly} \mid \text{Not joining}) \times \frac{P(\text{Not joining})}{P(\text{Frail elderly})} .$$

Dividing the above two equations results in the odds form of the Bayes's theorem:

$$\frac{P(\text{Joining} \mid \text{Frail elderly})}{P(\text{Not joining} \mid \text{Frail elderly})} = \frac{P(\text{Joining} \mid \text{Frail elderly})}{P(\text{Frail elderly} \mid \text{Not joining})} \times \frac{P(\text{Joining})}{P(\text{Not joining})} .$$

As the above has shown, the Bayes's theorem follows from very reasonable, simple assumptions. If beneficiaries are partitioned into the four groups, the numbers in each group are counted, and the probability of an event is defined as the count of the event divided by number of possibilities, then Bayes's theorem follows. Most readers will agree that these assumptions are reasonable and therefore that the implication of these assumptions (i.e., the Bayes's theorem) should also be reasonable.

Independence

In probabilities, the concept of independence has a very specific meaning. If two events are independent of each other, then the occurrence of one event does not reveal much about the occurrence of the other event. Mathematically, this condition can be presented as

$$P(A|B) = P(A).$$

This formula says that the probability of A occurring does not change given that B has occurred.

Independence means that the presence of one clue does not change the impact of another clue. An example might be the prevalence of diabetes and car accidents; knowing the probability of car accidents in a population will not reveal anything about the probability of diabetes.

When two events are independent, you can calculate the probability of both occurring from the marginal probabilities of each event occurring:

$$P(A \text{ and } B) = P(A) \times P(B).$$

Thus, you can calculate the probability of a person with diabetes having a car accident as the product of the probability of having diabetes and the probability of having a car accident.

Conditional Independence

A related concept is conditional independence. *Conditional independence* means that, for a specific population, the presence of one clue does not change the probability of another. Mathematically, this is shown as

$$P(A|B, C) = P(A|C).$$

The above formula reads that if you know that C has occurred, telling you that B has occurred does not add any new information to the estimate of probability of A. Another way of saying this is to say that in population C, knowing B does not reveal much about the chance for A. Conditional independence also allows you to calculate joint probabilities from marginal probabilities:

$$P(A \text{ and } B|C) = P(A|C) \times P(B|C).$$

The above formula states that among the population C, the probability of both A and B occurring together is equal to the product of probability of each event occurring.

It is possible for two events to be dependent, but they may become independent of each other when conditioned on the occurrence of a third event. For example, you may think that scheduling long shifts will lead to medication errors. This can be shown as follows (≠ means "not equal to"):

$$P(\text{Medication error}) \neq P(\text{Medication error}|\text{Long shift}).$$

At the same time, you may consider that in the population of employees that are not fatigued (even though they have long shifts), the two events are independent of each other:

$$P(\text{Medication error}|\text{Long shift, Not fatigued}) = P(\text{Medication error}|\text{Not fatigued}).$$

In English, this formula says that if the nurse is not fatigued, then it does not matter if the shift is long or short; the probability of medication error does not change. This example shows that related events may become independent under certain conditions.

Use of Independence

Independence and conditional independence are often invoked to simplify the calculation of complex likelihoods involving multiple events. It has already been shown how independence facilitates the calculation of joint probabilities. The advantage of verifying independence becomes even more pronounced when examining more than two events. Recall that the use of the odds form of Bayes's theorem requires the estimation of the likelihood ratio. When multiple events are considered before revising the prior odds, the estimation of the likelihood ratio involves conditioning future events on all prior events (Eisenstein and Alemi 1994):

$$P(C_1, C_2, C_3, \ldots, C_n|H_1) = P(C_1|H_1) \times P(C_2|H_1, C_1) \times P(C_3|H_1, C_1, C_2) \times P(C_4|H_1, C_1, C_2, C_3) \times \ldots \times P(C_n|H_1, C_1, C_2, C_3, \ldots, C_{n-1}).$$

Note that each term in the above formula is conditioned on the hypothesis, or on previous events. When events are considered, the posterior odds are modified and are used to condition all subsequent events. The first term is conditioned on no additional event; the second term is conditioned on the first event; the third term is conditioned on the first and second events, and so on until the last term that is conditioned on all subsequent $n - 1$ events. Keeping in mind that conditioning is reducing the sample size to the portion of the sample that has the condition, the above formula suggests a sequence for reducing the sample size. Because there are many events, the data has to be portioned in increasingly smaller sizes. In order for data to be partitioned so many times, a large database is needed.

Conditional independence allows you to calculate likelihood ratios associated with a series of events without the need for large databases. Instead of conditioning the event on the hypothesis and all prior events, you can now ignore all prior events:

$$P(C_1, C_2, C_3, \ldots, C_n | H_1) = P(C_1|H) \times P(C_2|H) \times P(C_3|H) \times P(C_4|H) \times \ldots \times P(C_n|H).$$

Conditional independence simplifies the calculation of the likelihood ratios. Now the odds form of Bayes's theorem can be rewritten in terms of the likelihood ratio associated with each event:

$$\frac{P(H|C_1, \ldots, C_n)}{P(N|C_1, \ldots, C_n)} = \frac{P(C_1|H)}{P(C_1|N)} \times \frac{P(C_2|H)}{P(C_2|N)} \times \ldots \times \frac{P(C_n|H)}{P(C_n|N)} \times \frac{P(H)}{P(N)}.$$

In other words, the above formula states

Posterior odds = Likelihood ratio of first clue × Likelihood ratio of second clue × . . . × Likelihood ratio of *n*th clue × Prior odds.

The odds form of Bayes's theorem has many applications. It is often used to estimate how various clues (events) may help revise prior probability of a target event. For example, you might use the above formula to predict the posterior odds of hospitalization for a frail elderly female patient if you accept that age and gender are conditionally independent of each other. Suppose the likelihood ratio associated with being frail elderly is $5/2$, meaning that knowing the patient is frail elderly will increase the odds of hospitalization by 2.5 times. Also suppose that knowing the patient is female reduces the odds for hospitalization by $9/10$. Now, if the prior odds for hospitalization is $1/2$, the posterior odds for hospitalization can be calculated using the following formula:

Posterior odds of hospitalization = Likelihood ratio associated with being frail elderly × Likelihood ratio associated with being female × Prior odds of hospitalization.

The posterior odds of hospitalization can now be calculated as

$$\text{Posterior odds of hospitalization} = \frac{5}{2} \times \frac{9}{10} \times \frac{1}{2} = 1.125.$$

For mutually exclusive and exhaustive events, the odds for an event can be restated as the probability of the event by using the following formula:

$$P = \frac{\text{Odds}}{1 + \text{Odds}}.$$

Using the above formula, you can calculate the probability of hospitalization:

$$P(\text{Hospitalization}) = \frac{1.125}{1 + 1.125} = 0.53.$$

Verifying Conditional Independence

There are several ways to verify conditional independence. These include (1) reducing sample size, (2) analyzing correlations, (3) asking experts, and (4) separating in causal maps.

Reducing Sample Size

If data exist, conditional independence can be verified by selecting the population that has the condition and verifying that the product of marginal probabilities is equal to the joint probability of the two events. For example, Table 3.3 presents 18 cases from a special unit prone to medication errors. The question is whether rate of medication errors is independent of length of work shift.

Using the data in Table 3.3, the probability of medication error is calculated as follows:

$$P(\text{Error}) = \frac{\text{Number of cases with errors}}{\text{Number of cases}} = \frac{6}{18} = 0.33,$$

$$P(\text{Long shift}) = \frac{\text{Number of cases seen by a provider in a long shift}}{\text{Number of cases}} = \frac{5}{18} = 0.28,$$

$$P(\text{Error and Long shift}) = \frac{\text{Number of cases with errors and long shift}}{\text{Number of cases}} = \frac{2}{18} = 0.11,$$

$$P(\text{Error and Long shift}) = 0.11 \neq .09 = 0.33 \times 0.28 = P(\text{Error}) \times P(\text{Long shift}).$$

TABLE 3.3 Medication Errors in 18 Consecutive Cases

Case	*Medication Error*	*Long Shift*	*Fatigue*
1	No	Yes	Yes
2	No	Yes	Yes
3	No	No	Yes
4	No	No	Yes
5	Yes	Yes	Yes
6	Yes	No	Yes
7	Yes	No	Yes
8	Yes	Yes	Yes
9	No	No	No
10	No	No	No
11	No	Yes	No
12	No	No	No
13	No	No	No
14	No	No	No
15	No	No	No
16	No	No	No
17	Yes	No	No
18	Yes	No	No

The previous calculations show that the probability of medication error and length of shift are not independent of each other. Knowing the length of the shift tells you something about the probability of error in that shift. However, consider the situation in which you are examining these two events among cases where the provider was fatigued. Now the population of cases you are examining is reduced to the cases 1 through 8. With this population, calculation of the probabilities yields the following:

$$P(\text{Error} \mid \text{Fatigued}) = 0.50,$$

$$P(\text{Long shift} \mid \text{Fatigued}) = 0.50,$$

$$P(\text{Error and Long shift} \mid \text{Fatigued}) = 0.25,$$

$$P(\text{Error and Long shift} \mid \text{Fatigued}) = 0.25 = 0.50 \times 0.50 = P(\text{Error} \mid \text{Fatigued}) \times P(\text{Long shift} \mid \text{Fatigued}).$$

Among fatigued providers, medication error is independent of length of work shift. The procedures used in this example, namely calculating the joint probability and examining it to see if it is approximately equal to the product of the marginal probability, is one way of verifying independence.

Independence can also be examined by calculating conditional probabilities through restricting the population size. For example, in the population of fatigued providers (i.e., in cases 1 through 8) there are several cases of working long shifts (i.e., cases 1, 2, 5, and 8). You can use this information to calculate conditional probabilities as follows:

$$P(\text{Error} \mid \text{Fatigue}) = 0.50,$$

$$P(\text{Error} \mid \text{Fatigue and Long shift}) = \frac{2}{4} = 0.50.$$

This again shows that, among fatigued workers, knowing that the work shift was long adds no information to the probability of medication error. The above procedure shows how independence can be verified by counting cases in reduced populations. If there is a considerable amount of data are available inside a database, the approach can easily be implemented by running a query that would select the condition and count the number of events of interest.

Analyzing Correlations

Another way to verify independence is to examine the correlations among the events (Streiner 2005). Two events that are correlated are dependent. For example, Table 3.4 examines the relationship between age and blood pressure by calculating the correlation between these two variables.

The correlation between age and blood pressure in the sample of data in Table 3.4 is 0.91. This correlation is relatively high and suggests that knowing something about the age of a person will tell you a great deal about the blood pressure. Therefore, age and blood pressure are dependent in this sample.

Partial correlations can also be used to verify conditional independence (Scheines 2002). If two events are conditionally independent from each other, then the partial correlation between the two events given the condition should be zero; this is called a *vanishing partial correlation*. Partial correlation between a and b given c can be calculated from pairwise correlations:

1. R_{ab} is the correlation between a and b.
2. R_{ac} is the correlation between events a and c.
3. R_{cb} is the correlation between event c and b.

Events a and b are conditionally independent of each other if the vanishing partial correlation condition holds. This condition states

$$R_{ab} = R_{ac} \times R_{cb}.$$

Using the data in Table 3.4, you can calculate the following correlations:

TABLE 3.4 Relationship Between Age and Blood Pressure in Seven Patients

Case	*Age*	*Blood Pressure*	*Weight*
1	35	140	200
2	30	130	185
3	19	120	180
4	20	111	175
5	17	105	170
6	16	103	165
7	20	102	155

$$R_{\text{age, blood pressure}} = 0.91,$$

$$R_{\text{age, weight}} = 0.82,$$

$$R_{\text{weight, blood pressure}} = 0.95.$$

Examination of the data shows that the vanishing partial correlation holds ($\approx$ means approximate equality):

$$R_{\text{age, blood pressure}} = 0.91 \approx 0.82 \times 0.95 = R_{\text{age, weight}} \times R_{\text{weight, blood pressure}}.$$

Therefore, you can conclude that, given a patient's weight, the variables of age and blood pressure are independent of each other because they have a partial correlation of zero.

Asking Experts

It is not always possible to gather data. Sometimes, independence must be verified subjectively by asking a knowledgeable expert about the relationship among the variables. Independence can be verified by asking the expert to tell if knowledge of one event will tell you a lot about the likelihood of another. Conditional independence can be verified by repeating the same task, but within specific populations. Gustafson and his colleagues (1973) described a procedure for assessing independence by directly querying experts as follows (see also Ludke, Stauss, and Gustafson 1977; Jeffrey 2004):

1. Write each event on a 3" × 5" card.
2. Ask each expert to assume a specific population in which the target event has occurred.
3. Ask the expert to pair the cards if knowing the value of one clue will alter the affect of another clue in predicting the target event.
4. Repeat these steps for other populations.
5. If several experts are involved, ask them to present their clustering of cards to each other.
6. Have experts discuss any areas of disagreement, and remind them that only major dependencies should be clustered.

7. Use majority rule to choose the final clusters. (To be accepted, a cluster must be approved by the majority of experts.)

Experts will have in mind different, sometimes wrong, notions of dependence, so the words "conditional dependence" should be avoided. Instead, focus on whether one clue tells you a lot about the influence of another clue in specific populations. Experts are more likely to understand this line of questioning as opposed to directly asking them to verify conditional independence.

Strictly speaking, when an expert says that knowledge of one clue does not change the impact of another, we could interpret this to mean

$$\frac{P(C_1|H, C_2)}{P(C_1|\text{Not } H, \text{Not } C_2)} = \frac{P(C_1|H)}{P(C_1|\text{Not } H)}$$

It says that the likelihood ratio of clue #1 does not depend on the occurrence of clue #2. This is a stronger condition that conditional independence because it requires conditional independence both in the population where event H has occurred and in the population where it has not. Experts can make these judgments easily, even though they may not be aware of the probabilistic implications.

Separate in Causal Maps

One can assess dependencies through analyzing maps of causal relationships (Pearl 2000; Greenland, Pearl, and Robins 1999). In a causal network, each node describes an event. The directed arcs between the nodes depict how one event causes another. Causal networks work for situations where there is no cyclical relationship among the variables; it is not possible to start from a node and follow the arcs and return to the same node. An expert is asked to draw a causal network of the events. If the expert can do so, then conditional dependence can be verified by the position of the nodes and the arcs. Several rules can be used to identify conditional dependencies in a causal network, including the following (Pearl 1988):

1. Any two nodes connected by an arrow are dependent. Cause and immediate consequence are dependent.
2. Multiple causes of same effect are dependent, as knowing the effect and one of the causes will indicate more about the probability of other causes.
3. If a cause always leads to an intermediary event that subsequently affects a consequence, then the consequence is independent of the cause given the intermediary event.
4. If one cause leads to multiple consequences, then the consequences are conditionally independent of each other given the cause.

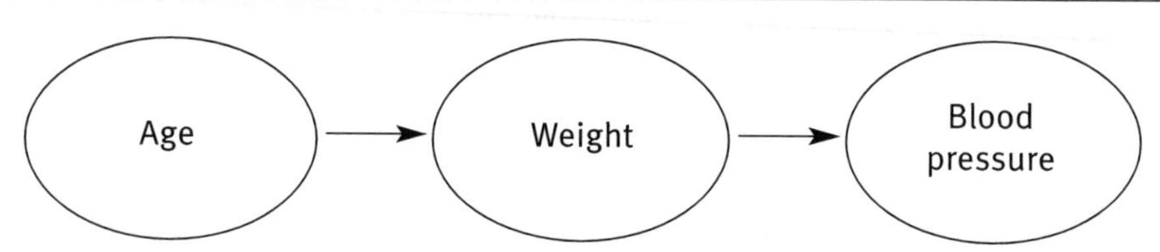

FIGURE 3.5 Causal Map for Age, Weight, and Blood Pressure

In the above rules, it is assumed that removing the condition will actually remove the path between the independent events. For example, think of event *A* leading to event *B* and then to event *C*. Imagine that the relationships are shown by a directed arrow from nodes *A* to *B* and *B* to *C*. If removal of node *C* renders nodes *A* and *B* disconnected from each other, then *A* and *B* are proclaimed independent from each other given *C*. Another way to say this is to observe that event *C* is always between events *A* and *B*, and there is no way of following the arcs from *A* to *B* without passing through *C*. In this situation, *A* is independent of *B* given *C:*

$$P(A|B, C) = P(A|C).$$

For example, an expert may provide the map in Figure 3.5 for the relationships among age, weight, and blood pressure.

In Figure 3.5, age and weight are shown to depend on each other. Age and blood pressure are show to be conditionally independent of each other, because there is no way of going from one to the other without passing through the weight node. Note that if there were an arc between age and blood pressure (i.e., if the expert believed there was a direct relationship between these two variables), then conditional independence would be violated. Analysis of causal maps can help identify a large number of independencies among the events being considered. More details and examples for using causal models to verify independence will be presented in Chapter 4.

Summary

One way of measuring uncertainty is through the use of the concept of probability. This chapter defines what probability is and how its calculus can be used to keep track of the probability of multiple events co-occurring, the probability of one or the other event occurring, and the probability of an event that is conditioned on the occurrence of other events. Probability is often thought of as an objective, mathematical process; however, it can also be applied to the subjective opinions and convictions of experts regarding the likelihood of events. Bayes's theorem is introduced as a means of revising subjective probabilities or existing opinions based upon new evidence. The concept of conditional probability is described in terms of reducing the sample space. Conditional independence makes the calculation of Bayes's thorem easier. The chapter provides different methods for testing for conditional independence, including graphical methods, correlation methods, and sample reduction methods.

Review What You Know

1. What is the daily probability of an event that has occurred once in the last year?
2. What is the daily probability of an event that last occurred 3 months ago?
3. What assumption did you make in answering question 2?
4. Using Table 3.5, what is the probability of hospitalization given that you are male?
5. Using Table 3.5, is insurance independent of age?
6. Using Table 3.5, what is the likelihood associated with being older than 65 years among hospitalized patients?
7. Using Table 3.5, in predicting hospitalization, what is the likelihood ratio associated with being 65 years old?
8. What are the prior odds for hospitalization before any other information is available?
9. Analyze the data in the Table 3.5 and report if any two variables are conditionally independent of each other in predicting probability of hospitalization? To accomplish this you need to calculate the likelihood ratio associated with the following clues:
   a. Male
   b. > 65 years old

TABLE 3.5
Sample Cases

Case	*Hospitalized*	*Gender*	*Age*	*Insured*
1	Yes	Male	> 65	Yes
2	Yes	Male	< 65	Yes
3	Yes	Female	> 65	Yes
4	Yes	Female	< 65	No
5	No	Male	> 65	No
6	No	Male	< 65	No
7	No	Female	> 65	No

c. Insured
d. Male and > 65 years old
e. Male and insured
f. > 65 years old and insured

Then you can see if adding a piece of information changes the likelihood ratio. Keep in mind that because the number of cases are too few, many ratios cannot be calculated.

10. Draw what causes medication errors on a piece of paper, with each cause in a separate node and arrows showing the direction of causality. List all causes and their immediate effects until the effects lead to a medication error. Repeat this until all paths to medication errors are listed. It would be helpful if you number the paths.
11. Analyze the graph you have produced and list all conditional dependencies inherent in the graph.

Audio/Visual Chapter Aids

To help you understand the concepts of measuring uncertainty, visit this book's companion web site at ache.org/DecisionAnalysis, go to Chapter 3, and view the audio/visual chapter aids.

References

Bayes, T. 1963. "Essays Toward Solving a Problem in the Doctrine of Changes." *Philosophical Translation of Royal Society* 53:370–418.

Eisenstein, E. L., and F. Alemi. 1994. "An Evaluation of Factors Influencing Bayesian Learning Systems." *Journal of the American Medical Informatics Association* 1 (3): 272–84.

de Finetti, B. 1937. "Foresight: Its Logical Laws, Its Subjective Sources." Translated by H. E. Kyburg, Jr. In *Studies in Subjective Probability*, edited by H. E. Kyburg, Jr. and H. E. Smokler, pp. 93–158. New York: Wiley, 1964.

Jeffrey, R. 2004. *Subjective Probability: The Real Thing*. Cambridge, England: Cambridge University Press.

Greenland, S., J. Pearl, and J. M. Robins. 1999. "Causal Diagrams for Epidemiologic Research." *Epidemiology* 10 (1): 37–48.

Gustafson, D. H., J. J. Kestly, R. L. Ludke, and F. Larson. 1973. "Probabilistic Information Processing: Implementation and Evaluation of a Semi-PIP Diagnostic System." *Computers and Biomedical Research* 6 (4): 355–70.

Ludke, R. L., F. F. Stauss, and D. H. Gustafson. 1977. "Comparison of Five Methods for Estimating Subjective Probability Distributions." *Organizational Behavior and Human Performance* 19 (1): 162–79.

Pearl, J. 1988. *Probabilistic Reasoning in Intelligent Systems: Networks of Plausible Inference.* San Francisco: Morgan Kaufmann.

———. 2000. *Causality: Models, Reasoning, and Inference.* Cambridge, England: Cambridge University Press.

Savage, L. 1954. *The Foundation of Statistics.* New York: John Wiley and Sons.

Scheines, R. 2002. "Computation and Causation." *Meta Philosophy* 33 (1 and 2): 158–80.

Streiner, D. L. 2005. "Finding Our Way: An Introduction to Path Analysis." *Canadian Journal of Psychiatry* 50 (2): 115–22.

Wallsten, T. S., and D. V. Budescu. 1983. "Encoding Subjective Probabilities: A Psychological and Psychometric Review." *Management Science* 29 (2) 151–73.

CHAPTER

4

MODELING UNCERTAINTY

Farrokh Alemi and David H. Gustafson

This chapter shows the use of Bayesian probability models in forecasting market demand for healthcare services. Bayesian probability models can be used to help decision makers manage their uncertainties about future events. This chapter builds on the material covered in Chapter 3. While the previous chapter mostly focused on mathematical formulas, this chapter has a behavioral focus and describes how to interact with the experts. It shows how probability models can be constructed from expert opinions and used to forecast future events.

Statisticians can predict the future by looking at the past; they have developed tools to forecast the likelihood of future events from historical trends. For example, future sales can be predicted based on historical sales figures. Sometimes, however, analysts must forecast unique events that lack antecedents. Other times, the environment has changed so radically that previous trends are irrelevant. In these circumstances, the traditional statistical tools are of little use and an alternative method must be found. This chapter provides a methodology for analyzing and forecasting events when historical data are not available. This approach is based on Bayesian subjective probability models.

To motivate this approach, suppose an analyst has to predict the demand for a new health maintenance organization (HMO). Employees in HMOs are required to consult a primary care physician before visiting a specialist; the primary care physician has financial incentives to reduce the inappropriate use of services. Experience with HMOs shows they can cut costs by reducing unnecessary hospitalization. Suppose an investigator wants to know what will happen if a new HMO is set up in which primary care physicians have e-mail contact with their patients. At first, predicting demand for the proposed HMO seems relatively easy because there is a great deal of national experience with HMOs. But the proposed HMO uses technology to set it apart from the crowd: The member will initiate contact with the HMO via the computer, which will interview the member and send a summary to the primary care physician, who would then consult the patient's record and decide whether the patient should

This book has a companion web site that features narrated presentations, animated examples, PowerPoint slides, online tools, web links, additional readings, and examples of students' work. To access this chapter's learning tools, go to ache.org/DecisionAnalysis and select Chapter 4.

1. wait and see what happens;
2. have specific tests done before visiting;
3. take a prescription, which would be phoned to a nearby pharmacy, and wait to see if the symptoms disappear;
4. come in for a visit; or
5. bypass the primary care system and visit a specialist.

When the decision is made, the computer will inform the patient about the primary care physician's recommendations. If the doctor does not recommend a visit, the computer will automatically call the member a few days later to see if the symptoms have diminished. All care will be supervised by the patient's primary care physician.

This is not the kind of HMO with which anyone has much experience, but let's blend a few more uncertainties into the mix. Assume that the local insurance market has changed radically in recent years—competition has increased, and businesses have organized powerful coalitions to control healthcare costs. At the federal level, national health insurance is again under discussion. With such radical changes on the horizon, even data that are only two years old may be irrelevant. As if these constraints were not enough, the analyst needs to produce the forecast in a hurry. What can be done? How can an analyst predict demand for an unprecedented product? The following sections present ten steps for using Bayesian probability models to accomplish this task.

Step 1: Select the Target Event

To use the calculus of probabilities in forecasting a target event, the analyst needs to make sure that the events of interest are mutually exclusive (i.e., the events cannot occur simultaneously) and exhaustive (i.e., one event in the set must happen). Thus, in regards to the proposed HMO, the analyst might start with the following list of mutually exclusive events:

- More than 75 percent of the employees will join the HMO.
- Between 51 percent and 75 percent of the employees will join the HMO.

- Between 26 percent and 50 percent of the employees will join the HMO.
- Fewer than 25 percent of the employees will join the HMO.

Note that the events listed above are exhaustive (they cover all possibilities) and exclusive (no two events can co-occur). When gathering experts' opinions, the events being forecasted should be related to the experts' daily experiences and should be expressed in terms they are familiar with. For example, benefit managers are more comfortable thinking about individuals; if you plan to tap the intuitions of a benefit manager about the proposed HMO, you should discuss the probability in terms of one employee. To accomplish this, the list of target events might change to the following:

- The employee will join the proposed HMO.
- The employee will not join the proposed HMO.

It makes no difference in the analysis if you estimate the probability of one employee joining or the percent of the entire population joining; these are mathematically equivalent. It may make a big difference to the experts, however, so be sure to define the events of interest in terms familiar to the experts. Expertise is selective; if you ask experts about situations even slightly outside of their specific area or frame of reference, they will give either no answer or erroneous responses. Expertise has its limits; for example, some weather forecasters might be able to predict tomorrow's weather but not the weather for two day after.

It is preferable to forecast as few events as possible. However, many analysts and decision makers tend to work with a great deal of complexity in real situations. More complex target events for the proposed HMO might include the following:

- The employee will never join the proposed HMO.
- The employee will not join the HMO in the first year, but will join in the second year.
- The employee will join the HMO in the first year, but will withdraw in the second year.
- The employee will join the HMO in the first year and will stay.

Again, the events are mutually exclusive and exhaustive, but now they are more complex. The forecasts deal not only with the applicants' decisions but also with the stability of those decisions. People may join when they are sick and withdraw when they are well. Turnover rates affect administration and utilization costs, so information about the stability of the risk pool is important. In spite of the utility of such a categorization, it is difficult to combine two predictions; therefore, for reasons of simplicity and accuracy, it is preferable to design a separate model for each event: one model to predict whether the employee will join the HMO, and another to predict whether an enrollee will remain a member.

The target events must be chosen carefully because a failure to minimize their number may indicate that the analyst has not captured the essence of the uncertainty. One way of ensuring that the underlying uncertainty is being addressed is to examine the link between the forecasted events and the actions the decision maker is contemplating. Unless these actions differ radically from one another, some of the events should be combined. A model of uncertainty needs to be based on no more than two events unless there are solid reasons for the contrary. Even then, it is often best to build multiple models to forecast more than two events.

In the example being followed here, the analyst was interested in predicting how many employees will join the HMO (and also how many will not join), because this was the key uncertainty that investors needed to judge the business plan. To predict the number of employees who will join, the analyst can calculate the probability that an individual employee will join, $P(\text{Joining})$. If the total number of employees is n, then the number who will join is $n \times P(\text{Joining})$. Likewise, the number of employees who will not join is $n \times [1 - P(\text{Joining})]$.

Step 2: Divide and Conquer

The demand for the proposed HMO could be assessed by asking experts, "Out of 100 employees, how many will join?" However, this question is somewhat rhetorical, and an expert might answer, "Who knows? Some people will join the proposed HMO, others will not—it all depends on many factors." If the question is posed in these terms, it is too general to have a reasonable answer. When the predictions are complex (i.e., many contradictory clues, or components, must be evaluated), experts' predictions can be way off the mark. When talking with experts, the first task is to understand whether they can make the desired forecast with confidence and without reservation. If they can, then the analyst can rely on their forecasts and can save time. When they cannot, however, the analyst can disassemble the forecasts into judgments about the individual clues and forecast from these clues.

Errors in predictions, or judgments, may be reduced by breaking complex judgments into several components, or clues. Then the expert can specify how each clue affects the forecast, and the analyst can judge individual situations based on the clues. It is not necessary to make a direct estimate of the probability of the complex event; its probability can be derived from the clues and their influences on the complex judgments.

Let's take the example of the online HMO to see how one might follow this proposed approach. Nothing is totally new, and even the most radical health plan has components that resemble aspects of established plans. Though the proposed HMO is novel, experience offers clues to help the analyst predict the reaction to it. The success of the HMO will depend on factors that have influenced demand for services in other circumstances. Experience shows that the plan's success depends on the composition of the potential enrollees. In other words, some people have characteristics that dispose them toward or against joining the HMO. As a first approximation, the plan might be more attractive to young employees who are familiar with computers, to high-salary employees who want to save time, to employees comfortable with delayed communications on telephone answering machines, and to patients who want more control over their care. If most employees are members of these groups, you might reasonably project a high demand.

One thing is for certain: Each individual will have some characteristics (i.e., clues) that suggest a likelihood to join the health plan and some that suggest the reverse. Seldom will all clues point to one conclusion. In these circumstances, the various characteristics should be weighted relative to each other before the analyst can predict if an employee will join the health plan. Bayes's probability theorem provides one way for doing this. As discussed in Chapter 3, *Bayes's theorem* is a formally optimal model for revising existing opinions (sometimes called prior opinions) in light of new evidence or clues. The theorem states

$$\frac{P(H \mid C_1, \ldots, C_n)}{P(N \mid C_1, \ldots, C_n)} = \frac{P(C_1, \ldots, C_n \mid H)}{P(C_1, \ldots, C_n \mid N)} \times \frac{P(H)}{P(N)},$$

where

- $P(\ )$ designates probability;
- H marks a target event or hypothesis occurring;
- N designates the same event not occurring;
- $P(H)$ is the probability of H occurring before considering the clues;
- $P(N)$ is the probability of H not occurring before considering the clues;

- $C_1, \ldots, C_n$ mark the clues 1 through n;
- $P(H|C_1, \ldots, C_n)$ is the posterior probability of hypothesis H occurring given clues 1 through n;
- $P(N|C_1, \ldots, C_n)$ is the posterior probability of hypothesis H not happening given clues 1 through n;
- $P(C_1, \ldots, C_n|H)$ is the prevalence (likelihood) of the clues among the situations where hypothesis H has occurred;
- $P(C_1, \ldots, C_n|N)$ is the prevalence (likelihood) of the clues among situation where hypothesis H has not occurred;
- $P(H|C_1, \ldots, C_n) \div P(N|C_1, \ldots, C_n)$ is the posterior odds for the hypothesis occurring given the various clues;
- $P(H|C_1, \ldots, C_n) \div P(N|C_1, \ldots, C_n)$ is the likelihood ratio that measures the diagnostic value of the clues; and
- $P(H) \div P(N)$ is referred to as the prior odds and shows the forecast before considering various clues.

In other words, Bayes's theorem states that

Posterior odds after review of clues =
Likelihood ratio associated with the clues × Prior odds.

Using Bayes's theorem, if C_1 through C_n reflect the various clues, the forecast regarding the HMO can be rewritten as

$$\frac{P(\text{Joining}|C_1, \ldots, C_n)}{P(\text{Not Joining}|C_1, \ldots, C_n)} = \frac{P(C_1, \ldots, C_n|\text{Joining})}{P(C_1, \ldots, C_n|\text{Not Joining})} \times \frac{P(\text{Joining})}{P(\text{Not joining})}.$$

The difference between $P(\text{Joining}|C_1, \ldots, C_n)$ and $P(\text{Joining})$ is the knowledge of clues C_1 through C_n. Bayes's theorem shows how an opinion about an employee's reaction to the plan will be modified by the knowledge of his characteristics. Because Bayes's theorem prescribes how opinions should be revised to reflect new data, it is a tool for consistent and systematic processing of opinions.

Step 3: Identify Clues

An analyst can work with an expert to specify the appropriate clues in a forecast. The identification of clues starts with the published literature. Even if the task seems unique, it is always surprising how much has been published about related topics. There is a great deal of literature on predicting decisions to join an HMO, and even though these studies do not concern HMOs with the unique characteristics of the HMO in this example, reading them can help the analyst think more carefully about possible clues.

One will seldom find exactly what is needed in the literature. Once the literature search is completed, one should use experts to help identify clues for a forecast. Even if there is extensive literature on a subject, an analyst cannot expect to select the most important variables or to discern all important clues without the assistance of an expert. In a few telephone interviews with experts, an analyst can determine the key variables, get suggestions on measuring each one, and identify two or three superior journal articles.

Experts should be chosen on the basis of accessibility and expertise. To forecast HMO enrollment, appropriate experts might be people with firsthand knowledge of the employees, such as benefit managers, actuaries in other insurance companies, and personnel from the local planning agency. It is useful to begin discussions with experts by asking broad questions designed to help the experts talk about themselves:

> Analyst: Would you tell me a little about your experience with employees' choice in health plans?

The expert might respond with an anecdote about irrational choices by employees, implying that a rational system cannot predict everyone's behavior. Or, the expert might mention how difficult it is to forecast or how many years she has spent studying these phenomena. The analyst should understand what is occurring here: In these early responses, the expert is expressing a sense of the importance and value of her experience and input. It is vital to acknowledge this hidden message and to allow ample time for the expert to describe their contributions.

After the expert has been primed by recalling these experiences, the analyst should ask about characteristics that might suggest an employee's decision to join or not join the plan:

> Analyst: Suppose you had to decide whether an employee is likely to join, but you could not contact the employee.
> I was chosen to be your eyes and ears. What should I look for?

After a few queries of this type, the analyst should ask more focused questions:

> Analyst: What is an example of a characteristic that would increase the chance an employee will join the HMO?

The second question is referred to as a *positive prompt* because it elicits clues that would increase the chance of joining. *Negative prompts* seek clues that decrease the probability. An example of a negative prompt is the following:

> Analyst: Describe an employee who is unlikely to join the proposed HMO.

Research shows that positive and negative prompts yield different sets of clues (Rothman and Salovey 1997; Rivers et al. 2005). Thus, modeling should start with clues that support the forecast, and then the clues that oppose it should be explored. Then responses can be combined so the model contains both sets of clues.

It is important to get opinions of several experts on what clues are important in the forecast. Each expert has access to a unique set of information; using more than one expert enables you to pool information and improve the accuracy of the recall of clues. At least three experts should be interviewed, each for about one hour. After a preliminary list of factors is collected during the interviews, the experts should have a chance to revise their lists, either by telephone, by mail, or in a meeting. If time and resources allow, the integrative group process is preferable for identifying the clues. This process is described in Chapter 6.

Suppose that the experts identified the following clues for predicting an employee's decision to join the new HMO:

- Age
- Income and value of time to the employee
- Gender
- Computer literacy
- Tendency to join an HMO

Step 4: Describe the Levels of Each Clue

A clue's *level* measures the extent to which it is present. At the simplest, there are two levels—presence or absence—but sometimes there are more. Gender has two levels: male and female. But age may be described in terms of six discrete levels, each corresponding to a decade: younger than 21 years, 21–30 years old, 31–40 years old, 41–50 years old, 51–60 years old, and older than 60 years.

In principle, it is possible to accommodate both discrete and continuous variables in a Bayesian model. *Discrete variables* have a determinable number of variables (e.g., gender has two levels: male and female).

Continuous variables have an infinite or near-infinite number of levels (e.g., age). In practice, discrete clues are used more frequently for two reasons:

1. Experts seem to have more difficulty estimating likelihood ratios associated with continuous clues.
2. In the health and social service areas, most clues tend to be discrete. Virtually all continuous clues can be transformed to discrete clues.

As with defining the forecast events, the primary rule for creating discrete levels is to minimize the number of categories. Rarely are more than five or six categories required, and frequently two or three suffice.

It is preferable to identify levels for various clues by asking the experts to describe a level at which the clue will increase the probability of the forecast events in question. Thus, the analyst may have the following conversation:

Analyst: What would be an example of an age that would favor joining the HMO?
Expert: Young people are more likely to join than older people.

Analyst: How do you define "young" employees?
Expert: Who knows? It all depends. But if you really push me, I would say younger than 30 years is different from older than 30 years. This is probably why the young used to say "never trust anybody over 30." This age marks real differences in life outlook.

Analyst: What age reduces the chance of joining the HMO?
Expert: Employees older than 40 years are different, too; they are pretty much settled in their ways. Of course, you understand we are just talking in general—there are many exceptions.

Analyst: Sure, I understand. But we are trying to model these general trends.

In all cases, each category or division should represent a different chance of joining the HMO. One way to check this is as follows:

Analyst: Do you think a 50-year-old employee is substantially less likely to join than a 40-year-old employee?
Expert: Yes, but the difference is not great.

After much interaction with the experts, the analyst might devise the following levels for each of the clues previously identified:

- Age: younger than 30 years old, 31–40 years old, and older than 41 years old
- Income and value of time to the employee: income over \$50,000, income between \$30,000 and \$50,000, and income less than \$30,000
- Gender: male and female
- Computer literacy: programs computers, frequently uses a computer, routinely uses output of a computer, and has no interaction with a computer
- Tendency to join an HMO: is enrolled in an HMO and is not enrolled in an HMO

In describing the levels of each clue, analysts also think through measurement issues. It is convenient to let the analyst decide on the measurement issues, but the measures should be reviewed by the expert to make sure they fit the expert's intentions. For example, income, hence hourly wage, can be used as a surrogate measure for "value of time to employee." But such surrogate measures may be misleading. If income is not a good surrogate for value of time, the analyst has wrecked the model by taking the easy way out. There is a story about a man who lost his keys in the street but was searching for them in his house. When asked why he was looking there, he responded with a certain pinched logic: "The street is dark; the light's better in the house." The lessons are that surrogate measures must be chosen carefully to preserve the value of the clue, and that the easy way is not always the best way.

Step 5: Test for Independence

Conditional independence is an important criterion that can streamline a long list of clues (Pearl 1988, 2000). Independence, as discussed in the previous chapter, means that the presence of one clue does not change the value of any other clue. Conditional independence means that for a specific population, such as employees who will join the HMO, the presence of one clue does not change the value of another. Conditional independence simplifies the forecasting task. The effect of a piece of information on the forecast is its likelihood ratio. Conditional independence allows you to write the likelihood ratio of several clues as a multiplication of the likelihood ratio of each clue. Thus, if C_1 through C_n are the clues in your forecast, the joint likelihood ratio of all the clues can be written as

$$\frac{P(C_1,\ldots,C_n \mid \text{Joining})}{P(C_1,\ldots,C_n \mid \text{Not Joining})} = \frac{P(C_1 \mid \text{Joining})}{P(C_1 \mid \text{Not Joining})} \times \frac{P(C_2 \mid \text{Joining})}{P(C_2 \mid \text{Not Joining})} \times \ldots \times \frac{P(C_n \mid \text{Joining})}{P(C_n \mid \text{Not Joining})}.$$

Assuming conditional independence, the effect of two clues is equal to the product of the effect of each clue. Conditional independence simplifies the number of estimates needed for measuring the joint influence of several pieces of information.

Let's examine whether age and gender are conditionally independent in predicting the probability of joining the HMO. Mathematically, if two clues (e.g., age and gender) are conditionally independent, then you should have

$$\frac{P(\text{Age} \mid \text{Gender, Joining})}{P(\text{Age} \mid \text{Gender, Not joining})} = \frac{P(\text{Age} \mid \text{Joining})}{P(\text{Age} \mid \text{Not joining})}.$$

This formula says that the effect of age on the forecast remains the same even when the gender of the person is known. Thus, the influence of age on the forecast does not depend on gender, and vice versa.

The chances for conditional dependence increase with the number of clues, so clues are likely to be conditionally dependent if the model contains more than six or seven clues. When clues are conditionally dependent, either one clue must be dropped from the analysis or the dependent clues must be combined into a new cluster of clues. If age and computer literacy were conditionally dependent, then either could be dropped from the analysis. As an alternative, the analyst could define a new cluster with the following combined levels:

- Younger than 30 years and programs a computer
- Younger than 30 years and frequently uses a computer
- Younger than 30 years and uses computer output
- Younger than 30 years and does not use a computer
- Older than 30 years and programs a computer
- Older than 30 years and frequently uses a computer
- Older than 30 years and uses computer output
- Older than 30 years and does not use a computer

There are statistical procedures for assessing conditional dependence. These procedures were reviewed in Chapter 3 and are further elaborated on in this chapter within the context of modeling experts' opinions. Experts will have in mind different, sometimes wrong, notions of dependence, so the words "conditional independence" should be avoided. Instead, analysts should focus on whether one clue indicates a lot about the influence of another clue. Experts are usually more likely to understand this line of questioning as opposed to understanding direct questions that ask them to verify conditional independence.

Analysts can also assess conditional independence through graphical methods (Pearl 2000). The decision maker is asked to list the possible causes and consequences (e.g., signs, symptoms, characteristics) of the condition being predicted. Only direct causes and consequences are listed, as indirect causes or consequences cannot be modeled through the odds form of Bayes's theorem. A target event is written in a node at the center of the page. All causes precede this node and are shown as arrows leading to the target node. All subsequent signs or symptoms are also shown as nodes that follow the target event node (arrows point from the target node toward the consequences). Figure 4.1 shows three causes and three consequences for the target event.

For example, in predicting who will join an HMO, you might draw the possible causes of people joining the HMO and the characteristics (consequences) that will distinguish people who have joined from those who have not. A node is created in the center and is labeled with the name of the target event. The decision maker might see time pressures and frequent travel as two reasons for joining an online HMO. The decision maker might also see that as a consequence of the HMO being joined by people who suffer time pressures and travel frequently, members of the HMO will be predominantly male, computer literate, and young. This diagram is shown in Figure 4.2.

To understand conditional dependencies implied by a graph, the following rules of dependence are applied:

1. *Connected nodes.* All nodes that are directly connected to each other are dependent on each other. The nodes in Figure 4.2 show how joining the HMO depends on the employee's time pressures, frequency of travel, age, gender, and computer usage. All five clues can be used to predict the probability of joining the HMO.
2. *Common effect.* If two or more causes that are not directly linked to each other have the same effect, then given the effect the causes are conditionally dependent on each other. Knowing that the effect was not influenced by one cause increases the probability of the remaining causes. For example, if employees who have joined the HMO have not done so because they travel often, then it is more likely that they joined because of time pressures.

The following rules apply to conditional independencies:

1. *Common cause.* If one cause has many effects, then given the cause the effects are conditionally independent from each other. This rule applies only if removing the cause would remove the link between the effects and the preceding nodes in the graph.

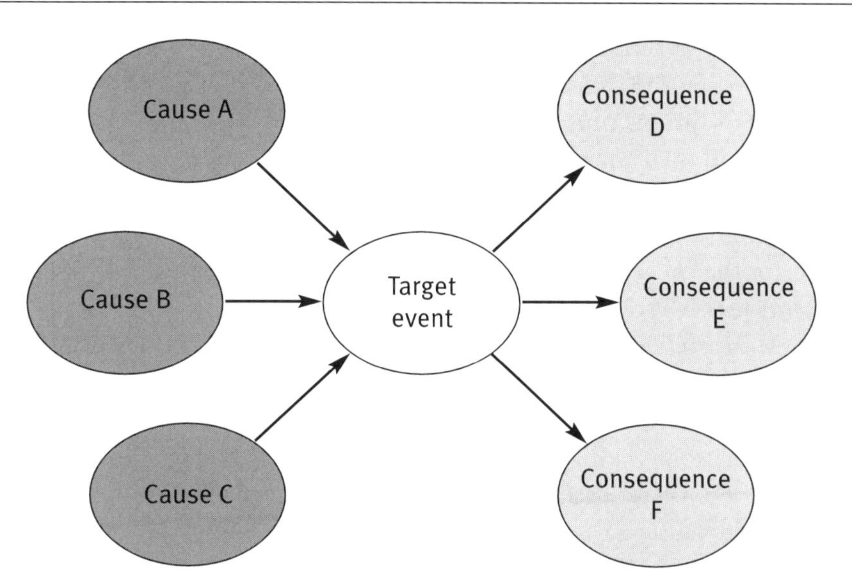

FIGURE 4.1 Causes and Consequences of Target Event Need to Be Drawn

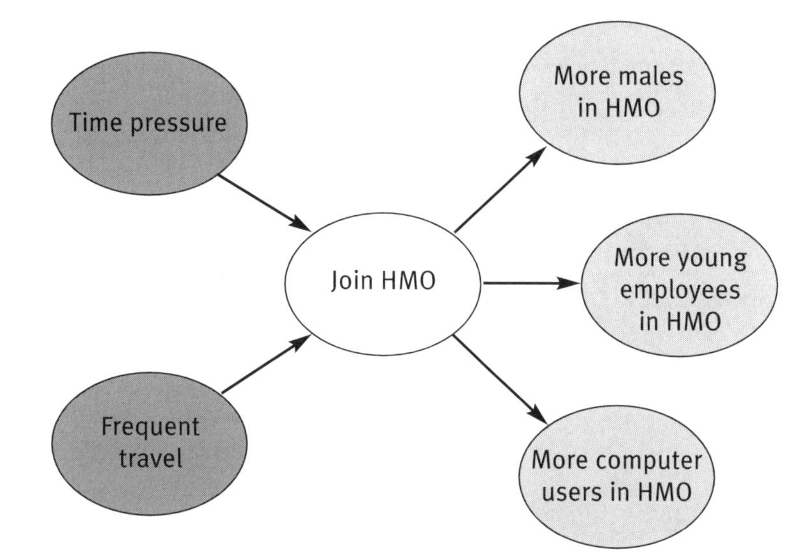

FIGURE 4.2 Causes and Three Signs (Consequences) of Joining the Online HMO

2. *Nodes arranged in a series.* For example, a cause leading to an intermediary event leading to a consequence can signal conditional independence of cause and consequence. For example, given the condition of joining the HMO, time pressure and age of employee are independent of each other because they are in a serial arrangement and removing the middle node (joining the HMO) will remove the connection between the two nodes.

If conditional dependence is found, the analyst has three choices. First, the analyst can ignore the dependencies among the clues. This would work well when the consequences depicted in the causal graph correspond directly with various causes in the graph. For example, employees who put high value on their time may select the HMO; as a consequence, the average salary of employees who join might be higher than those who do not join. In this situation, the cause can be ignored by including the consequence of the cause in the model. As consequences are conditionally independent, this will reduce the dependence among the clues in the model. Ignoring the dependencies in the clues will also work well when multiple clues point to the same conclusion and when the dependencies are small. But when this is not the case, ignoring the dependencies can lead to erroneous predictions.

Second, the analyst could help the decision maker revise the graph or use different causes or consequences so that the model has fewer dependencies. This is often done by better defining the clues. For example, an analyst could reduce the number of links among the nodes by revising the consequence so that it only occurs through the target event. If at all possible, several related causes should be combined into a single cause to reduce conditional dependencies among the clues used in predicting the target event.

Third, all conditionally dependent clues (whether cause or consequence) can be combined to predict the target event. Examples of how to combine two clues were provided earlier in this chapter. If one cause has n levels and another m levels, the new combined cause will have $n \times m$ levels. For each of these levels, separate likelihood ratios must be assessed.

For example, the Bayes's theorem for predicting the odds of joining the HMO can be presented as

$$\text{Posterior odds of joining} = \text{Likelihood ratio}_{\text{time pressure and travel frequency}} \times \text{Likelihood ratio}_{\text{age}} \times \text{Likelihood ratio}_{\text{gender}} \times \text{Likelihood ratio}_{\text{computer use}} \times \text{Prior odds of joining.}$$

Note that the likelihood ratio for the combination of time pressure and travel frequency refers to all possible combinations of levels of these two clues.

Step 6: Estimate Likelihood Ratios

This section explains how to estimate likelihood ratios from experts' subjective opinions (see also Van der Fels-Klerx et al. 2002; Otway and von Winterfeldt 1992). To estimate likelihood ratios, experts should think of the prevalence of the clue in a specific population. The importance of this point is not always appreciated. A likelihood estimate is conditioned on the forecast event, not vice versa. Thus, the effect of being young (younger than 30 years) on the probability of joining the HMO is determined by finding the number of young employees among joiners. There is a crucial distinction between this probability and the probability of joining if one is young. The first statement is conditioned on joining the HMO, the second on being young. The likelihood of individuals younger than 30 years joining is $P(\text{Young}|\text{Joining})$, while the probability of joining the HMO for a person younger than 30 years is $P(\text{Joining}|\text{Young})$. The two concepts are very different.

A likelihood ratio is estimated by asking questions about the prevalence of the clue in populations with and without the target event. For example, for forecasting the likelihood of joining the HMO, the analyst might ask the following:

> Analyst: Of 100 people who do join, how many are younger than 30 years? Of 100 people who do not join the HMO, how many are younger than 30 years?

The ratio of the answers to these two questions determines the likelihood ratio associated with being younger than 30 years. This ratio could be estimated directly by asking the expert to estimate the odds of finding the clue in populations with and without the target event:

> Analyst: Imagine two employees, one who will join the HMO and one who will not join. Who is more likely to be younger than 30 years? How many times more likely?

The likelihood ratios can be estimated by relying on experts' opinions, but the question naturally arises about whether experts can accurately estimate probabilities. Accurate probability estimation does not mean being correct in every forecast. For example, if you forecast that an employee has a 60 percent chance of joining the proposed HMO but the employee does not join, was the forecast inaccurate? Not necessarily. The accuracy of probability forecasts cannot be assessed by the occurrence of a single event. A better way to check the accuracy of a probability is to compare it against observed frequency counts. A 60 percent chance of joining is accurate if 60 of 100 employees join the proposed HMO. A single case reveals nothing about the accuracy of probability estimates.

Systematic bias may exist in subjective estimates of probabilities. Research shows that subjective probabilities for rare events are inordinately low, while they are inordinately high for common events. These results have led some psychologists to conclude that cognitive limitations of the assessor inevitably distorts subjective probability estimates.

Alemi, Gustafson, and Johnson (1986) argue that the accuracy of subjective estimates can be increased through three steps. First, experts should be allowed to use familiar terminology and decision aids. Distortion of probability estimates can be seen in a group of students, but not among real experts. For example, meteorologists seem to be good probability estimators. Weather forecasters are special because they assess familiar phenomena and have access to a host of relevant and overlapping objective information and judgment aids, such as computers and satellite photos. The point is that experts can reliably estimate likelihood ratios if they are dealing with a familiar concept and have access to their usual tools.

A second way of improving experts' estimates is to train them in selected probability concepts (Dietrich 1991). In particular, experts should learn the meaning of a likelihood ratio. Ratios larger than 1 support the occurrence of the forecast event; ratios less than 1 oppose the probability of the forecast event. A ratio of 1 to 2 reduces the odds of the forecast by half; a ratio of 2 doubles the odds.

The experts should also be taught the relationship between odds and probability. Odds of 2 to 1 mean a probability of 0.67; odds of 5 to 1 mean a probability of 0.83; odds of 10 to1 mean a probability of an almost certain event. The forecaster should walk the expert through and discuss in depth the likelihood ratio for the first clue before proceeding. The first few estimates of the likelihood ratio associated with a clue can each take 20 minutes because many things are discussed and modified. Later estimates often take less than a minute.

A third step for improving experts' estimates of probabilities is to rely on more than one expert (Walker et al. 2003) and on a process of estimation, discussion, and reestimation. Relying on a group of experts increases the chance of identifying major errors. In addition, the process of individual estimation, group discussion, and individual reestimation reduces pressures for artificial consensus while promoting information exchange among the experts.

Step 7: Estimate Prior Odds

According to Bayes's theorem, forecasts require two types of estimates: (1) likelihood ratios associated with specific clues, and (2) prior odds associated with the target event. Prior odds can be assessed by finding the historical prevalence of the event. In a situation without a precedent, prior odds can be estimated by asking experts to imagine the future prevalence of the event:

Analyst: Out of 100 employees, how many will join the HMO?

The response to this question provides the probability of joining, P(Joining), and this probability can be used to calculate the odds for joining:

$$\text{Odds for joining} = \frac{P(\text{Joining})}{1 - P(\text{Joining})}.$$

When no reasonable prior estimate is available and when a large number of clues is going to be examined, an analyst can arbitrarily assume that the prior odds for joining are 1 to 1 and then allow clues to alter posterior odds as the analyst proceeds with gathering information.

Step 8: Develop Scenarios

Decision makers use scenarios to think about alternative futures. The purpose of forecasting with scenarios is to make the decision maker sensitive to possible futures. The decision maker can work to change the possible futures. Many future predictions are self-fulfilling prophecies—a predicted event happens because steps are taken that increase the chance for it to happen. In this circumstance, predictions are less important than choosing the ideal future and working to make it come about. Scenarios help the decision maker choose a future and make it occur.

Scenarios are written as coherent and internally consistent narrative scripts. The more believable they are, the better. Scenarios are constructed by selecting various combinations of clue levels, writing a script, and adding details to make the group of clues more credible. An optimistic scenario may be constructed by choosing only clue levels that support the occurrence of the forecast event; a pessimistic scenario combines clues that oppose the event's occurrence. Realistic scenarios, on the other hand, are constructed from a mix of clue levels. In the HMO example, scenarios could describe hypothetical employees who would join the organization. A scenario describing an employee who is most likely to join is constructed by assembling all of the characteristics that support joining:

> A 29-year-old male employee earning more than $60,000. He is busy and values his time; he is familiar with computers and uses them both at work and at home. He is currently an HMO member, although he is not completely satisfied with it.

A pessimistic scenario describes the employees least likely to join:

A 55-year-old female employee earning less than $85,000. She has never used computers and has refused to join the firm's existing HMO.

More realistic scenarios combine other clue levels:

A 55-year-old female employee earning more than $60,000 has used computers but did not join the firm's existing HMO.

A large set of scenarios can be made by randomly choosing clue levels and then asking experts to throw out impossible combinations. To do this, first write each clue level on a card and make one pile for each clue. Each pile will contain all the levels of one clue. Randomly select a level from each pile, write it on a piece of paper, and return the card to the pile. Once a level for all clues are represented on the piece of paper, have an expert check the scenario and discard scenarios that are wildly improbable.

If experts are evaluating many scenarios (perhaps 100 or more), arrange the scenario text so they can understand them easily and omit frivolous detail. If experts are reviewing a few scenarios (perhaps 20 or so), add detail and write narratives to enhance the scenarios' credibility.

Because scenarios examine multiple futures, they introduce an element of uncertainty and prepare decision makers for surprises. In the HMO example, the examination of scenarios of possible members would help the decision makers understand that large segments of the population may not consider the HMO desirable. This leads to two possible changes. First, a committee could be assigned to examine the unmet needs of people unlikely to join and to make the proposal more attractive to segments not currently attracted to it. Second, another committee could examine how the proposed HMO could serve a small group of customers and still succeed.

Sometimes forecasting is complete after the decision maker has examined the scenarios. In these circumstances, making the decision maker intuitively aware of what might happen suffices. In other circumstances, decision makers may want a numerical forecast. To get to a numerical prediction, the analyst must take two more steps.

Step 9: Validate the Model

In the final analysis, any subjective probability model is just a set of opinions, and as such it should not be trusted until it passes vigorous evaluation. The evaluation of a subjective model requires answers to two related questions: Does the model reflect the experts' views? Are the experts' views accurate?

To answer the first question, design about 30 to 100 scenarios, ask the experts to rate each, and compare these ratings to model predictions. If the ratings and predictions match closely (a correlation above 0.7), then the model simulates the experts' judgments. For example, the analyst can generate 30 hypothetical employees and ask the experts to rate the probability that each will join the proposed HMO. To help the experts accomplish this, you should ask them to arrange the cases from more to less likely, to review pairs of adjacent employees to determine if the rank order is reasonable, and to change the rank orders of the employees if needed. Once the cases have been arranged in order, the experts would be asked to rate the chance of joining on a scale of 0 to 100. For each scenario, the analyst should use the Bayes's theorem to forecast whether the employee will join the HMO. Table 4.1 also shows the resulting ratings and predictions.

Next, compare the Bayes's theorem result to the average of the experts' ranking. If the rank-order correlation is higher than 0.70, the analyst may conclude that the model simulates many aspects of the experts' intuitions. Figure 4.3 shows the relationship between the model's predictions and the average experts' ratings.

The straight line of the graph shows the expected relationship. Some differences between the model's predictions and the experts' ratings should be expected, as the experts will show many idiosyncrasies and inconsistencies not found in the model. But the model's predictions and the experts' intuitions should not sharply diverge. One way to examine this is through correlations. If the correlation were lower than 0.7, then the experts' intuitions might not have been effectively modeled, in which case the model must be modified because the likelihood ratios might be too high or some important clues might have been omitted. In this example, the model's predictions and the average of the experts' ratings had a high correlation, which leads to the conclusion that the model simulate the experts' judgments.

The above procedure leaves unanswered the larger and perhaps more difficult question of the accuracy of the experts' intuitions. Experts' opinions can be validated if they can be compared to observed frequencies, but this is seldom possible (Howard 1980). In fact, if the analyst has access to observed frequencies, there is no need to consult experts to create subjective probability models. In the absence of objective data, what steps can an analyst take to reassure herself regarding her experts?

One way to increase confidence in experts' opinions is to use several experts. If the experts reach a consensus, then one should feel comfortable with a model that predicts that consensus. *Consensus* means that, after discussing the problem, experts independently rate the hypothetical

TABLE 4.1
Two Experts' Ratings and Bayes's Theorem on 30 Hypothetical Scenarios

Scenario Number	*Experts' Ratings*		*Average Rating*	*Model Predictions*
	Expert 1	*Expert 2*		
1	41	45	43.0	48
2	31	32	31.5	25
3	86	59	72.5	87
4	22	35	28.5	21
5	61	93	77.0	80
6	38	60	49.0	58
7	38	100	69.0	46
8	14	85	49.5	29
9	30	27	28.5	30
10	33	71	52.0	32
11	45	97	71.0	49
12	22	11	16.5	29
13	39	65	52.0	48
14	28	38	33.0	21
15	28	71	49.5	23
16	33	74	53.5	53
17	46	64	55.0	31
18	75	67	71.0	77
19	61	43	52.0	59
20	73	83	78.0	97
21	0	44	22.0	14
22	16	77	46.5	20
23	37	92	64.5	44
24	15	66	40.5	19
25	43	62	52.5	28
26	16	67	41.5	25
27	48	51	49.5	14
28	100	73	86.5	100
29	15	52	33.5	0
30	6	0	3.0	16

scenarios close to one another. One way of checking the degree of agreement among experts' ratings of the scenarios is to correlate the ratings of each pair of experts. Correlation values above 0.70 suggest excellent agreement; values between 0.50 and 0.70 suggest more moderate agreement. If the correlations are below 0.50, then experts differed, and it is best to examine their differences and redefine the forecast. In the previous example, the two experts had a high correlation, which suggests that they did not agree on the ratings of the scenarios.

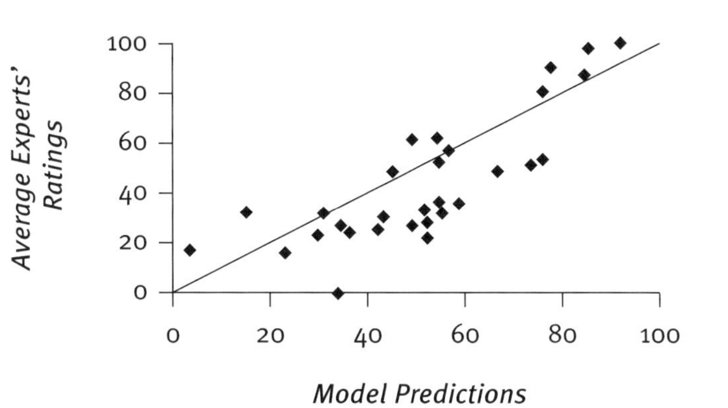

FIGURE 4.3 Validating a Model by Testing if it Simulates Experts' Judgments

Some investigators believe a model, even if it predicts the consensus of the best experts, is still not valid because only objective data can validate a model. According to this rationale, a model provides no reason to act unless it is backed by objective data. Although it is true that no model can be fully validated until its results can be compared to objective data, expert opinions are sufficient grounds for action in many circumstances. In some circumstances (e.g., surgery), people trust their lives to experts' opinions. If one is willing to trust one's life to expertise, one should be willing to accept expert opinion as a basis for business and policy action.

Step 10: Make a Forecast

To make a forecast, an analyst should begin by describing the characteristics of the situation at hand. The likelihood ratios corresponding to the situation at hand are used to make the forecast. In the HMO example, the likelihood ratios associated with characteristics of the employee are used to calculate the probability that an employee will join the HMO. Suppose you evaluated a 29-year-old man earning $60,000 who is computer literate but is not an HMO member. Suppose the likelihood ratios associated with these characteristics are 1.2 for being young, 1.1 for being male, 1.2 for having a high hourly wage, 3.0 for being computer literate, and 0.5 for not being a member of an HMO. Assuming prior odds were equal and the characteristics are conditionally independent, this employee's posterior odds of joining are calculated as follows:

$$\text{Odds of joining} = 1.1 \times 1.2 \times 3 \times 0.5 \times 1 = 1.98.$$

The probability of a mutually exclusive and exhaustive event A can be calculated from its odds using the following formula:

$$P(A) = \frac{\text{Odds}(A)}{1 + \text{Odds}(A)}$$

The above prediction then becomes

$$P(\text{Joining}) = \frac{1.98}{1 + 1.98} = 0.66.$$

The probability of joining can be used to estimate the number of employees likely to join the new HMO (in other words, the demand for the proposed product). If the analyst expects to have 50 of this type of employee, the analyst can forecast that 33 employees (50×0.66) will join. If one does similar calculations for other types of employees, one can calculate the total demand for the proposed HMO.

Analysis of demand for the proposed HMO shows that most employees would not join, but that 12 percent of the employed population might join. Careful analysis can allow the analyst to identify a small group of employees who could be expected to support the proposed HMO, showing that a niche is available for the innovative plan.

Summary

Forecasts of unique events are useful, but they are difficult because of the lack of data. Even when events are not unique, frequency counts are often unavailable, given time and budget constraints. However, the judgments of people with substantial expertise can serve as the basis of forecasts.

In predictions where many clues are needed for forecasting, experts may not function at their best; and as the number of clues increases, the task of forecasting becomes increasingly arduous. Bayes's theorem is a mathematical formula that can be used to aggregate the effect of various clues. This approach combines the strength of human expertise (i.e., estimating the relationship between the clue and the forecast) with the consistency of a mathematical model. Validating these models poses a problem because no objective standards are available, but once the model has passed scrutiny from several experts from different backgrounds, one can feel sufficiently confident about the model to recommend action based on its forecasts.

Review What You Know

Suppose you want to build a model that can predict a patient's breast cancer risk. You can interview an expert and thereafter use the model of the experts' judgment in evaluating patients' overall risk for breast cancer. Using the advice provided here, describe the process of getting the expert to identify clues (i.e., risk factors).

What will you ask an expert if you wish to estimate the likelihood ratio associated with the clue, "age < 9 years at menarche" in predicting a patient's breast cancer risk?

What will you ask from a primary care provider to estimate the prior odds for breast cancer among her patients?

In this chapter, it is suggested that instead of predicting probability of future events, it is sometimes sufficient to generate a number of future scenarios and have the decision maker evaluate these scenarios. Speculate under what circumstances you would stop at scenario generation and not proceed to a numerical estimation. Give an example of a situation in which only reviewing scenarios will be sufficient.

Rapid-Analysis Exercises

Construct a probability model to forecast an important event at work. Select an expert who will help you construct the model. Make an appointment with the expert and construct the model. Prepare a report that answers the following questions:

1. What are the assumptions about the problem and its causes?
2. What is the uncertain outcome?
3. Why would a model be useful and to whom would it be useful?
4. Conduct research to report if similar models or studies have been done by others.
5. What clues and clue levels can be used to make the prediction?
6. What are the likelihood ratios associated with each clue level?
7. Show the application of the model in a case or scenario.
8. What is the evidence that the model is valid?
   a. Is the model based on available data?
   b. Did the expert consider the model simple to use?
   c. Did the expert consider the model to be face valid?
   d. Does the model simulate the experts' judgment on at least 15 cases or scenarios?

   e. Graph the relationship between the model scores and the experts' ratings.
   f. Report the correlation between the model score and the experts' ratings.
9. If data are available, report whether the model corresponds with other measures of the same concept (i.e., construct validity)?
10. If data are available, report whether the model predicts any objective gold standard.

Audio/Visual Chapter Aids

To help you understand the concepts of modeling uncertainty, visit this book's companion web site at ache.org/DecisionAnalysis, go to Chapter 4, and view the audio/visual chapter aids.

References

Alemi, F., D. H. Gustafson, and M. Johnson. 1986. "How to Construct a Subjective Index." *Evaluation and the Health Professions* 9 (1): 45–52.

Dietrich, C. F. 1991. *Uncertainty, Calibration and Probability: The Statistics of Scientific and Industrial Measurement.* 2nd ed. Philadelphia, PA: Thomas and Francis.

Howard, R. A. 1980. "An Assessment of Decision Analysis." *Operations Research* 28 (1): 4–27.

Otway, H., and D. von Winterfeldt. 1992. "Expert Judgment in Risk Analysis and Management: Process, Context, and Pitfalls." *Risk Analysis* 12 (1): 83–93.

Pearl, J. 1988. *Probabilistic Reasoning in Intelligent Systems: Networks of Plausible Inference.* San Francisco: Morgan Kaufmann.

———. 2000. *Causality: Models, Reasoning, and Inference.* Cambridge, England: Cambridge University Press.

Rivers, S. E., P. Salovey, D. A. Pizarro, J. Pizarro, and T. R. Schneider. 2005. "Message Framing and Pap Test Utilization Among Women Attending a Community Health Clinic." *Journal of Health Psychology* 10 (1): 65–77.

Rothman, A. J., and P. Salovey. 1997. "Shaping Perceptions to Motivate Healthy Behavior: The Role of Message Framing." *Psychological Bulletin* 121 (1): 3–19.

Van der Fels-Klerx, I. H., L. H. Goossens, H. W. Saatkamp, and S. H. Horst. 2002. "Elicitation of Quantitative Data from a Heterogeneous Expert Panel: Formal Process and Application in Animal Health." *Risk Analysis* 22 (1): 67–81.

Walker, K. D., P. Catalano, J. K. Hammitt, and J. S. Evans. 2003. "Use of Expert Judgment in Exposure Assessment: Part 2. Calibration of Expert Judgments about Personal Exposures to Benzene." *Journal of Exposure Analysis and Environmental Epidemiology* 13 (1): 1–16.

CHAPTER

5

DECISION TREES

Farrokh Alemi and David H. Gustafson

This chapter introduces decision trees, which are tools for choosing among alternatives. Tools for measuring a decision maker's value and uncertainty were introduced in chapters 2 through 4. Those tools are useful for many problems, but their usefulness is limited when a series of intervening events is likely. When a sequence of events must be analyzed, decision trees provide a means to consider both value and uncertainty.

The first part of this chapter defines decision trees, shows how they are constructed, and describes how they can be analyzed using mathematical expectations. The middle part of the chapter introduces the concept of "folding back," which is useful for analyzing decision trees. The last part of the chapter extends the discussion from a single consequence (i.e., healthcare costs to an employer) to an analysis of multiple consequences. Simple decisions involve one consequence of interest; in the simplest decisions, that is cost. If a decision maker's attitudes toward risk affect the decision, then costs must be transferred to a utility scale. If the decision involves multiple consequences, then the analyst needs to develop an MAV model to transfer the consequences to one scale. These extensions of the method are discussed in the last part of the chapter. In addition, the chapter ends with a discussion of the importance of analyzing the sensitivity of conclusions to input, a topic that will repeatedly be returned to in this and other chapters (e.g., Chapter 8).

The Benefit Manager's Dilemma

This chapter focuses on a dilemma faced by the benefits manager of a bank with 992 employees, all of them covered by an indemnity health insurance program. The benefit manager wants to analyze if a preferred provider arrangement will save the bank healthcare funds. Currently, employees can seek care from any physician and, after satisfying an annual deductible, must pay only a copayment, with the employer paying the remainder. A preferred provider organization (PPO) has approached the benefits manager and has

This book has a companion web site that features narrated presentations, animated examples, PowerPoint slides, online tools, web links, additional readings, and examples of students' work. To access this chapter's learning tools, go to ache.org/DecisionAnalysis and select Chapter 5.

offered to discount services to those employees who use its clinic and hospital. As an inducement, the PPO wants the bank to increase the deductible and/or copayment of employees who use other providers. Employees would still be free to seek care from any provider, but it would cost them more.

The logic of the arrangement is simple: The PPO can offer a discount because it expects a high volume of sales. Nevertheless, the benefits manager wonders what would happen if employees started using the PPO. In particular, an increase in the rate of referrals and clinic visits could easily eat away the savings on the price per visit. A change of physicians could also alter the employees' place of and rate of hospitalization, which would likewise threaten the potential savings.

Before proceeding, some terminology should be clarified. *Discount* refers to the proposed charges at the PPO compared to what the employer would pay under its existing arrangement with the current provider. *Deductible* is a minimum sum that must be exceeded before the health plan picks up the bill. *Copayment* is the portion of the bill the employee must pay after the deductible is exceeded.

Describing the Problem

A decision tree is a visual tool that shows the sequence of events tells the central line of the story. If the analysis ignores these intervening events, then the sequence and the related story are lost. It would be like reading the beginning and ending of a novel; it may be effective at getting the message across but not at communicating the story.

Imagine a tree with a root, a trunk, and many branches. Lay it on its side, and you have an image of a decision tree. The word "tree" has a special meaning in graph theory. Branches of the decision tree do not lead to the root, trunk, or other branches. Thus, a decision tree is not circular; you cannot begin at one place, travel along the tree, and return to the same place. Because a decision tree shows the temporal sequence—events to the left happen before events to the right—it is described as starting with the leftmost node.

The first part of the decision tree is the *root.* The root of the decision tree, placed to the left and shown as a small square, represents a decision. There are at least two lines emanating from this decision node. Each line corresponds to one option. In Figure 5.1, two lines represent the options of signing a contract with the PPO or continuing with the current plan.

The second component of a decision tree consists of the *chance nodes.* These nodes show the events over which the decision maker has no direct control. From a chance node, several lines are drawn, each showing a different possible event. Suppose, for example, that joining the PPO will change the utilization of hospital and outpatient care. Figure 5.2 portrays these events.

Note that the chance nodes are identified by circles. The distinction between circles and boxes indicates whether the decision maker has control over the events that follow a node. Figure 5.2 suggests that, for people who join the PPO, there is an unspecified probability of hospitalization, outpatient care, or no utilization. These probabilities are shown as P_1, P_2, . . . , P_6; it is the practice to place probabilities above the lines leading to the events they are concerned with.

The third element in a decision tree consists of the *consequences.* While the middle of the decision tree shows events following the decision, the right side (at the end of the branches) shows the consequences of these events. Suppose, for the sake of simplicity, that the benefits manager is only interested in costs to the employer, which exclude copayments and deductibles paid by the employee. Hospital and clinic charges are labeled C_1, C_2, . . . , C_6 and are shown in Figure 5.3.

Figure 5.3 represents the three major elements of a decision tree: decisions, possible events, and consequences (in this case, costs). Also, it is important to keep in mind that a decision tree contains a temporal sequence—events at the left precede events on the right.

Solicitation Process

A decision tree, once analyzed and reported, indicates a preferred option and the rationale for choosing it. Such a report communicates the nature of the decision to other members of the organization. The decision tree and the final report on the preferred option are important organizational documents that can influence people, for better or worse, long after the original decision makers have left.

While the analysis and the final report are important by themselves, the process of gathering data and modifying the decision tree are equally important—perhaps more so. The process helps in several ways:

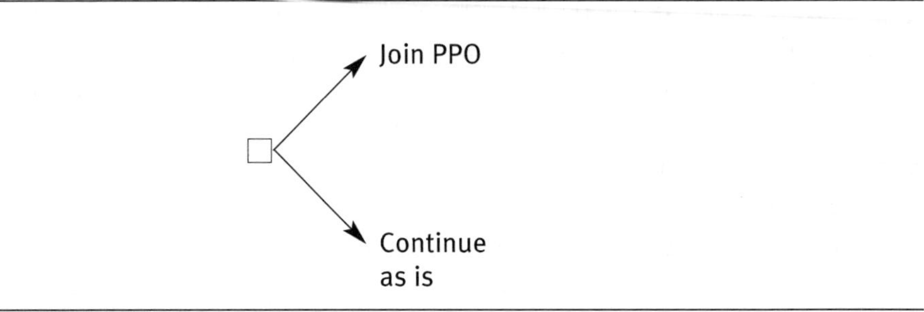

FIGURE 5.1 An Example of a Decision Node

FIGURE 5.2 Possible Events Are Placed to the Right of the Decision Node

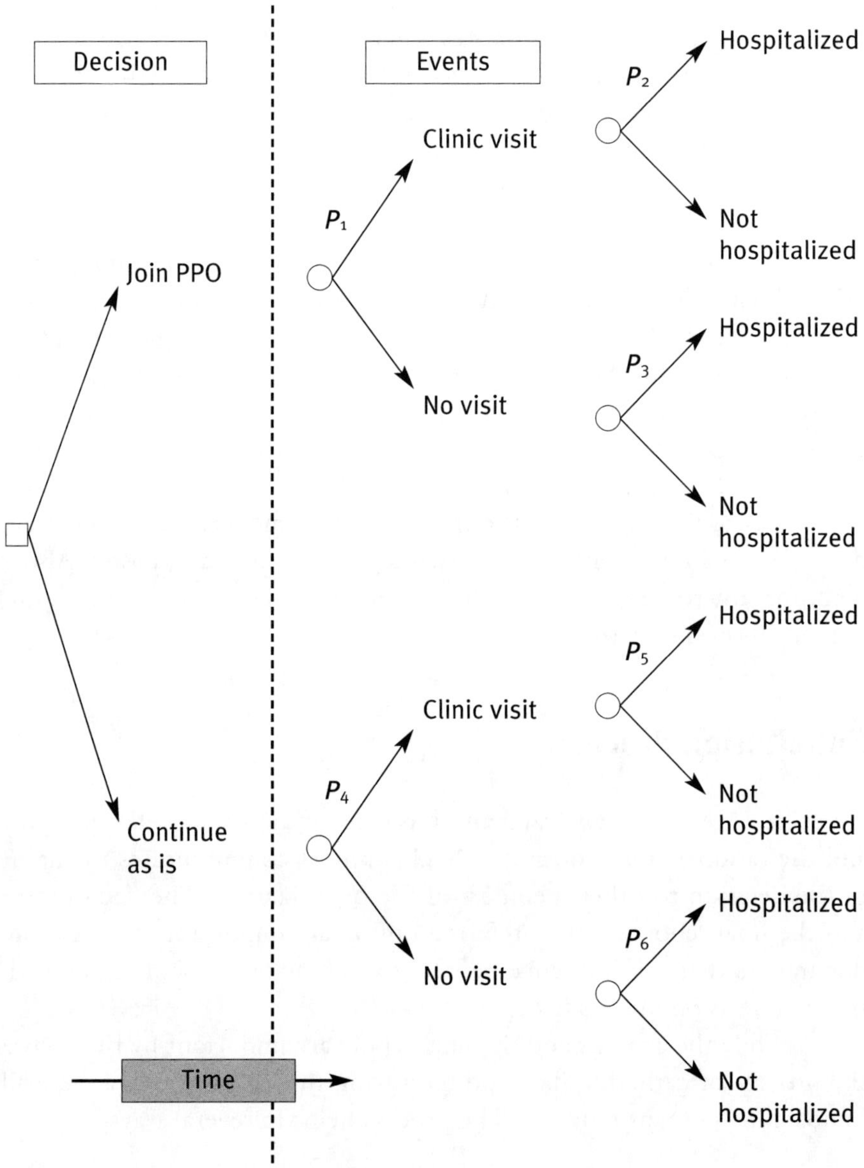

Decision

Events

Join PPO

Continue as is

P_1 Clinic visit

No visit

P_2 Hospitalized

Not hospitalized

P_3 Hospitalized

Not hospitalized

P_4 Clinic visit

No visit

P_5 Hospitalized

Not hospitalized

P_6 Hospitalized

Not hospitalized

Time

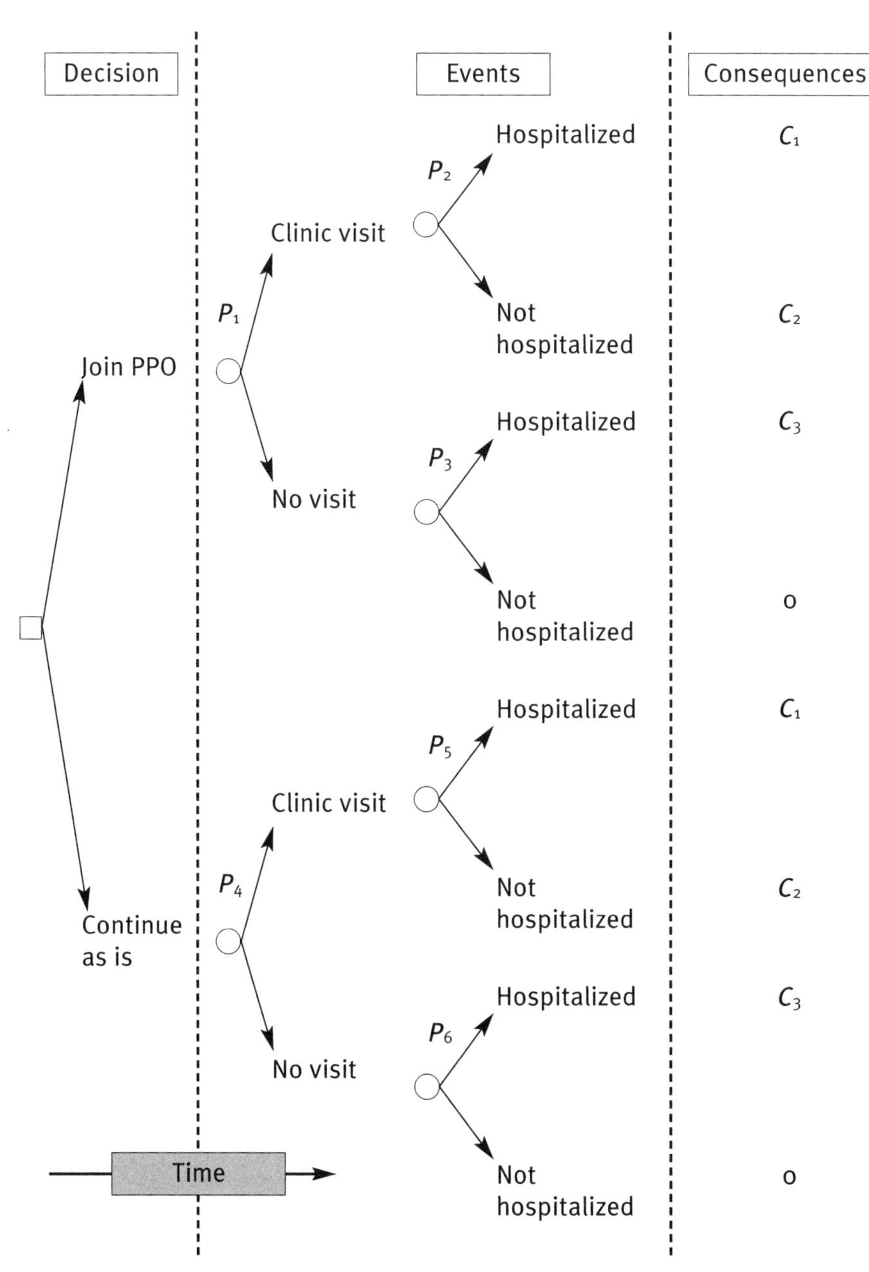

FIGURE 5.3 Consequences Are Placed to the Right of the Decision Tree

1. Decision makers are informed that a decision is looming and that they must articulate their concerns before it is completed.
2. Clients are reassured that the analysis is fair and open.
3. New insights are provided while facilitating discussion of the decision.
4. Decision makers at various levels are removed from day-to-day concerns, allowing them to ponder the impending changes. As decision makers put more thought into the decision, they develop more insight into their own beliefs.

5. Discussions among decision makers will produce further information and insights. If the analysis was done without their involvement, the positive atmosphere of collaboration would be lost.

Once a basic decision-tree structure has been organized, it is important to return to the decision makers and see if all relevant issues have been modeled. When the analyst showed Figure 5.3 to the decision makers, for example, they pointed out the following additional changes:

1. The analysis should separate general outpatient care from mental health care, because payments for the latter are capped and payments for the former are not.
2. The analysis should concentrate on employees who file claims, because only they incur costs to the employer.

The analyst revised the model to reflect these issues, and in subsequent meetings the client added still more details, particularly about the relationships among the copayment, discount, and deductible. This is important because the order in which these terms are incorporated changes the value of the different options. Negotiations between the employer and the PPO suggested that the discount is on the first dollar, before the employee pays the copayment. Employees had a $200 individual and a $500 family deductible for costs paid for clinics or hospitalization. The insurance plan required employees to meet the deductible before the copayment. Once these considerations were incorporated, the revised model presented in Figure 5.4 was created.

Note that for ease of presentation some nodes have been combined, and as a consequence, the sums of some probabilities may add up to more than 1.

In summary, the development of the decision tree proceeds toward increased specification and complexity. The early model is simple, later models are more sophisticated, and the final one may be too complicated to show all elements and is used primarily for analytical purposes. Each step toward increasing specification involves interaction with the decision maker—an essential element to a successful analysis.

Estimating the Probabilities

In a decision tree, each probability is conditioned on the events preceding it. Thus, P_1 in Figure 5.4 is not the probability of hospitalization but the probability of hospitalization given that the person has met the deductible

FIGURE 5.4 Revised Decision Tree

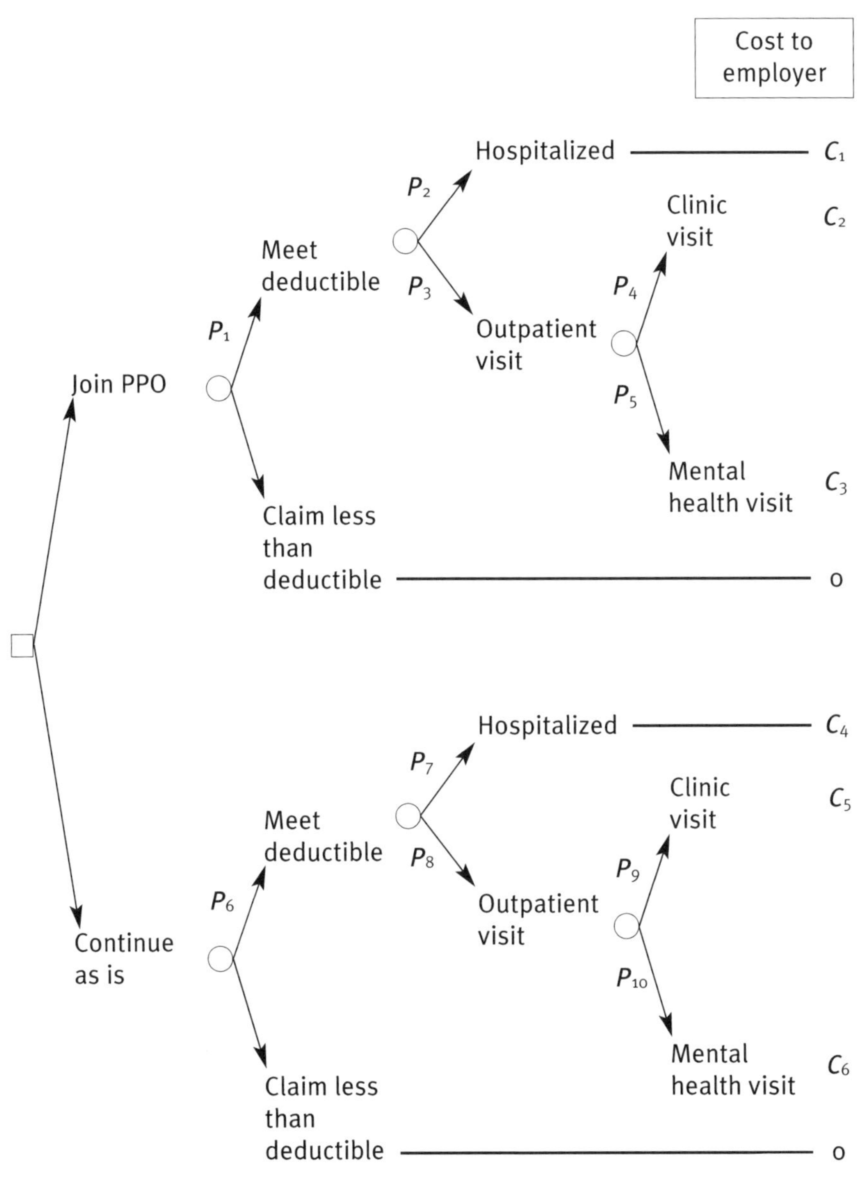

and has joined the PPO. It is important not to confuse conditional probabilities with marginal probabilities, as discussed in Chapter 3.

Conditional probabilities for the decision tree can be estimated by either analyzing objective data or obtaining subjective opinions of the experts (see Chapter 3). The probabilities needed for the lower part of the decision tree, P_4 through P_6, can be assessed by reviewing the employer's current experiences. The analyst reviewed one year of the data from the employer's records and estimated the various probabilities needed for the lower part of the decision tree.

The probabilities for the upper part of the decision tree are more difficult to assess because they require speculation regarding what might happen if employees use the preferred clinic. The decision maker identified several factors that might affect future outcomes:

1. The preferred clinic might have less efficient practices, leading to more hospitalizations and eventually more costs. The validity of this claim was examined by looking at PPO practice patterns and estimating the probabilities from these patterns.
2. Employees who join the PPO might overutilize services because they have lower copayments. If this is the case, the probabilities associated with the use of services will go up.
3. Employees moving from solo practices to group practices may lead to overutilization of specialists. Again, this will show in the probability of the utilization of services.
4. Clinicians may generate their own demand, especially when they have few visits.

To estimate the potential effect of these issues on the probability of hospitalization, the analyst reviewed the literature and brought together a panel of experts familiar with practice patterns of different clinics. The analyst asked them to assess the difference between the preferred clinic and the average clinic. The analyst then used the estimates available through the literature to assess the potential effect of these differences on utilization rates. Table 5.1 provides a summary of the synthetic estimate of what might happen to hospitalization rates by joining the PPO.

This estimate shows how the effect of joining the PPO was gauged by combining the expert's assessments with the published research literature. Although these estimates are rough, they are usually sufficient. Keep in mind that the purpose of these numbers is not to answer precisely what will happen but to determine whether one option is roughly better than the other. The assumptions made in the analysis can be tested by conducting a *sensitivity analysis*—a process in which one or two estimates are changed slightly to see if it would lead to entirely different decisions. In this example, the analysis was not sensitive to small changes in probabilities but was sensitive to the cost per hospitalization.

TABLE 5.1 Increase in Hospitalization Rates Projected at the PPO Clinic

	Difference Between PPO and Others	*Effect of 1% Change*	*Net Effect of Change*
Occupancy rate of primary hospital	−5.0%	−0.43	2.15%
Number of patients seen per day	2.50%	−0.65	−1.63%
Group versus solo practice	20.00%	0.007	0.14%
Effect of copayment reduction	+10.0%	+0.1	1.00%
Total effect of change to PPO			1.67%

Estimating Hospitalization Costs

In estimating cost per hospitalization, the analyst started with the assumption that the employees will incur the same charges as current patients at the preferred hospital. Because the provider, as a large referral center, treats patients who are extremely ill, an adjustment needed to be made. Bank employees are unlikely to be as sick, and thus will not incur equally high charges, so charges should be adjusted to reflect this difference.

This adjustment is made by using a system developed by Medicare to measure differences in the case mix of different institutions. In this system, each group of diseases is assigned a cost relative to the average case. Patients with diseases requiring more resources have higher costs and are assigned values greater than 1. Similarly, patients with relatively inexpensive diseases receive a value less than 1. As Figure 5.5 shows, each healthcare organization is assumed to have different frequency of diseases.

The case mix for an institution is the cost of treating the disease weighted by the frequency of occurrence of the disease at that institution. Suppose Medicare has set the cost of ith diagnosis-related group (DRG) to be C_i, and P_{ij} measures the frequency of occurrence of DRG i at hospital j, then

$$\text{Case mix for hospital } j = \sum_{i=1,\ldots,n} P_{ij} \times C_i.$$

The ratio of two case-mix calculations at two different institutions is called a *case-mix factor*. It shows how the two institutions are different. A case-mix factor of 1 suggests that the two institutions have patients of similar diseases. Tertiary hospitals tend to have a case-mix factor that is above 1 when compared to community hospitals, indicating that tertiary hospitals see sicker patients.

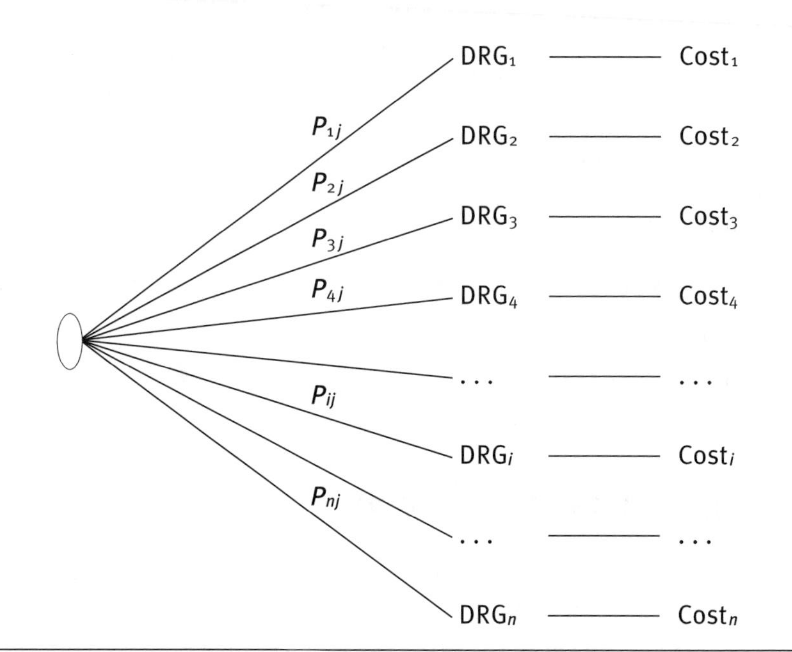

FIGURE 5.5 A Decision-Tree Structure for Calculating the Case Mix at Hospital *J* Based on DRGs

To measure the cost that bank employees would have at the preferred hospital, the analyst reviewed employee records at the bank and patient records at the preferred hospital. The analyst constructed a case-mix index for each. Employees had a case-mix factor of 0.90, suggesting that these employees were not as sick as the average Medicare enrollees; the case-mix index at the preferred hospital that year was 1.17, suggesting that patients at the preferred hospital were sicker than the average Medicare patient. The ratio of the two was calculated as 1.3. This suggested that the diseases treated at the preferred hospital were about 30 percent more costly than those typically faced by employees, so the analyst proportionally adjusted the average hospitalization charges at the preferred hospital. The average hospitalization cost at the preferred hospital was $4,796. Using the case-mix difference, the analysis predicted that if bank employees were hospitalized at the preferred hospital, they would have an average hospitalization cost of $4,796 ÷ 1.3, or roughly 30 percent less cost.

Figure 5.6 shows the estimated costs for the lower and upper parts of the decision tree. Costs reported in Figure 5.6 reflect the cost per employee's family per year.

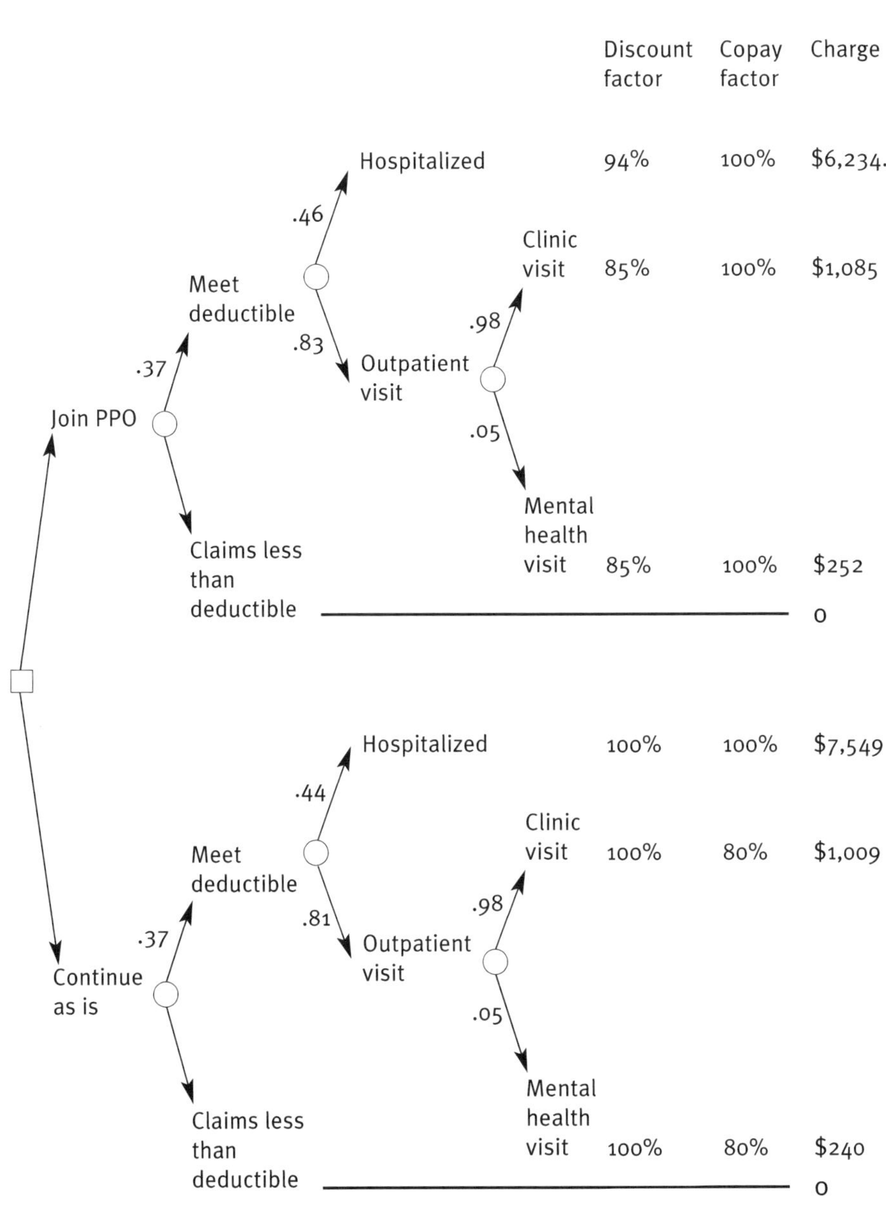

FIGURE 5.6 A Decision Tree with Estimated Costs and Probabilities Costs

Analysis of Decision Trees

The analysis of decision trees is based on the concept of expectation. The word "expectation" suggests some sort of anticipation about the future rather than an exact formula. In mathematics, the concept of *expectation* is more precise. If you believe costs $C_1, C_2, \ldots, C_n$ may happen with probabilities $P_1, P_2, \ldots, P_n$, then the mathematical expectation is

$$\text{Expected cost} = \sum_{i=1,\ldots,n} P_i \times C_i.$$

Each node of a decision tree can be replaced by its expected cost in a method called *folding back*. The expected cost at a node is the sum of the costs weighted by the probability of their occurrence. Consider, for example, the node for employees who in the current situation meet their deductibles and have outpatient visits. They have a 98 percent chance of having an outpatient visit costing \$1,009 per year per person (80 percent of which is charged to the employer, and the rest of which is paid by the employee). They also have a 5 percent chance of having a mental health visit costing \$240 (80 percent of which is charged to the employer, and the rest to the employee). The expected cost to the employer for outpatient visits per employee per year is then calculated as

$$\text{Employer's expected cost for outpatient visits} = \\ (0.98 \times 0.80 \times \$1{,}009) + (0.05 \times 0.80 \times \$240) = \$800.66.$$

This expected cost can replace the node for outpatient visits in the "continue as is" situation in the decision tree. Likewise, the process can now be repeated to fold back the decision tree further and replace each node with its expected cost. Figure 5.7 shows the calculation of the expected cost of continuing as is through three steps.

The employer's expected cost for joining the PPO was calculated to be \$871.08 per employee's family per year. This is \$597.86 per employee's family per year less than the current situation. As the firm has 992 employees, the analysis suggests that switching to the PPO will result in cost savings of almost half million dollars per year.

The problem with the folding-back method is that it is not easy to represent the calculation in formulas with programs such as Excel; too much of the information is visual. However, there is another way of analyzing a decision tree that takes advantage of the decision tree's structure and does not require folding-back procedures. First, all the probabilities for each path in the decision tree are multiplied together to find the joint probability of the path. For example, after joining the PPO, the joint probability of meeting the deductible and being hospitalized is provided by multiplying 0.37 (the probability of meeting the deductible for people who join the PPO) by 0.46 (the probability of being hospitalized if the person has joined the PPO and meets the deductible). To calculate the expected cost/value, the joint probability of each path is multiplied by the corresponding cost/value and summed for each option. Table 5.2 shows each

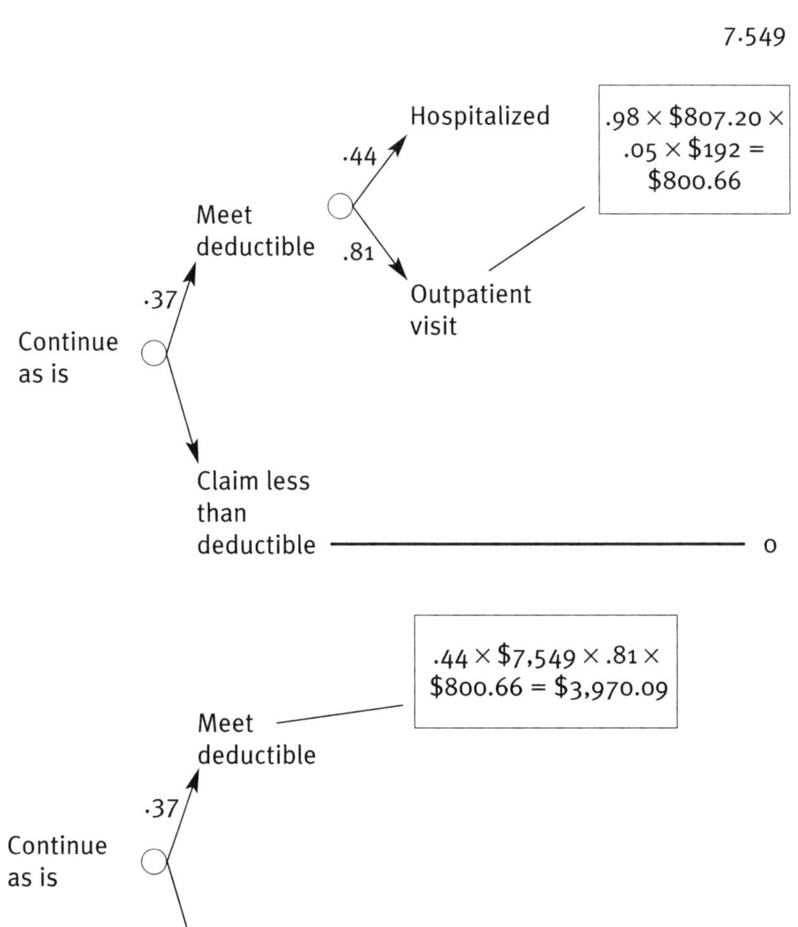

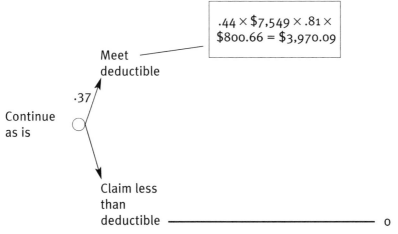

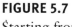

FIGURE 5.7 Starting from the Right, Each Node Is Replaced with its Expected Value

of the paths in the upper part of the decision tree in Figure 5.7, the corresponding joint probability of the sequence, and its associated costs.

This information can be used to calculate the expected cost by multiplying the cost and the probability of each path and summing the results. Using the terms introduced in Figure 5.4, the expected cost of joining the PPO can be calculated using the following formula:

TABLE 5.2 Using the Paths in a Decision Tree to Calculate Expected Cost

Path Depicting the Sequence of Events After Joining the PPO	Formula Using Terms in Figure 5.4	Joint Probability of Sequence	Cost of Sequence	Probability of Sequence Times its Cost
Meet deductible, Hospitalization	P_1P_2	0.17	\$3,467.88	\$590.23
Meet deductible, Outpatient visit, Clinic visit	$P_1P_3P_4$	0.30	\$922.25	\$277.56
Meet deductible, Outpatient visit, Mental health visit	$P_1P_3P_5$	0.02	\$214.20	\$3.29
Expected cost of joining PPO				\$871.08

$$\text{Expected cost (Joining PPO)} = (P_1 \times P_2 \times C_1) + (P_1 \times P_3 \times P_4 \times C_2) + (P_1 \times P_3 \times P_5 \times C_3).$$

Note that the above formula does not show situations that lead to zero cost (not meeting the deductible or meeting the deductible but not having any additional healthcare utilization). If you wanted to show the path leading to zero cost for employees who do not meet the deductible, you would have to add the following term to the above formula: $+ (1 - P_1) \times 0$.

The expected cost of continuing as is can be calculated as

$$\text{Expected cost (Continuing as is)} = (P_6 \times P_7 \times C_4) + (P_6 \times P_8 \times P_9 \times C_5) + (P_1 \times P_6 \times P_8 \times C_6).$$

When expected cost is expressed as a formula, it is possible to enter the formula into Excel and ask a series of "what if" questions. The analyst can change the values of one variable and see the effect of the change on the expected-cost calculations.

Sensitivity Analysis

Some analysts mistakenly stop the analysis after a preferred option has been identified. This is not the point to end the analysis but the start of real understanding of what leads to the choice of one option over another. As previously mentioned, the purpose of an analysis is to provide insight and not to produce numbers. One way to help decision makers better understand the structure of their decision is to conduct a sensitivity analysis on the data to see if the conclusions are particularly sensitive to some inputs. Many decision makers are skeptical of the numbers used in the analysis and wonder if the conclusions could be different if the estimated numbers were different. *Sensitivity analysis* is the process of changing the input parameters until the output (the conclusions) is affected. In other words, it is the process of changing the numbers until the analysis falls apart and the conclusions are reversed.

Sensitivity analysis starts with changing a single estimate at a time until the conclusions are reversed. Two point estimates are calculated, one for the best possible scenario and the other for the worst possible scenario. For example, in estimating the costs associated with joining the PPO, the probability of hospitalization given that the person has met the deductible is an important estimate about which the decision maker may express reservations. To understand the sensitivity of the conclusions to this probability, three estimates are obtained: (1) the probability set to maximum (when everyone is hospitalized), (2) the probability set to minimum (when no one is hospitalized), and (3) the initial expected value, or the *base case* (see Table 5.3).

Changing this conditional probability leads to a change in the expected cost of joining the PPO. To understand whether the conclusions are sensitive to the changes in this conditional probability, analysts typically plot the changes. The *x*-axis will show the changing estimate—in this case, the conditional probability of hospitalization for employees who meet the deductible and have joined the PPO. The *y*-axis shows the value of the decision options—in this case, either the expected cost of joining the PPO or the expected cost of continuing as is. A line is drawn for each option. Figure 5.8 shows the resulting sensitivity graph.

Note that in Figure 5.8, joining the PPO is preferred, for the most part, to continuing as is. Only at very high probabilities of hospitalization, which the decision maker might consider improbable, is the situation reversed. The conclusions are reversed at 0.93, which is called the *reversal*, or *break-even, point.* If the estimate is near the reversal point, then the

TABLE 5.3
Effect of Changing the Probability of Hospitalization

	Probability	*Join PPO*	*Continue As Is*
Maximum	1.00	$1563.96	$1,468.93
Estimated	0.46	$871.08	$1,468.93
Minimum	0.00	$280.85	$1,468.93

FIGURE 5.8 Sensitivity of Conclusions to Conditional Probability of Hospitalization

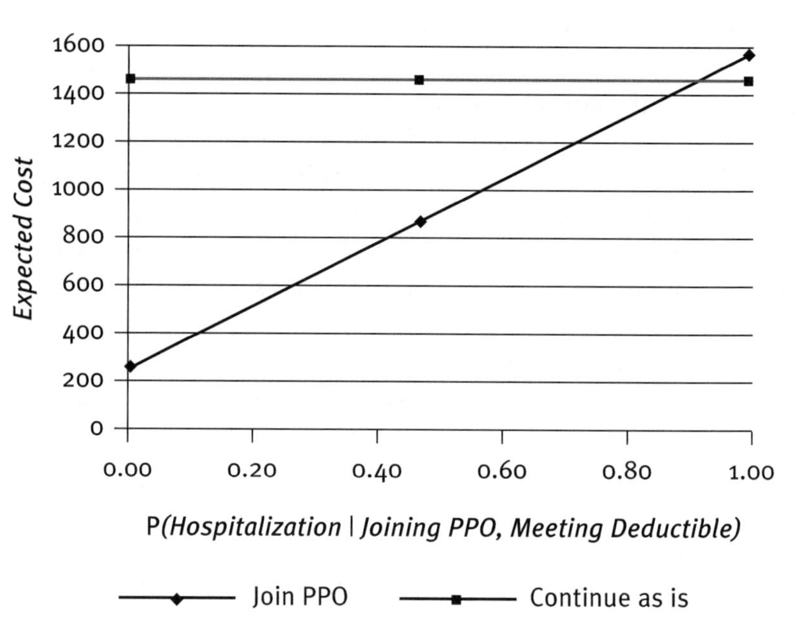

analyst will be concerned. If the estimate is far away, the analyst will be less concerned. The distance between the current estimate of 0.37 and the reversal point of 0.93 suggests that small inaccuracies in the estimation of the probability will not matter in the final analysis. What will matter? The answer can be found by conducting a sensitivity analysis on each of the parameters in the analysis to find one in which small changes will lead to decision reversals.

The analysis calculates the cost of hospitalization for employees from current hospital costs at the preferred hospital. PPO hospitalization costs are reduced by a factor of 1.3 to reflect the case mix of the employed population. It assumes that the employed population is less severely sick than the general population at the preferred hospital. The reversal point for the estimate of case mix is 0.65, at which point the cost of hospitalization for the employees at the preferred hospital would be estimated to be $6,935. This seemed unlikely, as it would have claimed that the bank's employees needed to be significantly sicker than the current patients at the preferred hospital, which is a national referral center.

It is important to find the reversal points for each of the estimates in a decision tree. This can be done by solving an equation in which the variable of interest is changed to produce an expected value equal to the alternative option. This can also be done easily in Excel using the goal-seeking tool, which finds an estimate for the variable of interest that would make the difference between the two options become zero.

So far, changing one estimate to see if it leads to a decision reversal has been discussed. What if analysts change two or more estimates simultaneously? How can the sensitivity of the decision to changes in multiple estimates be examined? For example, what if both the estimates of probability of hospitalization and the cost of hospitalization were wrong? To assess the sensitivity of the conclusions to simultaneous changes in several estimates, the technique of *linear programming* must be used. This technique allows the minimization of an objective subject to constraints on several variables. The absolute difference between the expected value of the two options is minimized subject to constraints imposed by the low and high ranges of the various estimates.

For example, you might minimize the difference between the expected cost of joining the PPO and continuing as is subject to a case mix ranging from 1 to 1.4 and the conditional probability of hospitalization ranging from 0.3 to 0.5. Mathematically, this shown as follows:

Minimize objective = Expected cost (Joining HMO) – Expected cost (Continue as is),

where

- $1 <$ Case mix of PPO to bank employees < 1.4; and
- $0.3 < P(\text{Hospitalization}|\text{Joining PPO, Meeting deductible}) < 0.5$.

It is difficult to solve linear programs by hand. One possibility is to solve for the worst-case scenario. In this situation, the assumption is that joining the PPO will lead to the worst rate of hospitalization (0.5) and the worst cost of hospitalization (case mix of 1). Even in this worst-case scenario, joining the PPO remains the preferred option. In addition to using the worst-case scenarios, it is also possible to use Excel's solver tool as a relatively easy way to use linear programming. Using the solver tool, the analyst found that there are no solutions that would make the difference between joining the PPO and continuing as is become zero subject to the above constraints. Therefore, even with both constraints changing at the same time, there is no reversal of conclusions.

Missed Perspectives

The purpose of any analysis is to provide insight. Often when decision makers review an analysis, they find that important issues are missed. In the

PPO example, one decision maker believed the potential savings were insufficient to counterbalance the political and economic costs of instituting the proposed change. The current healthcare providers were customers of the client, and signing a contract with the PPO might alienate them and induce them to take their business elsewhere. Incorporating the risk of losing customers would improve the calculations and help the bank decide whether the savings would counterbalance the political costs (more on this in the next section).

Furthermore, additional discussion leads to another critical perspective: Would it be better to wait for a better offer from a different provider? The consequences of waiting could have been incorporated into the analysis by placing an additional branch from the decision node, marked as "wait for additional options." This would have provided a more comprehensive analysis of the decision.

New avenues often open when an analysis is completed. It is important to remember that one purpose of analysis is to help decision makers understand the components of their problem and to devise increasingly imaginative solutions to it. Therefore, there is no reason to act defensively if a client begins articulating new options and considerations while the analyst presents the findings. Instead, the analyst should actively encourage the clients to discuss their concerns and consider modifying the analysis to include them.

A serious shortcoming with decision trees is that many clients believe they show every possible option. Actually, there is considerable danger in assuming that the problem is as simple as a decision tree makes it seem. In this example, many other options may exist for reducing healthcare costs aside from joining the PPO; but perhaps because they were not included in the analysis, they will be ignored by the decision maker, who (like the rest of us) is victim to the "out of sight, out of mind" fallacy (Silvera et al. 2005; Fischhoff, Slovic, and Lichtenstein 1978).

The "myth of analysis" can explain why things not seen are not considered. This myth is the belief that analysis is impartial and rests on proper assumptions and that it is robust and comprehensive. Perpetuating this myth prevents further inquiry and imaginative solutions to problems. Decision trees could easily fall into this trap, because they appear so comprehensive and logical that decision makers fail to imagine any course of action not explicitly included in them.

The final presentation of a decision-tree analysis is broken into two segments. First, the report summarizes the results of the decision tree and the sensitivity analysis. The report of the analysis should have these examinations in the appendix and the base-case, best-case, and worst-case solutions in the main report. The section containing the recommendation of the reports should refer to the sensitivity of the conclusions to changes in the input. Second, the analyst should ask the clients to share their ideas about options and considerations not modeled in the analysis. If one does not explicitly search for new alternatives, the analysis might do more harm than good. Instead of fostering creativity, it can allow the analyst and decision maker to hide behind a cloak of missed options and poorly comprehended mathematics.

Expected Value or Utility

Sometimes the consequences of an event are not just additional cost or savings, and it is important to measure the utility associated with various outcomes. In these circumstances, one measures the value of each consequence in terms of its utility and not merely its costs. To fold back the decision tree, expected utility is used instead of the expected cost.

When Bernoulli (1738) was experimenting with the notion of expectation, he noticed that people did not prefer the alternative with the highest expected monetary value; people are not willing to pay a large amount of money for a gamble with infinite expected return. In explanation, Bernoulli suggested that people maximize utility rather than monetary value, and costs should be transformed to utilities before expectations are taken. He named this model *expected utility*.

According to expected utility, if an alternative has n outcomes with costs $C_1, \ldots, C_n$ associated probabilities of $P_1, \ldots, P_n$, and if each cost has a particular utility to the decision maker of $U_1, \ldots, U_n$, then

$$\text{Expected utility} = \sum_{i=1,\ldots,n} P_i \times U_i.$$

Bernoulli resolved the paradox of why people would not participate in a gamble with infinite return by arguing that the first dollar gained has a greater utility than the millionth dollar. The beauty of a utility model is that it allows the marginal value of gains and losses to decrease with their magnitude. In contrast, mathematical expectation assigns every dollar the same value. When the costs of outcomes differ considerably—say, when one outcome costs $1,000,000 and another $1,000—one can prevent small gains from being overvalued by using utilities instead of costs.

Utilities are also better than costs in testing whether benefits meet the client's goals. Using costs in the PPO analysis, joining the PPO would lead to expected savings of about half a million dollars. Yet, when the bank had not acted six months after completing the analysis, it became clear that this savings was not sufficient to cause a change because nonmonetary issues were involved. The analyst could have uncovered this problem if, instead of monetary returns, he had used utility estimates.

Chapter 2 describes how to measure utility over many dimensions, both monetary and nonmonetary, was described. In the PPO example, cost was not the sole concern—the bank had many objectives for changing its healthcare plan. If it wanted only to lower costs, it could have ceased providing healthcare coverage entirely, or it could have increased the copayment. The bank was concerned about the employees' reactions, which it anticipated would be based on concerns for quality, accessibility, and, to a lesser extent, cost to employees. A utility model should have been constructed for these concerns, and the model should have been used to assess the value of each consequence.

Utility is also preferable for clients who must consider attitudes toward risk. This is because expected utility, in contrast to expected cost, reflects attitudes toward risk. A risk-neutral individual bets the expected monetary value of a gamble. A risk taker bets more on the same gamble because she associates more utility to the high returns. A risk-adverse individual cares less for the high returns and bets less. Research shows that most individuals are risk seeking when they can choose between a small loss and a gamble for a large gain, and they are risk adverse when they must choose between a small gain and a gamble for a large loss (Kahneman and Tversky 1979).

A client, especially when trying to decide for an organization, may exclude personal attitudes about risk and request that the analysis of the decision tree be based on expected cost and not expected utility. Thus, the client may prefer to assume a risk-neutral position and behave as if every dollar of gain or loss were equivalent. The advantage of making the risk attitudes explicit is that it leads to insights about one's own policies; the disadvantage is that such policies may not be relevant to other decision makers.

Transformation of costs to values/utilities is important in most situations. But when the analysis is not done for a specific decision maker, monetary values are paramount, the marginal value of a dollar seems constant across the range of consequences, and attitudes toward risk seem irrelevant, then it may be reasonable to explicitly measure the cost and implicitly consider the nonmonetary issues.

When asked, the executives raised the issue that money was not the sole consideration. Many of the hospitals' CEOs were on the bank's executive board. The bank was concerned that by preferring one healthcare provider, they may lose their goodwill and, at an extreme, the current providers may shift their funds to a competing bank. Figure 5.9 shows the resulting dilemma faced by the bank.

Figure 5.9 shows that the bank faces the loss of half a million dollars per year for continuing as is. Alternatively, it can join the PPO but faces a chance of losing its healthcare customer's goodwill. To further analyze this decision tree, it is necessary to assess the probability of losing the healthcare organization's goodwill and the value or utility associated with the overall affect of both cost and goodwill. If attitudes toward risk do not matter in this analysis, then the analyst can focus on measuring overall value using MAV models discussed in Chapter 2. Assume that goodwill is given a weight of 0.75, and cost savings of half a million dollars per year is given a weight of 0.25. Also assume that the probability of healthcare organizations shifting their funds to other banks is considered to be small—say, 1 percent. Figure 5.10 summarizes these data.

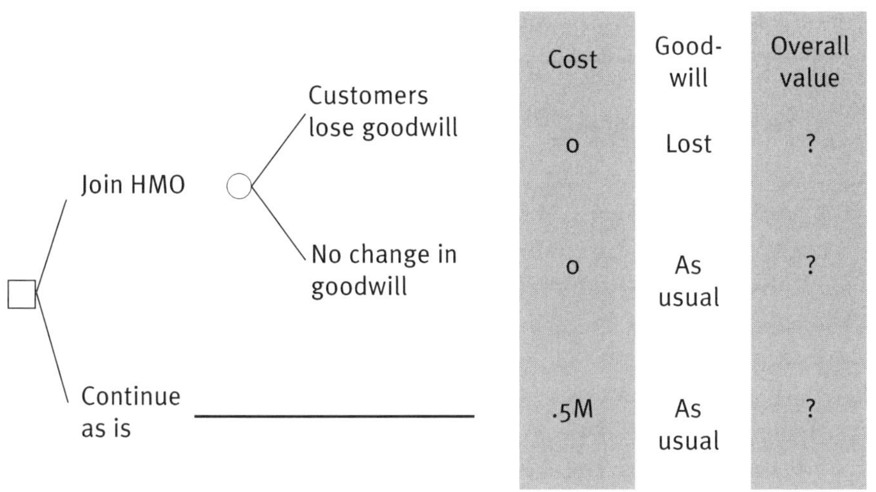

FIGURE 5.9 A Decision Tree Showing Bank's Concern over Losing Healthcare Customers

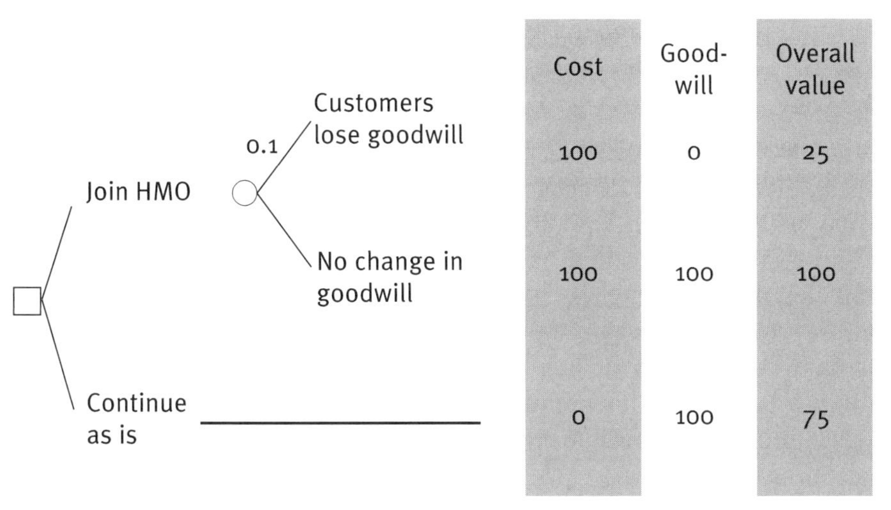

FIGURE 5.10 Value Associated with Cost and Losing Goodwill

The expected value for joining the PPO can be calculated by folding back, starting with the top right side. There is a probability of 1 percent of having an overall value of 25 versus a probability of 99 percent of having a value of 100. The expected value for this node is $(0.01 \times 25) + (0.99 \times 100) = 99.25$. The expected value for the continuing as is node is shown as 75. Therefore, despite the small risk of losing goodwill with some healthcare bank customers, the preferred course of action is to go ahead with the change.

The analyst can conduct a sensitivity analysis to see at what probability of losing goodwill is joining the PPO no longer reasonable (see Figure 5.11). As the probability of losing goodwill increases, the value of joining the PPO decreases. At probabilities higher than 0.35, joining the PPO is no longer preferred over continuing as is.

Sequential Decisions

There are many situations in which one decision leads to another. A current decision must be made with future options in mind. For example, consider a risk-management department inside a hospital. After a sentinel event in which a patient has been hurt, the risk manager can step in with several actions to reduce the probability of a lawsuit. The patient's bill can be written off, or a nurse might be assigned to stay with the patient for the remainder of the hospitalization. Whether the risk manager takes these steps depends on the effectiveness of the preventive strategy. It also depends on what the hospital will do if it is sued. For example, if sued, the risk manager faces the decision to settle out of court or to wait for the verdict. Thus, the two decisions are related. The first decision of preventing the lawsuit is related to the subsequent decision of the disposition of the lawsuit after it occurs. This section describes how to model and analyze interrelated decisions.

As before, the most immediate decision is put to the left of a decision tree, followed by its consequences to the right. If there are any related subsequent decisions, they are entered as nodes to the right of the decision tree, or after specific consequences. For example, the decision to prevent lawsuits is put to the left in Figure 5.12. If the lawsuit occurs, a subsequent decision needs to be made about what to do about the lawsuit. Therefore, following the link that indicates the occurrence of the lawsuit, a node is entered for how to manage the lawsuit. To analyze a decision tree with multiple decisions in it, the folding back process is used with one new exception: All nodes are replaced with their expected value/cost as before,

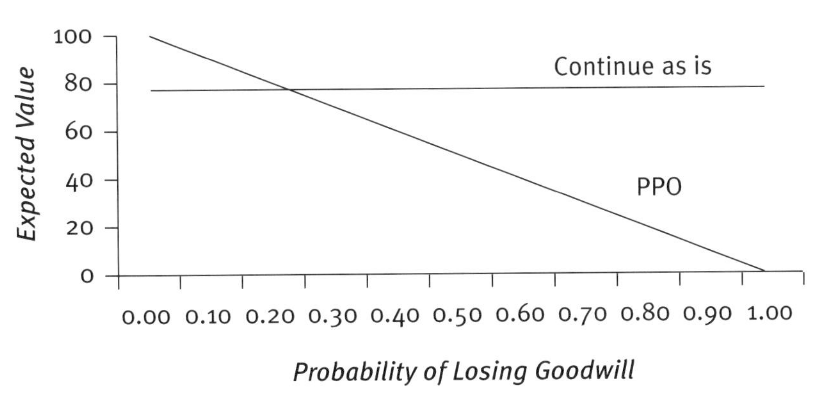

FIGURE 5.11 Sensitivity of Conclusions to Probability of Losing Goodwill After Joining the PPO

but the decision node is replaced with the minimum cost or maximum utility/value of the options available at that node. This is done because, at any decision node, the decision maker is expected to maximize his value/utilities or minimize cost.

In the book *Quick Analysis for Busy Decision Makers*, Behn and Vaupel (1982) suggest how decision-tree analysis can be applied to the problem of settling out of court. Here, their suggestions are applied to a potential malpractice situation. As Figure 5.12 shows, the cost of forgoing the hospital bill and assigning a dedicated nurse to the patient is estimated at $30,000. If the case is taken to the court, there is an estimated $25,000 legal cost. If the hospital loses the case, the verdict is assumed to be for $1 million. Figure 5.12 summarizes these costs. The question is whether it is reasonable to proceed with the preventive action. To answer this question, three probabilities are needed:

1. The probability that the person will file a lawsuit if no preventive action is taken.
2. The probability of a lawsuit if preventive action is taken.
3. The probability of a favorable verdict if the case goes to court.

The estimation of these probabilities and the cost payments need to be appropriate to the situation at hand. Figure 5.12 provides rough estimates for these probabilities and costs, but in reality the situation should be tailored to the nature of the patient, the injury, and experiences with such lawsuits. The published data in the literature can be used to tailor the analysis to the situation at hand. Following are some examples of where the numbers might come from:

FIGURE 5.12 The Decision to Prevent a Malpractice Lawsuit

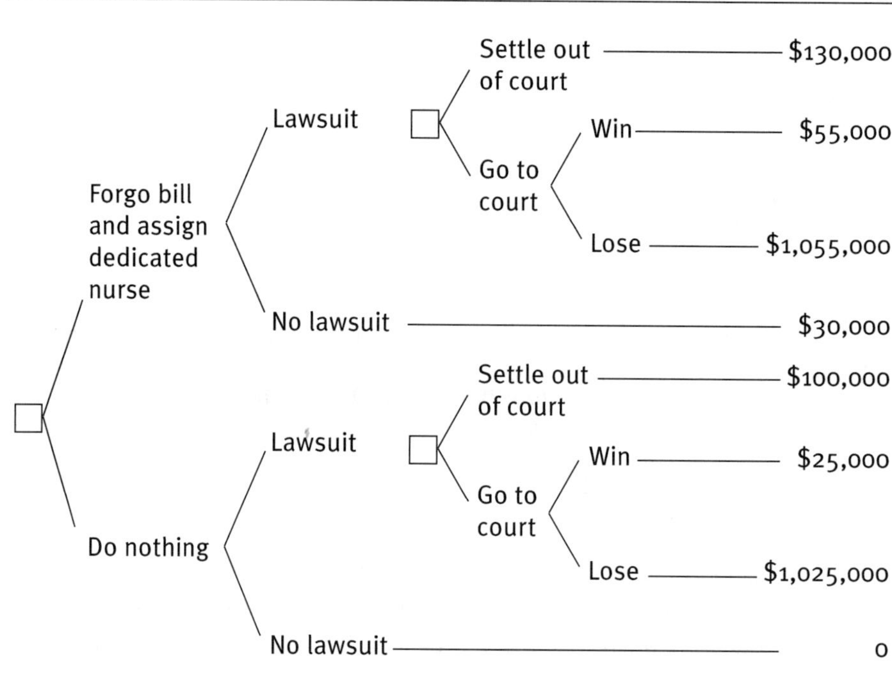

- Driver and Alemi (1995) provide an example of estimating probability of lawsuits from patients' characteristics and circumstances surrounding the incidence. They built a Bayesian probability model for predicting whether the patient will sue from data such as the patient's age, gender, family income, and length of relationship with the doctor; the severity of injury; the patient's attribution of cause of the event; the number of mishaps; the patient's legal or healthcare work experience; and the type of sentinel event.
- Selbst, Friedman, and Singh (2005) provide objective data on epidemiology and etiology of lawsuits involving children. They show that, in 1997, hospitals settled in 93 percent of cases involving mostly diagnostic errors in emergency departments for meningitis, appendicitis, arm fracture, and testicular torsion. Among the costs not settled, the courts found in favor of the hospital in 80 percent of cases and in favor of the patient in 20 percent of cases. The payout depended on the nature of injury. In 1997, average payout was $7,000 for emotional injury, $149,000 for death of the patient, $300,000 for major permanent injury, and $540,000 for quadriplegic injury.
- Bors-Koefoed and colleagues (1998) provide statistical models for assessing the probability of an unfavorable outcome for a lawsuit and the likely amount of payout for obstetrical claims. They showed that

> Indicators of increased indemnity payment were: non-reassuring intrapartum fetal heart rate tracing, later year of delivery, intensity of long-term care required, and participation of a particular defense law firm. Perinatal or childhood death, the use of pitocin, and settlement date increasingly removed from the occurrence date were the determinants of decreased payments in this model. Finally, the presence of major neurological deficits, the prolongation of a case, and the involvement of multiple law firms and defense witnesses increased the expense charged to and paid by the insurance company.

Many similar articles exist in the Medline literature from which both the maximum payout and the probability of these payouts can be assessed. If the probability of winning in court for the case at hand is 60 percent, and the probability of lawsuit is 15 percent and is reduced to 5 percent after the preventive action, then the optimal decision under these assumptions can be calculated.

To fold back the decision tree, start from the top right side and first fold back the node associated with the court outcomes. The expected cost for going to the court is (0.6 × $55,000) + (0.4 × $1,055,000) = $455,000. At this point, the decision tree is pruned as shown in Figure 5.13.

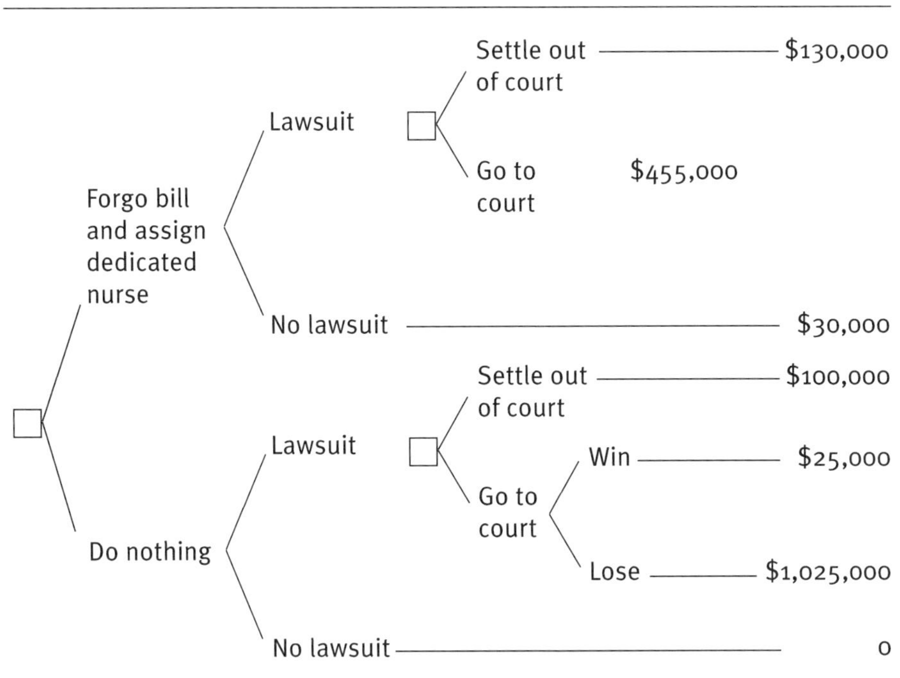

FIGURE 5.13 Replacing the Court Outcomes with Their Expected Costs

Settlement out of court will cost \$130,000 and is preferred to going to court. Therefore, the expected cost for a lawsuit is \$130,000. Note that in a decision node, always use the minimum expected cost associated with the options available at that node. This now reduces the decision tree as shown in Figure 5.14.

Next, calculate the expected cost for preventive action as $(0.05 \times \$130{,}000) + (0.95 \times \$30{,}000) = \$35{,}000$. This results in the final decision tree shown in Figure 5.15.

FIGURE 5.14 The Expected Cost for the Decison Node Is the Option with Minimum Cost

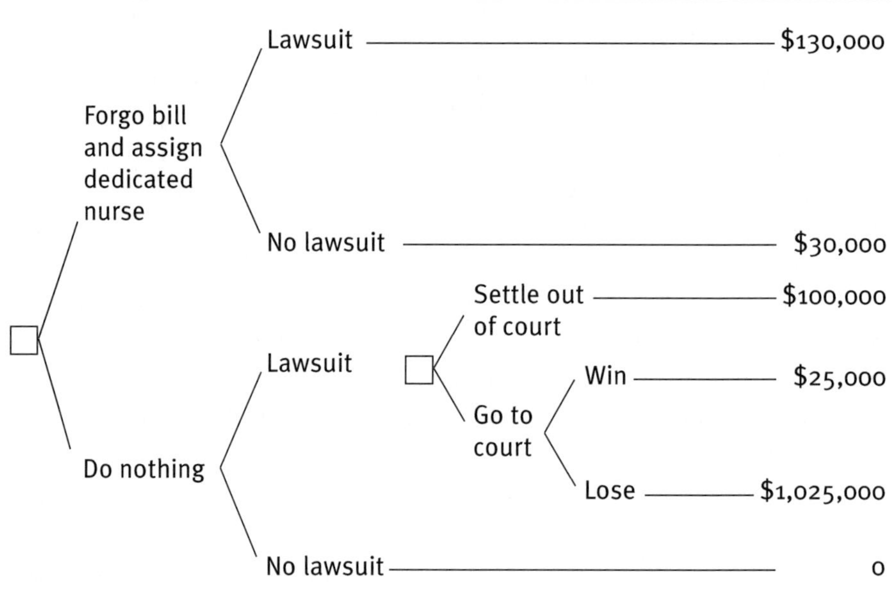

FIGURE 5.15 The Expected Cost of Preventing a Lawsuit

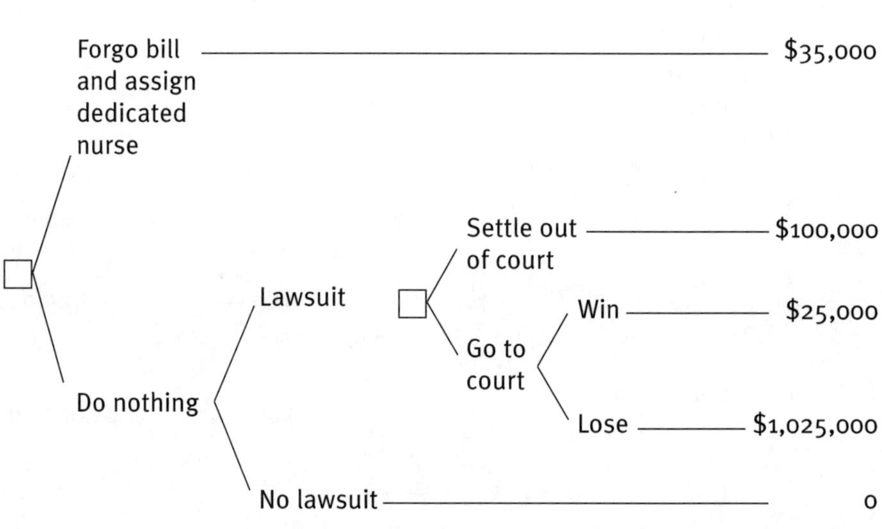

A similar set of calculations can be carried out for the option of doing nothing. In these circumstances, the expected cost associated with the court case is (0.6 × \$25,000) + (0.4 × \$1,025,000) = \$425,000. The preferred option is to settle out of court for \$100,000. The expected cost for a lawsuit is \$100,000. The expected cost for doing nothing is (0.15 × \$100,000) + (0.85 × 0) = \$15,000, which is lower than the expected cost of taking preventive action. For this situation (given the probabilities and costs estimated) the best course of action is to not take any preventive action. A sensitivity analysis can help find the probabilities and costs at which point conclusions are reversed.

Summary

Previous chapters have presented several useful tools a decision analyst can use in modeling decisions, such as how to quantify the values of stakeholders and how to systematically include a consideration of uncertain events in making decisions. This chapter presents another tool for modeling decisions—decision trees. Decision trees are useful in situations when making a decision is dependent on a series of events occurring. These situations include both subjective value and uncertainty, and decision trees are able to accommodate such simultaneous considerations in making decisions. A decision tree models a temporal sequence of events, beginning with the root, which represents a particular decision. Chance nodes emanate from the root of the decision tree and represent all the possible events that follow from a given decision. The final element of a decision tree is the consequences, or the potential effects or results of the various chance nodes.

A decision tree, once constructed, can provide decision makers with a preferred option. This is done by calculating an expected value through the folding back of the tree, where each node is replaced with its expected value. The decision-making process that utilizes decision trees does not end with the identification of a preferred option. Sensitivity analysis is done to see if conclusions can be changed with minor changes in the estimates.

Review What You Know

1. Define the following terms.
   a. Decision node

   b. Event node
   c. Decision tree
   d. Sensitivity analysis
   e. Folding back
   f. Expected cost
   g. Expected value
   h. Sequential decisions
2. What is the expected cost in a gamble that has a 10 percent chance of losing $10,000? Draw the node and calculate the expected cost.
3. Recalculate the expected cost of assigning a dedicated nurse as a preventive action if instead of the potential loss of $1,250,000 the maximum award was $250,000.
4. Recalculate the expected cost of joining the PPO if hospitalization rate for the preferred hospital was underestimated and the correct rate was 0.54 rather than 0.44.
5. When the probabilities of arcs coming out of a node do not add up to 1, what does this mean in terms of the existence of mutually exclusive and exhaustive events?
6. Does calculating case-mix index involve calculating an expected value? What events and which probabilities are involved in this calculation?
7. What is a risk-averse person?
8. Using the decision tree for joining the PPO, calculate the probability of each pathway that comes out of the node for doing nothing.

Rapid-Analysis Exercises

Option 1: Analyzing Local Universal Health Insurance

Evaluate what will happen if your county chooses to self-insure all residents, both employed and unemployed, who have lived in the county for at least two years. The worksheet shown in Figure 5.16 supplies a decision tree to help you analyze this decision. The premiums for the new plan (node C) can be estimated as the current costs of hospital and clinic services minus the following factors: (1) administrative healthcare costs go down in single payer systems; (2) uncompensated care costs are reduced when almost everyone is insured; and (3) the federal government will pay the equivalent of the current employer's tax subsidy to the county. Use the first part of Figure 5.16 to determine the estimated premiums for the new plan. Then, use these premiums as input on the second part of Figure 5.16, which evaluates the plan's impact on taxes.

FIGURE 5.16 Worksheet for Analyzing Local Universal Health Insurance

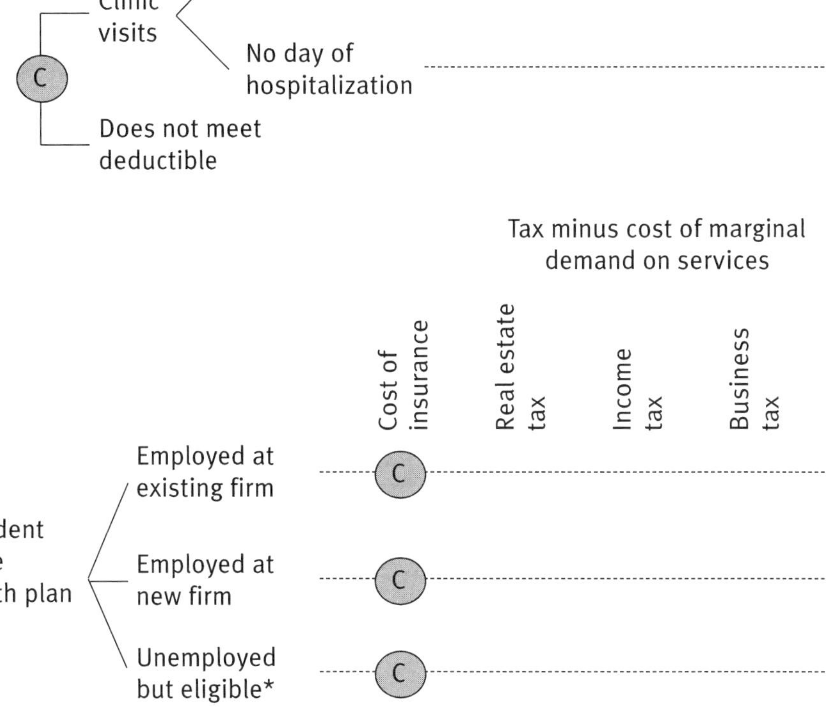

* Residents are eligible for coverage after they have lived in the country for at least two years.

When a region has health insurance for every resident, employers' costs of insurance will be lower. Therefore, more employers will move to the county to take advantage of these savings. These new employers will pay a business tax, thus enhancing the tax base of the county. New employers need new employees, so more residents will move to the county. These new residents will contribute to the county's income tax and will pay real estate taxes. Offering free health insurance to all residents will also attract the unemployed and the chronically sick, though they may be deterred by a required waiting period of two years. Use the second part of the decision tree in Figure 5.16 to determine these costs.

In your analysis, be sure to calculate the impact of this health insurance plan as per resident, not per business, per year. Include data from literature or from knowledgeable experts in your analysis. Multiply the impact of the program (per resident) times the projected number of residents to calculate the total costs of or the savings associated with the program.

Option 2: Analyzing Fetal and Maternal Rights

A clinician is facing an important dilemma of choosing between fetal and maternal rights. The patient is a 34-year-old woman with a 41-week intrauterine pregnancy. The mother is refusing induction of labor. Without the labor induction, the fetus may die. Despite this risk, the mother wants to pursue a vaginal delivery. What should the clinician do?

Model the clinician's decision when the mother refuses to undergo a necessary life-saving cesarean for the infant. Make sure that your analysis is based on the viability of the infant as well as the intrusiveness of the clinician's intervention. Create a decision tree and solicit the utility of various courses of action under different probabilities (see Mohaupt and Sharma 1998).

Audio/Visual Chapter Aids

To help you understand the concepts of decision trees, visit this book's companion web site at ache.org/DecisionAnalysis, go to Chapter 5, and view the audio/visual chapter aids.

References

Behn, R. D., and J. W. Vaupel. 1982. *Quick Analysis for Busy Decision Makers.* New York: Basic Books.

Bernoulli, D. 1738. "Spearman theoria novai de mensura sortus." *Comettariii Academiae Saentiarum Imperialses Petropolitica* 5:175–92. Translated by L. Somner. 1954. *Econometrica* 22:23–36.

Bors-Koefoed, R., S. Zylstra, L. J. Resseguie, B. A. Ricci, E. E. Kelly, and M. C. Mondor. 1998. "Statistical Models of Outcome in Malpractice Lawsuits Involving Death or Neurologically Impaired Infants." *Journal of Maternal-Fetal Medicine* 7 (3): 124–31.

Driver, J. F., and F. Alemi. 1995. "Forecasting Without Historical Data: Bayesian Probability Models Utilizing Expert Opinions." *Journal of Medical Systems* 19 (4): 359–74.

Fischhoff, B., P. Slovic, and S. Lichtenstein. 1978. "Fault Trees: Sensitivity of Estimated Failure Probabilities to Problem Presentation." *Journal of Experimental Psychology Human Perception and Performance* 4 (2): 330–34.

Kahneman, D., and A. Tversky. 1979. "Prospect Theory: An Analysis of Decisions Under Risk." *Econometrica* 47: 263–91.

Mohaupt, S. M., and K. K. Sharma. 1998. "Forensic Implications and Medical-Legal Dilemmas of Maternal Versus Fetal Rights." *Journal of Forensic Science* 43 (5): 985–92.

Selbst, S. M., M. J. Friedman, and S. B. Singh. 2005. "Epidemiology and Etiology of Malpractice Lawsuits Involving Children in US Emergency Departments and Urgent Care Centers." *Pediatric Emergency Care* 21 (3): 165–9.

Silvera, D. H., F. R. Kardes, N. Harvey, M. L. Cronley, and D. C. Houghton. 2005. "Contextual Influences on Omission Neglect in the Fault Tree Paradigm." *Journal of Consumer Psychology* 15 (2): 117–26.

CHAPTER

6

MODELING GROUP DECISIONS

David H. Gustafson and Farrokh Alemi

There are many occasions in which a group, rather than an individual, has to make a decision. A good example is the board of director's decision about a major capital purchase. Conflict can arise in these decisions, and there are at least three ways to reduce this conflict:

1. *Majority rule.* This group model includes any aspect that the majority of the group has included in their individual models.
2. *Average differences.* This group model is defined as the average of the parameters of each individual model.
3. *Behavioral consensus.* This group model is based on unanimous agreement reached through discussions and without the use of majority rule, averaging, or any other mathematical resolution of differences.

This chapter discusses how an analyst can bring about a behavioral consensus around a model of a group decision. A model of a group of decision makers could be thought of as an average of the individual models of various members of the group. In this way, a model is built for each member, and the parameters of the models are averaged to represent the group. But groups are not just a collection of individuals; there is a synergy of thought and ideas that emerges from successful groups. Mathematical aggregation of the individuals' models into a group model loses the real advantage of having the group, which is to arrive at better decisions than the best member of the group could arrive at alone. To effectively model a group's decision, one should create a model that reflects the group's behavioral consensus, which may be very different from the average of each individual's input.

Decision analysts have for some time focused on mathematical methods of aggregating the judgment of various experts or decision makers (Jacobs 1995; Meyer and Booker 1991). This chapter does not review the literature on mathematical aggregation of experts' opinions. Instead, this chapter focuses on the behavioral methods of getting a group to come to a consensus around a model. The goal of this chapter is to design a process

This book has a companion web site that features narrated presentations, animated examples, PowerPoint slides, online tools, web links, additional readings, and examples of students' work. To access this chapter's learning tools, go to ache.org/DecisionAnalysis and select Chapter 6.

where group members can, after reasonable deliberation, agree about a specific model and its parameters.

The processes described in this chapter can be used to help the group generate, share, discuss, and prioritize ideas to reach a final decision. Decision making is more than choosing among alternatives. Often, the choice itself is the tip of the iceberg. Much more needs to be done to articulate the options available and to clarify the process of decision making. This is especially important in group decision making, where key ideas belong to different people; there should be an organized and systematic effort to solicit and arrange these ideas in ways that help the deliberation of the group. This chapter helps an analyst go beyond immediate choices and build a model of the group's collective insights and reasoning. Much of the advice provided in this chapter focuses on how to help group members articulate their ideas.

The task of structuring a decision and estimating the parameters of the model requires a great deal of input from the group. Most decision makers see the process of building models as awkward and artificial. The questions posed by the analyst may seem to be a contorted way of looking at the decision at hand. The analyst's frequent interruptions to structure and assess various estimates may interfere with the group's free-flowing deliberations. If a group's decision has to be modeled effectively, then a process needs to be found that constructs a model without interfering with the group's interactions. This chapter provides one such group process.

The chapter starts with a history of commonly used approaches to structured group meetings. After the history, a new approach called *integrative group process* (IGP) will be presented. This approach borrows from many of the existing methods of improving group processes.

A Short History of Consensus Building

Research on group processes started in earnest in the late 1960s and early 1970s. It has grown in recent years to studies of group decision-support systems, in which computers are used to facilitate meetings. Note that this review of approaches is selective as the literature is vast.

Group Communication Strategy

To understand what works in group processes, this review starts with one of the simplest group processes, the *group communication strategy*. This approach originates from a set of normative instructions proposed by Hall and Watson (1970). Before a group meeting starts, members are instructed to

1. avoid arguing;
2. avoid win-lose statements;
3. avoid changing opinions to reduce conflict;
4. avoid conflict-reducing techniques, such as majority votes and bargaining; and
5. view differences of opinion as natural and initial agreements as suspect.

No other process changes are made. Group members talk freely about topics they choose, with no break in how or when various components of the meeting are accomplished. During these conversations, the analyst constructs a model of the group, with each member contributing at will and commenting on what is relevant. After the start of the meeting, group members may or may not follow the recommended rules for interaction. The expectation is that most will follow these simple instructions if reminded to do so at start of the meeting.

In the decade following Watson and Hall's work, a number of studies evaluated their recommendations. Their findings suggested that when there are large status differences, group members weigh the opinions and suggestions of high-status persons more heavily (Forsyth 1998; Pagliari and Grimshaw 2002). In these groups, the group communication strategy may not do well. Furthermore, little is known about the success of normative instructions in situations in which group members are in conflict or have substantial stakes in the final group judgment.

Nominal Group Process

Another approach to helping groups talk through their differences is the *nominal group process* (Gallagher et al. 1993). This is a generic name for face-to-face group techniques in which group members are instructed not to interact with each other except at specific steps in the process. The following are the steps in the process:

1. Silent idea generation
2. Round-robin sharing of ideas
3. Feedback to the group
4. Explanatory group discussion
5. Individual reassessment
6. Mathematical aggregation of revised judgments

The nominal group process produces a prioritized list of ideas as well as numerical estimates in a short time frame. For example, an analyst can use this process to solicit attributes for a value model and then repeat the process to solicit weights for the attributes. This approach remains popular despite the fact that it has been more than 30 years since its inception (Moon 1999; Carney, McIntosh, and Worth 1996). It is one of the key group processes used to develop treatment algorithms and consensus panels (Cruse et al. 2002). Research on the nominal group process is extensive. A recent review (Black et al. 1999) shows that in numerous circumstances the process produces better results than unstructured group interactions. The performance of the nominal group process may depend on the task structure, selection of participants, presentation of the scientific information available to the group, structure of the group interaction, and method of synthesizing individual judgments. Given the various factors that affect the performance of the nominal group process, analysts should rely on it when the process makes sense for the situation at hand. Three components of the nominal group process may explain the success of the process.

1. Ideas should not be evaluated one at a time. The analyst should collect many ideas before any one of them is evaluated. Postponing evaluation increases creative solutions.
2. In estimating numbers, rethinking improves the accuracy of the numbers. A sort of bootstrapping occurs, where the group members better themselves by listening to other group members and revising their own opinions.
3. Individual generation of ideas leads to more creative ideas than generating ideas while listening to other group members.

Despite widespread use of the nominal group process in consensus panels (Jones and Hunter 1995), the process is not without serious problems. In tasks that require judging the worth of several alternatives, for example, in developing a multi-attribute value (MAV) model, this technique may produce judgments inferior to the judgment of the most knowledgeable group member. But by far, the most serious problem with the process is that participants feel awkward about restrictions in their interactions. After the group meeting, they may feel that the conclusions were forced through the process and not through group interaction. Therefore, they may not be committed to the group's consensus. When acceptance of the group's decision is crucial in determining whether the model is put to use, less structured group processes produce more widely accepted group decisions (Rotondi 1999).

Delphi Process

Another technique widely used by consensus groups in healthcare settings is the *Delphi process* (Jones and Hunter 1995). This process was designed as a procedure for aggregating group members' opinions without face-to-face interaction. It is frequently used with e-mail or other web-based platforms. When using this technique, group members answer three interrelated questionnaires; the analyst summarizes the responses from each survey and mails the synthesis back to the same or other groups for further comment (Ryan et al. 2001). For example, the first questionnaire may ask the group members to describe the attributes in a value model; the second may present the attributes, ask for revisions, and request weighting of the relative importance of the attributes; and the third may continue with the revisions of the model, present a set of scenarios, and ask the respondents to rate them. In some applications, such as in forecasting technological changes based on insights of a large group of experts, the Delphi process has proven useful. The Delphi process is also useful in situations in which conflict or status differences among group members are so strong as to render the group dysfunctional. The most insightful feature of the Delphi process is that a meeting of minds can occur without an actual face-to-face meeting.

Nevertheless, studies have been that face-to-face interaction is superior to Delphi's remote and private opinion gathering (Cho, Turoff, and Hiltz 2003; Woudenberg 1991). Even limited interaction can help improve the Delphi process. In one study, for example, the Delphi process's remote feedback was compared to the nominal group process's in-person feedback. The Delphi process's remote feedback reduced the accuracy of the group members' estimates (Gustafson et al. 1973).

Social Judgment Analysis

Difficulty with existing group processes has led a number of investigators to design their own modeling process that can be used in group settings. These approaches often use computers to help model the decision maker in a group setting. In the 1990s, many studies were published regarding what affects the performance of group decision-support systems (see, for example, Fjermestad and Hiltz 1998). The *social judgment analysis* is a group process that uses computers to model each member as they interact with each other (see Toseland and Rivas 1984). It was designed to reduce the pressure for group members to comply with the group's mind-set just to feel more accepted by the group. Following are the steps in the process:

1. Group members meet in face-to-face meetings, in which they have access to a computer.
2. Each group member rates a series of scenarios. A scenario is a combination of clues that affect a judgment. For example, in judging creditworthiness of companies, the clues may be last year's profit, changes in market share, and management changes. A scenario is constructed by varying levels of these three clues. In the first scenario, the company was not profitable last year, has gained a significant market share, and has stable management. In the second scenario, the company was profitable last year, has a small market share, and has stable management. More scenarios can be constructed by using different levels of each clue.
3. The computer analyzes the group members' ratings to see which factors most affect the judgment. This is usually done through regressing the scenario ratings on the elements of, or the clues in, the scenarios.
4. The group members review the results of the computer analysis. The computer analysis indicates that the way group members rated the scenarios suggests that certain clues are most important in their judgment. The analysis then lists these clues.
5. Group members often do not agree with the results of the analysis and revise their ratings of the scenarios so that the ratings best fit with what they consider most important.
6. Once group members come to terms with the way they wish to judge the scenarios, a consensus model is developed and used to represent the group's judgment.

Computer-facilitated meetings in general and social judgment analysis in particular may seem to be too much work for some meetings. But with the growing use of computers, many meetings are occurring through computers anyway. Many decision makers are in different locations and must use the computer to collaborate. In these settings, group decision-support systems can help improve the self-insight of individual group members and eventually the quality and speed of arriving at group consensus. The value of this technique is demonstrated in recent studies focused on helping clinicians understand their own judgments (Holzworth and Wills 1999). Social judgment analysis works well because it focuses the decision maker's attention on why an alternative is preferred rather than on which alternative is preferred. It provides group feedback that helps decision makers focus their reasoning. Data show that people change their opinions to conform to group norms. Although this behavior is healthy for keeping the peace in the group, it is counterproductive if ideas are being judged based on their popularity as opposed to their merits. Rohrbaugh's (1979) study showed that when feedback focused on why an idea was preferred as opposed to which idea was more popular, the group's final judgment was more accurate. Rohrbaugh also showed that social judgment analysis is more accurate than the Delphi process and the nominal group process.

Cognitive Mapping

Interest in the use of computers in group processes has led to many innovations. Eden, Jones, and Sims (1983) were among the first to develop a process for modeling how a group arrives at its judgments through *cognitive mapping*. This process starts with constructing two parallel statements of the problem: one showing the factors leading to the problem, the other showing the factors leading to a satisfactory solution. For example, the problem may be stated as "high labor costs," and the solution may be stated as "lowering the labor cost." The causes of high labor cost and the factors leading to lowering labor costs are also organized. For example, a cause of the problem may be a "shortage of qualified workers." A solution may be "more availability of qualified workers." Causes of the problem and factors leading to the solutions are related—usually, the solution can be produced by rephrasing the causes. Through linguistic manipulation of the statement of the problem, cognitive mapping hopes to stimulate new ideas.

Eden and colleagues, when they use cognitive mapping, often collect the group members' ideas about the problem and its solutions separately and then revise these ideas in a face-to-face meeting. Occasionally, they quantify the influence of causes and effects through a round-robin process, where group members write down their estimates and share them afterwards. They then simulate how changing one factor may affect the problem. These simulations may lead to new insights into the problem. Cognitive mapping of groups of decision makers continues to be an active area of research (Vennix 2000).

Computer-Facilitated Group Process

Social judgment analysis and cognitive mapping were the start of many innovative methods of computer-facilitated collaboration. McLeod (1992) summarized the group decision-support literature and found that *computer-facilitated group process* increased the quality of the decision and led to more equal participation by group members, more focus on task, and less focus on social networking and support. At the same time, McLeod identified that computer-facilitated group interaction decreased consensus and member satisfaction with the group meeting. The reduction in member satisfaction with computer-facilitated group process might be attributable to the central role of a facilitator in controlling who speaks when in group processes (Austin, Liker, and McLeod 1993). Strauss (1997) showed that computer-facilitated groups have lower cohesiveness and group satisfaction than face-to-face groups, primarily because of the rate with which the group members interact. Even a simple technology such as teleconferencing has been shown to have detrimental effects on group discussion and processes (Alemi et al. 1997). Face-to-face meetings, when possible and when they are run well, are more efficient at getting ideas across to group members; as a consequence of this improved efficiency, group members think others have heard their point of view.

Lessons Learned

Many group processes can be used to model a group's decision. A review of some of these processes creates a bewildering number of methods of teamwork. This section reviews key lessons learned from research on effective team processes. Three and half decades of research on effective group work point to the following lessons:

1. *Postpone evaluation.* It is best to separate idea generation from idea evaluation. When evaluation is postponed, more ideas and more creative ideas emerge.
2. *Think again.* It is best to think through the decision again, especially when numerical estimates are involved. In repetition, people gain confidence in what they are doing and can see pitfalls they missed previously.
3. *Meet before the meeting.* It is useful to get input from group members individually, before they can influence each other. This can often occur through use of computers and might be one way of combining computer-facilitated decision support with face-to-face meetings.
4. *Judge the merit of ideas.* It is important to evaluate ideas based on their merit and not based on their popularity. Successful group processes separate ideas from the originator of the idea. In this fashion, ideas are judged on the basis of their merits rather than on who proposed them.
5. *Instruct the group to behave.* It is best to instruct group members to keep calm and accept conflict as productive. Simple instructions at the start of the meeting can set the tone of the group discussions to come.

6. *Use computers to facilitate components of the meeting.* It is best to use technology to help groups arrive at a consensus, but such use should not reduce the rate of the exchange of ideas or the ease with which members interact.

Integrative Group Process

Integrative group process (IGP) is designed to model a group's decision while helping the group come to a behavioral consensus. This is an eclectic group process based on more than 30 years of research on teamwork and group interaction literature:

- Like the nominal group process, IGP postpones the evaluation of ideas until the analyst has collected the ideas of all members. In addition, both approaches improve estimates of relative importance of ideas through repetition (i.e., both require the group member to assess, discuss, and revise their numerical estimates).
- Like the Delphi process, IGP obtains remote and private opinions. But unlike Delphi, these remote contributions are followed by face-to-face interactions.
- Like the group communication strategy, IGP sets ground rules for free-form group interaction.
- Like social judgment analysis and cognitive mapping, IGP focuses discussion on the group members' reasoning rather than the group's decision. Thus, group members can better understand why they disagree on a point, if they come to see each other's reasoning.
- Like computer-facilitated group processes, IGP collects ideas from group members via computers: typically by e-mails. Integrative group process and computer-facilitated group process differ in what occurs after the initial collection of ideas; IGP emphasizes face-to-face meetings after computer-facilitated collection of ideas.

Integrative group process has six steps:

1. Select the best experts, despite their conflicts.
2. Meet before the meeting to make a "straw model."
3. Redo the straw model during the meeting.
4. Estimate the model's parameters.
5. Discuss major differences and reestimate the parameters.
6. Ignore small differences and prepare a report.

The output from IGP is a mathematical model (e.g., MAV model, Bayesian probability model). Some administrators tend to use the ideas behind IGP to guide a committee's or a group's decision making when there is no need for a mathematical model. In these circumstances, all aspects of IGP are followed, but no parameters for the model are estimated. Such uses of the process are encouraged.

Step 1: Select the Best Experts

The composition of the group is an important and generally controllable aspect of the group. Occasionally, an analyst may avoid putting too many high-status members in the group, fearing that they will not be able to work together—this is a mistake. The best experts and decision makers must be invited to participate in the meeting; without them, crucial information will be missing from the meeting, and the quality of the decision may be affected. Instead of avoiding conflict, the IGP process helps manage conflict among group member so that productive quality work can be accomplished despite status differences or a prior history of conflict.

The analyst needs to think about what portion of the group should come from inside versus outside the organization. If employees closest to the process are invited to join the decision-making group, then the group's decisions are more likely to be implemented. If people removed from the process, perhaps experts outside the organization, are engaged, then more radical solutions may be proposed and more rapid change may occur. In the end, a balance needs to be struck between the percentage of the group that is selected from inside and outside the organization.

There is very little data regarding ideal size for a team. In general, there are two considerations: (1) the more people, the more difficult it is to manage the team; (2) the fewer the people, the smaller the pool of ideas that the team has access to (de Dreu 2006). Teams of three to seven people are the most common size. The size of the group should depend on its purpose. Experiments with groups of various sizes have shown that if the quality of the group's solution is of considerable importance, it is useful to include a large number of members (e.g., seven to nine) so that many inputs are available to the group in making its decision. If the degree of consensus is of primary importance, it is useful to choose a smaller group (e.g., five or six) so that members' opinions can be considered and discussed. It is a general rule of thumb that the group size should not be smaller than three to five. Groups that meet face-to-face should not have more than nine members, or each member may not be able to participate adequately. A recent study showed that groups of five are more likely to have dialog and groups of ten are more likely to have monologs (Fay, Garrod, and Carletta 2000). If the purpose is to encourage interaction among group members, then groups of five seem more practical.

Heterogeneity of the group's background is closely related to the size of the group and is another important aspect of the design of successful groups. A necessary, though not sufficient, requirement for adequate group judgments is to have an appropriate knowledge pool in the group. Because no one person is an expert in all aspects of a problem, diverse backgrounds and expertise are imperative. Involving people from different functional units of the organization helps bring different expertise to the problem. Differences in background and knowledge could, however, accentuate the conflict between the group members. If neither originality nor quality are criteria for evaluating the team's work, the analyst should select group members to minimize differences in their backgrounds.

Getting people to devote their time to a meeting is difficult. Many people remember wasted efforts in other meetings and avoid new meetings. The analyst can take several steps to increase participation. First, the analyst should examine the purpose of the meeting. If it is difficult to obtain participation, perhaps the problem being addressed is not important. People who are close to a problem invariably care about it and are willing to address it. But if they think the problem is not real, or the search for a solution is only a formality, they are less likely to participate.

Second, the analyst can improve meeting participation by clear communications concerning the meeting logistics and expectations. The communication should clarify why the meeting is important, why it is useful to model the task, and what can be expected at the end of the meeting. It should clarify the logistics of the meeting (i.e., when, where, and how) and emphasize that the meeting is an ad hoc group.

Third, it may be useful to remind the invited group members about who else is being invited. People are more likely to come to meetings if people they admire will be present. The analyst should emphasize (1) who nominated the potential group member and (2) that very few people were asked to participate. It should be clear that the group member's contribution is unique and valued. Finally, it helps if group members are reimbursed for their time with an honorarium.

Step 2: Meet Before the Meeting

Before a face-to-face meeting, group members are individually interviewed and modeled. If group members live far apart, the interviews are done by phone, via a series of e-mails, or through computer connections. Whether done remotely or face-to-face, the interviews are scheduled before the meeting. During each interview, which takes roughly one hour, the analyst explains the group's task, elicits the participant's model (i.e., attributes or clues), asks the participant to estimate utilities or probabilities, and walks the participant through the steps in the IGP process so there will be no surprises in the actual meeting. The bulk of the interview time, however, is spent listening to the group member and trying to model the reasoning behind her choices.

For example, if the group is to create a decision tree, the analyst asks the member to do so and listens to why specific steps are important in the decision. If the group's task is to suggest alternative solutions to a problem, the analyst obtains a list of viable alternatives and tries to understand which evaluation criteria are important for evaluating these alternatives. If the group member's opinions depend on many rules, the analyst solicits these rules and makes sure that the mathematical model reflects them. The point is that no matter what the task is, the analyst tries not only to accomplish the task but also to understand the reasoning behind it.

Keep in mind that while the bulk of interview time is spent structuring the decision, the analyst must also assess utilities and probabilities so that the participant understands what is going to happen at the meeting. A brief training in probability concepts might also be useful before assessing probabilities. See Chapter 3 for an introduction on probabilities.

After interviewing each group member individually, the analyst collates the responses of all participants and creates a *straw model*, which is a decision model that is designed to be redone. The face-to-face meeting starts with a presentation of the straw model and proceeds with a request for improvements. Constructing the model before the group meeting has three advantages:

1. Creating a straw model increases the accuracy of the group's judgment by ensuring that the group process will not prevent an individual from presenting his ideas.
2. The interviews before the meeting save the group some working time by collecting members' ideas before the meeting.
3. Because the straw model serves as a blueprint to guide the group's discussion, it saves additional time by partitioning the group's task into smaller, more manageable discussions.

Step 3: Redo the Straw Model

The analyst explains the basic structure of the straw model (e.g., the attributes used in the evaluation task, the decision events used in a tree structure, the clues used in a forecast) on flip charts—one component per chart. The flip charts are spread around the room so that any member can see what has been said to date. The group convenes to revise the straw model.

The analyst introduces herself, explains the group's task and agenda, restates the importance of the task, and asks members to introduce themselves. These introductions are an important part of the group process. If members are not explicitly introduced, they will do so implicitly throughout their deliberations.

The analyst presents the straw model, asks the group to revise the model, and focuses the group's attention on one of the components in the straw model as a starting point. The focus on one component at a time is an important way of managing the group's time and conflicts. As group members suggest new ideas or modifications, the analyst records them on the appropriate pages in front of the group. Thus, the analyst serves as a secretary to the group, making sure that ideas are not lost. Recording the comments reassures the group members that their ideas are being put in front of the group for further consideration. The process continues until the group identifies, discusses, and revises all relevant components in the decision structure.

Through active listening (e.g., nodding, asking for clarification) and recording group members' ideas on the flip charts, the analyst plays the important role of directing the discussion, preventing premature closure of ideas (Van de Ven and Delbecq 1974), focusing the group on task-related activities, distributing the group's time over different aspects of the task, postponing evaluation of ideas, and separating people from ideas so that ideas are judged on their own merits. The analyst uses the instructions developed for the group communication strategy as guidelines for this phase of interaction. The analyst should not participate in the content of the discussions and should not restate what has been said in her own words.

Step 4: Estimate the Model's Parameters

In this step of IGP, the analyst helps the group put numbers to the decision components (e.g., assess weights for the utility models, assess likelihood ratios associated with various clues). This task is done individually and without discussion until a major difference between the group members is identified. While working individually, the group remains in the presence of one another. Seeing each other working helps the group members exert more effort on the task at hand. As the group proceeds, the analyst collects the group's responses and puts the answers on a flip chart. The scores are listed on the flip chart in a manner that does not identify who has said them.

Step 5: Discuss Major Differences

IGP focuses the group's discussion on the group's logic. Instead of discussing differences in numerical ratings, the group discusses the reasons behind their ratings. This approach to discussion has been shown to reduce conflict among group members (Rohrbaugh 1979). Disagreements among group members have different sources. Some disagreements are caused by unclear problem specification; these disagreements are reduced through clarifying the assumptions behind group member's perspectives. Still other disagreements are caused by differences in knowledge and experience; discussion may reduce these conflicts if group members succeed in communicating the rationale for their judgments. Some group members may raise considerations that others have missed or may see flaws in the logic. Other disagreements are attributable to value differences or fatigue. Better communication may not reduce this type of conflict; IGP reduces conflicts that are caused by misconceptions and miscommunications and accepts other conflicts as inherent to the task.

To save the group's time, the analyst should identify major differences among members and focus the group's attention on them. Small differences are probably because of errors in estimating numbers and not substantive issues. When there are major differences in numerical ratings, the analyst should stop the group members from working individually and ask for a discussion. This is done without identifying the group average (norm) or whose ratings differed from the average. Disclosures of the members involved could have ill effects by polarizing the group. The existence of the disagreement and the need to resolve it through discussion are more important than which members differed in their ratings.

After the group members have discussed their differences, the analyst asks group members to individually reestimate the model parameters. This process of estimating, discussing, and reestimating leads to more accurate results than the use of other processes that eliminate any one of the three steps (Gustafson et al. 1973).

Step 6: Ignore Small Differences

Although the analyst encourages group members to resolve their differences through discussion, at some point it is necessary to stop the interaction and mathematically resolve minor group differences, such as by averaging the estimates from various group members. If major differences remain, it is necessary to report these differences. In a few days after the meeting has ended, a report is written about the meeting. This report contains several different topics, including the following:

- Why the meeting was convened
- Methods used to facilitate the meeting and analyze the findings
- A detailed description of the consensus model structure

- Whether group participants arrived at a consensus regarding model parameters
- Extent of agreement in the final numerical ratings of various group members
- The average parameters assessed by the group
- Conclusions and next steps in the group's task

A document about the group's deliberation is important not only to people who were in the meeting but also to people who were not. Vinokur and Burnstein (1978) had individual subjects list the persuasiveness of pro and con arguments. The net balance of the persuasiveness of the arguments correlated with attitude changes produced by group discussion. But more importantly, other individuals not present in the group discussion, who were exposed to the same arguments, changed their attitudes in the same way. These results show that the information content of group discussion is important in convincing people outside the group. Similar results have been reported in patients' decisions to conduct breast examination. The more persuasive the arguments for breast examination are, the more likely it is that a patient will do it (Ruiter et al. 2001). Similarly, a well-documented decision model can help convince others.

Summary

There are many occasions in which a group, rather than an individual, has to make a decision. A good example is a board of director's decision about a major capital purchase. This chapter discusses how to build a model for a group's decision. Our approach is based on creating a group consensus around the parameters of the model. There are many different approaches to help a group arrive to a consensus. The group communication strategy instructs group members on the ground rules for discussion and then invites group members to talk freely about topics from which the analyst constructs the decision model. The nominal group process differs in that group members only interact at specific steps in the decision-making process. Discussion is postponed until all ideas are listed. The outcome of the process is a prioritized list of ideas and corresponding numerical estimates. The Delphi process relies on aggregation of group members' opinions without face-to-face interaction. Interrelated questionnaires are sent to decision makers to query them about their choices and their reasons for their choices. Difficulty exists with these established group processes. As a result, researchers have begun to design novel modeling processes for use in group settings. Many of these procedures, such as social judgment analysis, utilize computers to aid in the modeling process. The discovery of the usefulness of computers in modeling decisions has led to several innovations, including the use of cognitive mapping for making decisions. The result of newly established methods for modeling processes is a computer-facilitated group process, which has increased decision quality, equal participation among members, and focus on task.

This chapter discusses these various methods for how an analyst can model a group's decision and discusses empirical support and criticism for each method. The chapter also synthesizes key aspects of these various processes into a new process called integrative group process (IGP). Like group communication strategy, IGP instructs group members about avoiding certain behaviors. Like nominal group process, it delays discussion until all ideas are on the table. Like Delphi process, it gathers group's ideas before the face-to-face meeting. And like social judgment and cognitive mapping, it constructs a mathematical model of the decision maker's ideas.

Review What You Know

1. List the steps in the nominal group process.
2. How is the IGP different from the nominal group process?
3. Of all the processes you have learned about here, which process or component of a process can you use at work? Be specific about why you prefer one approach to another.
4. In which group processes is there a delay in the evaluation of ideas? Why would postponing evaluation help the group process?
5. If experts have conflicts among them, or if employees have sharp status differences, should you avoid having them in the same group?
6. What is the point of asking for utility or probability assessments before the group meets?
7. Is it better to change the group's meeting process or to instruct group members to stay on task and avoid falling into conflicts?
8. In what steps within the IGP do group members work with numbers? In what steps in the IGP do group members specify the structure of the decision model?
9. What is a straw model?

Rapid-Analysis Exercises

Using your classmates or work colleagues, conduct an IGP on a decision topic of your choice. One classmate should be the facilitator, and two or three others should be the experts in the group. Select the topic in a manner that your classmates have expertise in. Conduct all the steps in IGP, including the construction of a straw model and the numerical estimation of the mode. Make sure you allocate sufficient time for each component: a week to interview classmates and create a straw model, half a day to review the straw model, four to six hours to generate the scenarios, and half a day to conduct the numerical estimation and related discussion. Prepare a report analyzing the agreement among the experts as well as between the experts and the model.

Audio/Visual Chapter Aids

To help you understand the concepts of modeling group's decisions, visit this book's companion web site at ache.org/DecisionAnalysis, go to Chapter 6, and view the audio/visual chapter aids.

References

Alemi, F., M. Jackson, T. Parren, L. Williams, B. Cavor, S. Llorens, and M. Mosavel. 1997. "Participation in Teleconference Support Groups: Application to Drug-Using Pregnant Patients." *Journal of Medical Systems* 21 (2): 119–25.

Austin, L. C., J. K. Liker, and P. L. McLeod. 1993. "Who Controls the Technology in Group Support Systems? Determinants and Consequences." *Human-Computer Interaction* 8 (3): 217–36.

Black, N., M. Murphy, D. Lamping, M. McKee, C. Sanderson, J. Askham, and T. Marteau. 1999. "Consensus Development Methods: A Review of Best Practice in Creating Clinical Guidelines." *Journal of Health Services Research and Policy* 4 (4): 236–48.

Carney, O., J. McIntosh, and A. Worth. 1996. "The Use of the Nominal Group Technique in Research with Community Nurses." *Journal of Advanced Nursing* 23 (5): 1024–9.

Cho, H. K., M. Turoff, and S. R. Hiltz. 2003. "The Impacts of Delphi Communication Structure on Small and Medium Sized Asynchronous

Groups." *Proceedings of the 36th Hawaii International Conference on System Sciences*, 171.

Cruse, H., M. Winiarek, J. Marshburn, O. Clark, and B. Djulbegovic. 2002. "Quality and Methods of Developing Practice Guidelines." *BMC Health Services Research* 2 (1): 1.

de Drue, C. K. W. 2006. "When Too Little or Too Much Hurts: Evidence for a Curvilinear Relationship Between Task Conflict and Innovation in Teams." *Journal of Management* 32 (1) 83–107.

Eden, C., S. Jones, and D. Sims. 1983. *Messing About in Problems.* Oxford, England: Pergamon Press.

Fay, F., S. Garrod, and J. Carletta. 2000. "Group Discussion as Interactive Dialogue or as Serial Monologue: The Influence of Group Size." *Psychological Science* 11 (6): 481–6.

Fjermestad, J., and S. R. Hiltz. 1998. "An Analysis of the Effects of Mode of Communication on Group Decision Making." *HICSS* 1 (1): 17.

Forsyth, D. R. 2005. *Group Dynamics.* 4th ed. Belmont, CA: Thompson Wadsworth Publishing.

Gallagher, M., T. Hares, J. Spencer, C. Bradshaw, and I. Webb I. 1993. "The Nominal Group Technique: A Research Tool for General Practice?" *Family Practice* 10 (1): 76–81.

Gustafson, D. H., R. U. Shukla, A. Delbecq, and G. W. Walster. 1973. "A Comparative Study of Differences in Subjective Likelihood Estimates Made by Individuals Interacting Groups, Delphi Process, and Nominal Groups." *Organizational Behavior and Human Performance* 9 (2): 280–91.

Hall, J., and W. H. Watson. 1970. "The Effects of a Normative Intervention on a Group Decision Making Performance." *Human Relations* 23 (2): 299–317.

Holzworth, R. J., and C. E. Wills. 1999. "Nurses' Judgments Regarding Seclusion and Restraint of Psychiatric Patients: A Social Judgment Analysis." *Research in Nursing and Health* 22 (3): 189–201.

Jacobs, R. A. 1995. "Methods for Combining Experts' Probability Assessments." *Neural Computation* 7 (5): 867–88.

Jones, J., and D. Hunter. 1995. "Consensus Methods for Medical and Health Services Research." *BMJ* 311 (7001): 376–80.

McLeod, P. L. 1992. "An Assessment of the Experimental Literature on Electronic Support of Group Work: Results of a Meta-Analysis." *Human-Computer Interaction* 7 (3): 257–80.

Meyer, M., and J. Booker. 1991. *Eliciting and Analyzing Expert Judgment: A Practical Guide.* Vol. 5, *Knowledge-Based Systems.* London: Academic Press.

Moon, R. H. 1999. "Finding Diamonds in the Trenches with the Nominal Group Process." *Family Practice Management* 6 (5): 49–50.

Pagliari, C., and J. Grimshaw. 2002. "Impact of Group Structure and Process on Multidisciplinary Evidence-Based Guideline Development: An Observational Study." *Journal of Evaluation in Clinical Practice* 8 (2): 145–53.

Rohrbaugh, J. 1979. "Improving the Quality of Group Judgment: Social Judgment Analysis and the Nominal Group Technique." *Organizational Behavior and Human Performance* 28 (2): 272–88.

Rotondi, A. J. 1999. "Assessing a Team's Problem Solving Ability: Evaluation of the Team Problem Solving Assessment Tool (TPSAT)." *Health Care Management Science* 2 (4): 205–14.

Ruiter, R. A., G. Kok, B. Verplanken, and J. Brug. 2001. "Evoked Fear and Effects of Appeals on Attitudes to Performing Breast Self-Examination: An Information-Processing Perspective." *Health Education Research* 16 (3): 307–19.

Ryan, M., D. A. Scott, C. Reeves, A. Bate, E. R. van Teijlingen, E. M. Russell, M. Napper, and C. M. Robb. 2001. "Eliciting Public Preferences for Healthcare: A Systematic Review of Techniques." *Health Technology Assessment* 5 (5): 1–186.

Straus, S. G. 1997. "Technology, Group Process, and Group Outcomes: Testing the Connections in Computer-Mediated and Face-to-Face Groups." *Human-Computer Interaction* 12 (3): 227–66.

Toseland, R. W., and R. F. Rivas. 1984. "Structured Methods for Working with Task Groups." *Administration in Social Work* 8 (2): 49–58.

Van de Ven, A. H., and A. Delbecq. 1974. "The Effectiveness of Nominal, Delphi, and Interacting Group Decision Making Process." *Academy of Management Journal* 17 (4): 605–21.

Vennix, J. A. M. 2000. "Group Model-Building: Tackling Messy Problems." *System Dynamics Review* 15 (4): 379–401.

Vinokur, A., and E. Burnstein. 1978. "Novel Argumentation and Attitude Change: The Case of Polarization Following Group Discussion." *European Journal of Social Psychology* 8 (3): 335–48.

Woudenberg, F. 1991. "An Evaluation of Delphi." *Technological Forecasting and Social Change* 40: 131–50.

CHAPTER

7

ROOT-CAUSE ANALYSIS

Farrokh Alemi, Jee Vang, and Kathryn Laskey

Root-cause and failure-mode analyses are commonly performed in hospitals to understand factors that contribute to errors and mistakes. Despite the effort that healthcare professionals put into creating these analyses, few models of root causes are validated or used to predict future occurrences of adverse events. This chapter shows how the assumptions and conclusions of a root-cause analysis can be verified against observed data. This chapter builds on Chapter 3 and Chapter 4.

Root-cause analysis, according to the Joint Commission on Accreditation of Healthcare Organizations (JCAHO) (2005) is a "process for identifying the basic or causal factors that underlie variation in performance, including the occurrence or possible occurrence of a sentinel event." *Sentinel events* include medication errors, patient suicide, procedure complications, wrong-site surgery, treatment delay, restraint death, assault or rape, transfusion death, and infant abduction. Direct causes bring about the sentinel event without any other intervening event, and most direct causes are physically proximate to the sentinel event. However, the direct causes are themselves caused by root causes. Because of accreditation requirements and renewed interest in patient safety, many hospitals and clinics are actively conducting root-cause analyses.

When a sentinel event occurs, most employees are focused on the direct causes that have led to the event. For example, many will claim that the cause of medication error is a failure to check the label against the patient's armband. But this is just the direct cause. To get to the real reason, one should ask *why* the clinician did not check the label against the armband. The purpose of a root-cause analysis is to go beyond the direct and somewhat apparent causes to figure out the underlying reasons for the event (i.e., the root causes). The objective is to force one to think harder about the source of the problem. It is possible that the label was not checked against the armband because the label was missing. Furthermore, it is also possible that the label was missing because the computer was not printing the labels. Then, the direct cause is the failure to check the label against the armband and the root cause is computer malfunction. Exhorting employees

This book has a companion web site that features narrated presentations, animated examples, PowerPoint slides, online tools, web links, additional readings, and examples of students' work. To access this chapter's learning tools, go to ache.org/DecisionAnalysis and select Chapter 7.

to check the armband against the label is a waste of time if there is no label to check in the first place. A focus on direct causes may prevent a sentinel event for a while, but sooner or later the root cause will lead to a sentinel event. Inattention to root causes promotes palliative solutions that do not work in the long run. The value of root-cause analyses lies in identifying the true, underlying causes. An investigation that does not do this at best is a waste of time and resources and at worst can exacerbate the problems it was intended to fix. But how can one know if the speculations about the root causes of an event are correct?

One way to check the accuracy of a root-cause analysis is to examine the time to the next sentinel event. Unfortunately, because sentinel events are rare, one has to wait a long time to see them occur again, even if no changes were made. An alternative needs to be found to check the accuracy and consistency of a root-cause analysis without having to wait for the next sentinel incident.

Many who conduct root-cause analyses become overconfident about the accuracy of their own insights. No matter how poorly an analysis is carried out, because there is no easy way of proving a person wrong, people persist in their own fallacies. Some people are even incredulous about the possibility that their imagined causal influences could be wrong. They insist on the correctness of their insights because those insights seem obvious. However, a complex problem that has led to a sentinel event and that has been left unaddressed by hundreds of smart people for years is unlikely to have an obvious solution. After all, if the solution was so obvious, why was it not adopted earlier? The search for obvious solutions contradicts the elusiveness of correcting for sentinel events. If a sound and reliable method existed for checking the accuracy and consistency of a root-cause analysis, then employees might correct their misperceptions and not be so overconfident.

Simple methods for checking the accuracy of root-cause analyses have not been available to date (Boxwala et al. 2004). This chapter suggests a method for doing so. As before, clinicians propose a set of causes. But now several additional steps are taken. First, probabilities are used to quantify the relationship between causes and effects. Then, the laws of probability and causal diagrams are examined to see if the suggested causes are consistent with the clinician's other beliefs and with existing objective data. Through a cycle of testing model assumptions and conclusions against observed data, one improves the accuracy of the analysis and gains new insights into the causes of the sentinel event.

Bayesian Networks

Bayesian causal networks can be used to validate root-cause analyses. A *Bayesian causal network* is a mathematical model of causes and effects. It consists of a set of nodes, typically pictured as ovals, connected by directed arcs. Each node represents a mutually exclusive and collectively exhaustive set of possible events. For example, Figure 7.1 shows a Bayesian network with two nodes. The node labeled "armband legible?" has three possible values, of which exactly one must occur and two cannot coincide. These values are "no armband," "poor legibility," and "good legibility." The other node, labeled "armband checked?" has two possible values: "sure" and "not sure." A node with two possible values is called a *binary node*. Binary nodes are common in root-cause analyses.

A Bayesian network is a cyclical directed graph, meaning that you cannot start from a node and follow the arcs to arrive back to where you started. In a Bayesian network, the relationships among any three nodes can be described as having one of the following three structures: serial, diverging, or converging. Each of these graph structures can be verified through tests of conditional independence and are further explained through the examples below.

The relationship between the armband being legible and its being checked in Figure 7.1 is a direct causal relationship. Bayesian networks can also represent indirect causal relationships through the concept of conditional independence, as shown in Figure 7.2. Figure 7.2 illustrates a *serial* graph structure, in which the sentinel event is independent of the root cause given the known value for the direct cause. In this example, the root cause labeled "understaffing" is an indirect cause of the sentinel event; there is no direct arc from this root cause to the sentinel event. This means that the action of the root cause on the sentinel event is indirect, operating through an intermediate cause. The direct cause of a medication error is a fatigued nurse. The root cause, understaffing, is conditionally independent of the sentinel event given the intermediate cause. This means that if you intervene in any given instance to relieve a fatigued nurse, you can

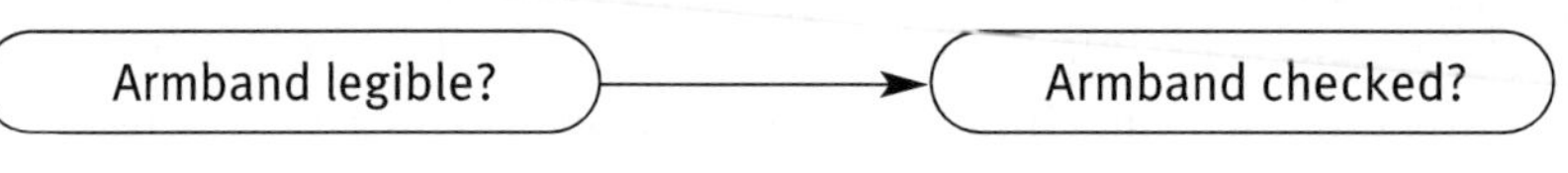

Armband legible	Armband checked? Done	Not done
No armband	0%	100%
Poor legibility	80%	20%
Good legibility	99%	1%

FIGURE 7.1 A Bayesian Causal Model with a Local Probability Table

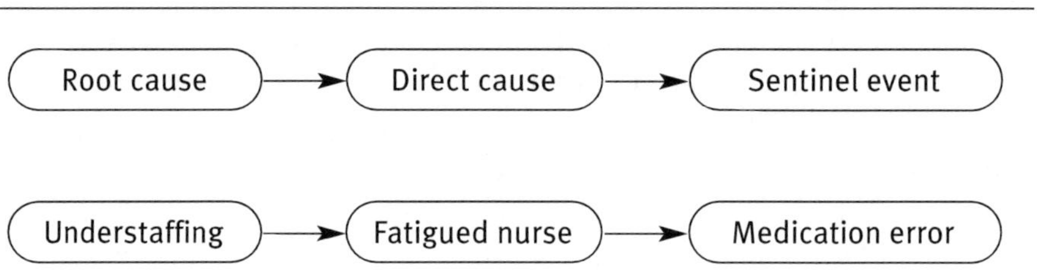

FIGURE 7.2 Serial Example of Direct and Root Causes of Medication Error

break the link from the root cause to the sentinel event, thus reducing the probability of the sentinel event to its nominal level. However, this solution is a palliative one and will not produce a long-term solution unless the root cause is addressed.

Another type of conditional independence occurs when a cause gives rise independently to two different effects, as depicted in Figure 7.3. This type of graph structure is known as *diverging*. In this example, high blood pressure and diabetes are conditionally independent given the value of weight gain, but they are correlated because of the influence of the common cause. That is, the two effects typically either occur together (when the common cause is present) or are both absent (when the common cause is absent). This type of conditional independence relationship is quite useful for diagnosing the presence of root causes that can lead to multiple independent effects that each influence different sentinel events. For example, understaffing might lead to several different intermediate causes, each of which could be a precursor of different sentinel events. If several of these precursor events were to be observed, one could infer that the understaffing problem was sufficiently severe to affect patient care. Proactive remediation could then be initiated before serious adverse medical outcomes occur.

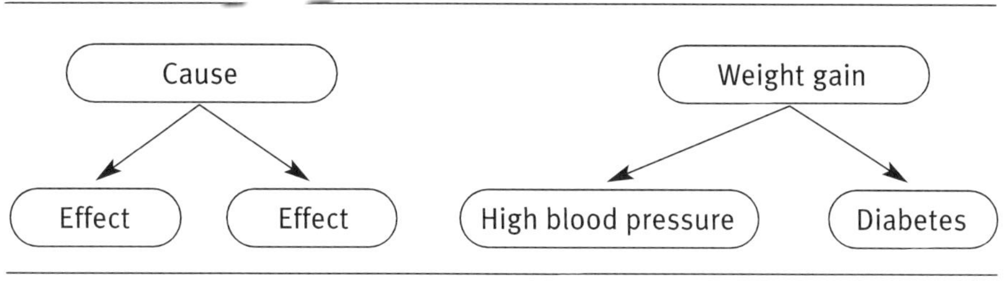

FIGURE 7.3 Conditional Independence Is Assumed in a Diverging Structure

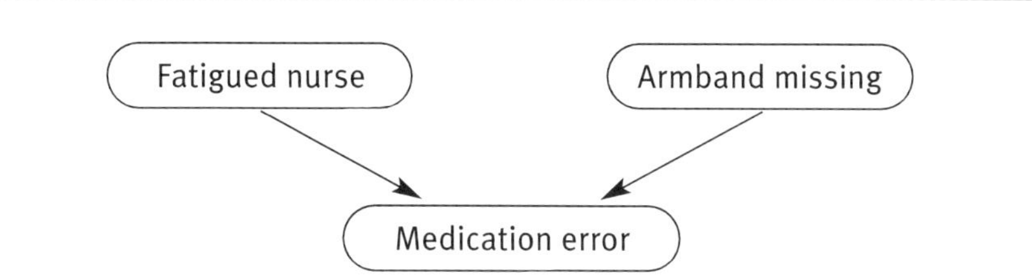

FIGURE 7.4 Two Causes Converging into a Common Effect

Figures 7.2 and 7.3 illustrate serial and diverging causal structures, respectively. As you have seen, a serial structure represents the action of an indirect causal relationship, and a diverging structure represents multiple independent effects of a single cause. In both of these cases, the two terminal nodes are conditionally independent of each other given the middle node. A different kind of causal structure, *converging*, is shown in Figure 7.4. A converging structure occurs when two different causes can produce a single effect, as when either a fatigued nurse or a missing armband can cause a medication error. Notice that in this case, the terminal nodes are not conditionally independent given the middle node. For example, if the sentinel event is known to occur, and you learn that the armband was present, this will increase the probability that the nurse was unacceptably fatigued. Likewise, if you find that the armband was missing, this will reduce the likelihood that the problem was caused by fatigue.

Data can be used, if available, to validate the graph structure of a Bayesian causal network. As noted above, when a connection is serial or diverging, the terminal nodes are conditionally independent given the intermediate node. In general, a node in a Bayesian network is conditionally independent of all its nondescendents given its parents. This general condition implies a set of correlations that should be equal to zero if the causal assumptions correct. Although it is tedious to verify all of these relationships by hand, it is straightforward to automate the verification process, and computer programs have been written to accomplish the task.

Given a causal graph, one can read off the assumed conditional independencies. Conditional independencies are identified by examining serial or diverging graphs in causal models so that removing the condition would sever the directional flow from the cause to the effect. Often, a complicated root-cause analysis can be broken into smaller components containing serial and diverging structures. If these structures are observed, and if removing the condition in these structures would sever the link between the other two nodes, then a conditional dependency has been identified. Careful examination of conditionally independent relationships is an important element of specifying and validating a Bayesian network for root-cause analyses.

Validation of Conditional Independence

Once conditional independencies have been identified, the assumptions can be verified by examining data or by querying experts. If data are available, the correlations in a serial structure between the root cause and the sentinel event should equal the correlation between the root cause and the direct cause times the correlation between the direct cause and the sentinel event:

$$R_{\text{root cause, sentinel event}} = R_{\text{root cause, direct cause}} \times R_{\text{direct cause, sentinel event}},$$

where

- $R_{\text{root cause, sentinel event}}$ is the correlation between the root cause and the sentinel event,
- $R_{\text{root cause, direct cause}}$ is the correlation between the root cause and the direct cause, and
- $R_{\text{direct cause, sentinel event}}$ is the correlation between the direct cause and the sentinel event.

In a diverging structure, a similar relationship should hold. In particular, correlation between the two effects should be equal to the multiplication of the correlation between the cause and each effect:

$$R_{\text{effect1, effect2}} = R_{\text{cause, effect1}} \times R_{\text{cause, effect2}},$$

where

- $R_{\text{effect1, effect2}}$ is the correlation between the two effects,
- $R_{\text{cause, effect1}}$ is the correlation between the cause and the first effect, and
- $R_{\text{cause, effect2}}$ is the correlation between the cause and the second effect.

If data are not available, the analyst can ask the investigative team to verify assumptions of conditional independence based on their intuitions. For example, in the serial structure in Figure 7.2, if you know that the nurse was fatigued, would information about staffing add much to your estimate of the probability of medication error? If the answer is no, then the assumption of conditional independence has been verified. Another way to ask the same questions is, does understaffing affect medication errors only by creating a fatigued nurse? In this method, the exclusivity of the mechanism of change is checked. Still another way of verifying conditional independence is by asking for estimates of various probabilities:

Question: What do you think is the probability of medication error when the nurse is fatigued?
Answer: It is higher than when the nurse is not fatigued but still relatively low.

Question: What do you think is the probability of medication error when the nurse is fatigued and working in an understaffed unit.
Answer: Well, I think understaffing leads to a fatigued nurse, but you are not asking about that, are you?

Question: No, I want to know about the probability of medication error in these circumstances.
Answer: I would say it is similar to the probability of medication error among fatigued nurses.

If conditional independence is violated, then the serial or diverging structures in the graph are incorrect. If these conditions are met, then the causal graph is correct.

Let's look at slightly more complicated sets of causes. Figure 7.5 shows four proposed causes for medication error: understaffing, fatigued nurse, vague communications, and similar medication bottles. Two root causes (understaffing and vague communications) are shown to precede the direct cause of a fatigued nurse. Removing the node labeled "fatigued nurse" would stop the flow from these two root causes to the medication

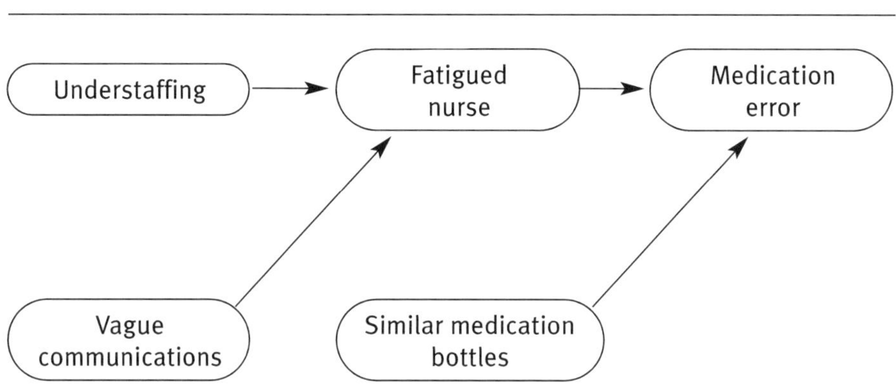

FIGURE 7.5 Four Possible Causes of Medication Error and Their Relationships

error. Therefore, a conditional independence is assumed. This assumption can be verified either through data or through experts' judgments. Assume that if you know that the nurse is fatigued, understaffing adds no additional information to the probability of medication error; therefore, this independence is verified. But suppose that even when the nurse is not fatigued, vague communications may lead to medication errors. Therefore, the assumption of the conditional independence of vague communications and medication error is not met.

Because the assumptions of the model are not correct, the causal network needs to be modified. Further exploration may indicate that vague communications, similar medication bottles, and a fatigued nurse directly affect medication errors. This example shows how verifying conditional independence could help revise root-cause analyses.

Predictions from Root Causes

The causal model behind root-cause analyses can be used to predict the probability of a sentinel event, and this probability can then be compared to the intuitions of the investigative team. The probability of the sentinel event can be calculated from each of the direct causes, and the probability of direct causes can be calculated from their root causes:

$$P(\text{Sentinel} \mid \text{event} \mid \text{Various causes}) = P(\text{Sentinel event} \mid \text{Direct causes}) \times P(\text{Direct causes} \mid \text{Root causes}) \times P(\text{Root causes}).$$

To calculate the probability of sentinel event S given a set of different unobserved (C_U) and observed causes (C_i), you can use the following formula:

$$P(S \mid C_1, C_2, \ldots, C_n) = \sum_{C_U} P(S \mid C_1, C_2, \ldots, C_n) + P(C_{U_1}) + P(C_{U_2}) + \ldots + P(C_{U_N}).$$

The above formula requires careful tracking of numerous probabilities. Because these calculations are tedious, investigative teams can use widely available software, such as Netica, to simplify the calculations. An example can demonstrate how such calculations are made using this software. Suppose Figure 7.6 shows root causes for wrong-site surgery in a hospital. First, note that the root causes listed are poor physician training and understaffing as it contributes to a fatigued nurse. These are the root causes because they are independent of the sentinel event given the various direct causes. The direct causes listed are the nurse marking the patient wrong, the surgeon not following the markings, and the patient providing

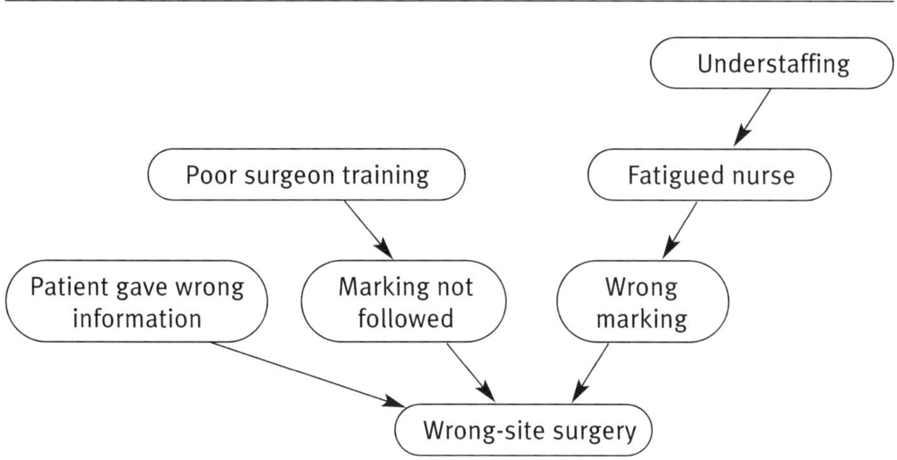

FIGURE 7.6 Root Causes for Wrong-Site Surgery

wrong information. These are direct causes because an arc connects them to the sentinel event.

Given the root-cause analysis in Figure 7.5, the next step is to estimate the probability of the various causes and effects. These probabilities are obtained by asking the expert to assess the conditional probabilities implied in the graph (Ludke, Stauss, and Gustafson 1977; Spizzichino 2001). Each node is conditioned on its direct causes. For example, to estimate the probability of having a fatigued nurse, the investigators need to ask the expert the following two questions:

1. In 100 occasions in which a unit is understaffed, what is the frequency of finding a fatigued nurse?
2. In 100 occasions in which a unit is not understaffed, what is the frequency of finding a fatigued nurse?

Obviously, estimates of probabilities from experts are subjective and therefore may be unreliable. But if experts are provided with tools (e.g., calculators, paper, pencils), brief training in the concept of conditional probabilities, and available objective data (e.g., JCAHO's reports on prevalence of various causes), and if experts are allowed to discuss their different estimates, then experts' estimates are usually accurate and reliable. These probabilities may not be accurate to the last digit, but can provide for a test of consistency. Suppose that through interviewing experts or through analyzing hospital data, the investigative team has estimated the following probabilities:

$$P(\text{Understaffing}) = .40$$
$$P(\text{Patient provided wrong information}) = .05$$
$$P(\text{Poor surgeon training}) = .12$$

P(Fatigued nurse | Understaffing) = .30
P(Fatigued nurse | No understaffing) = .05
P(Nurse marked patient incorrectly|Fatigued nurse) = .17
P(Nurse marked patient incorrectly|Not fatigued nurse) = 0.01
P(Surgeon did not follow markings|Poor training) = 0.10
P(Surgeon did not follow markings|Good training) = 0.01
P(Wrong-site surgery | Patient gave wrong information, Nurse marked patient incorrectly and Surgeon did not follow markings) as given as in Table 7.1

Using these estimates, you can use Netica software to calculate the probability of wrong-site surgeries when no information about any causes is present as 0.06 (see Figure 7.7 to see these calculations with Netica software). Does this seem reasonable to the investigative team? If the probability is significantly higher than what the investigative team expected, then perhaps important constraints that prevent wrong-site surgeries have been missed. If it is too low, then an important cause or mechanism by which wrong-site surgeries occur might have been missed. If the probability is in the ballpark but not exactly what was expected, then perhaps the estimated probabilities might be wrong. In any case, when there is no correspondence between the probability of the sentinel event and the investigative team's intuition, it is time to rethink the analysis and its parameters.

Other probabilities can also be calculated and compared to the experts' intuitions. Suppose on a particular unit on a particular day, you find the nurse was fatigued but the clinician was well-trained and the patient provided accurate information. Given the above estimates and the root cause in Figure 7.6, the probability of wrong-site surgery on this day is

TABLE 7.1 Estimated Probabilities of Wrong-Site Surgery Given Various Conditions

Conditions			*Probability of Wrong-Site Surgery Given Conditions*
Patient Provided Wrong Information	*Surgeon Did Not Follow Markings*	*Nurse Marked Patient Incorrectly*	
True	True	True	0.75
True	True	False	0.75
True	False	True	0.70
True	False	False	0.60
False	True	True	0.75
False	True	False	0.70
False	False	True	0.30
False	False	False	0.01

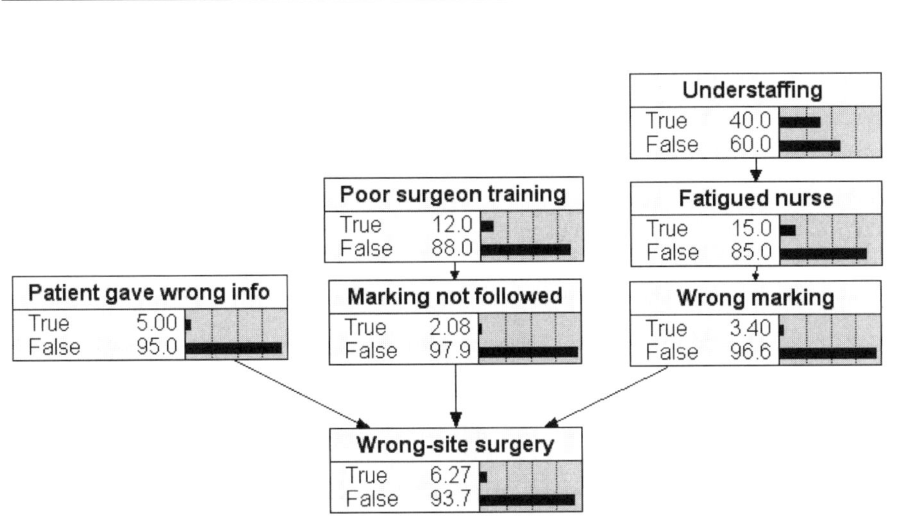

FIGURE 7.7 Application of Netica Software to Root-Cause Analysis from Figure 7.6

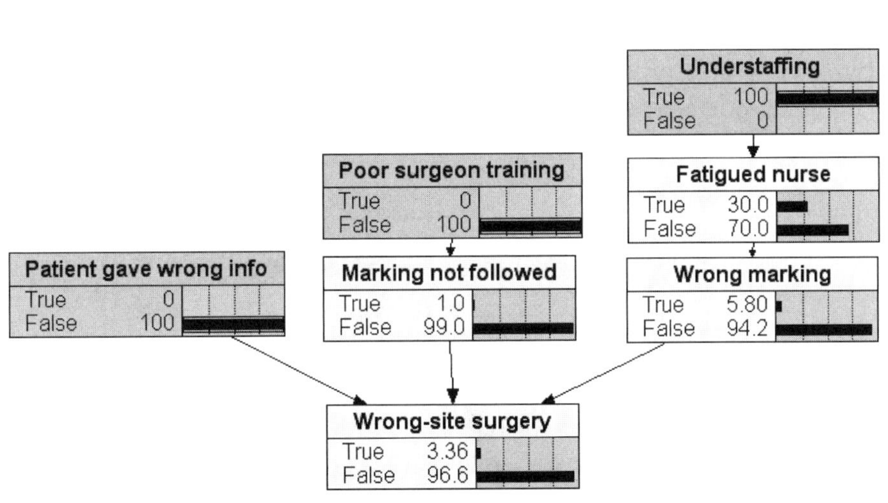

FIGURE 7.8 Probability of Wrong-Site Surgery

calculated as 0.03 using Netica (see Figure 7.8). If this corresponds to the investigative team's expectation, then the analysis is consistent and one can proceed. If not, one needs to examine why not and look for adjustments that would fit the model predictions to experienced rates.

Reverse Predictions

The Bayesian network can also be used to calculate the probability of observing a cause given that an effect has occurred. This is the reverse of how most people think about causes and effects. Most people start with a cause and want to predict the probability of the effect. Bayesian probability models allow you to do the reverse. One can start with known sentinel events and ask about the prevalence of a particular cause among them. Because causes are not as rare as sentinel events, this procedure allows one to check on the adequacy of the analysis without having to wait a long time for the reoccurrence of the sentinel event. To make things easier, JCAHO publishes the prevalence of categories of causes among sentinel events (see http://www.jcipatientsafety.org). Despite limitations (Boxwala et al. 2004), these data can be used to examine the consistency of a root-cause analysis done in one organization against the industry patterns roughly reported through JCAHO's voluntary system. A large discrepancy between observed prevalence of causes among sentinel events and assumed prevalence of causes in the investigative team's model suggest errors in assignments of probabilities as well as possible missed causes or constraints.

Netica software can calculate the prevalence of understaffing in the model of wrong-site surgeries. First, the probability of wrong-site surgery is set to 100%. The software then reports the prevalence of understaffing.

The software calculated that understaffing was present in 44 percent of wrong-site surgeries (see Figure 7.9). But is this a reasonable estimate?

FIGURE 7.9 Root Causes of Sentinel Events, 1995–2004

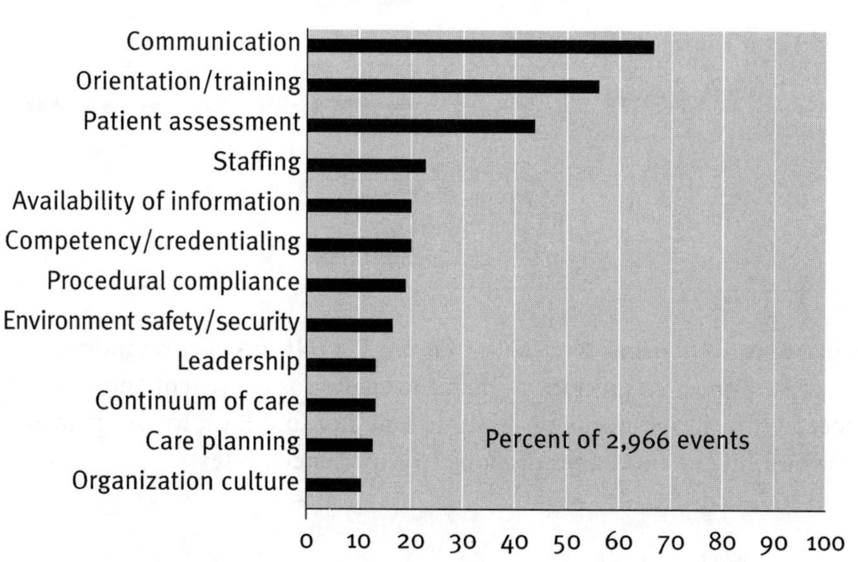

SOURCE: Joint Commission on Accreditation of Healthcare Organizations. 2005. "Sentinel Event Statistics." [Online information; retrieved 6/16/05]. http://www.jcaho.org/accredited+ organizations/ambulatory+care/sentinel+events/root+causes+of+sentinel+event.htm.

In contrast, JCAHO reports staffing levels to be a cause of sentinel event in fewer than 20 percent of surgeries (see Figure 7.10). Obviously, there are many reasons for a healthcare organization to differ from other aggregate data reported by JCAHO. But JCAHO's data can be used as a rough benchmark. Because the two probabilities differ considerably, these differences suggest the need to rethink the analysis.

Overview of Proposed Method for Root-Cause Analyses

Sentinel events can be reduced if healthcare organization create a blame-free environment, conduct a root-cause analysis, and take concrete actions in response to the analysis. Conduct a verifiable root-cause analysis by completing the following steps:

1. Before a sentinel event occurs, an investigative team is organized. The team should include a facilitator and a team leader. The facilitator's responsibility is to organize tasks, serve as staff to the team, and conduct team meetings in an efficient and effective method (see Chapter 6) for details). The facilitator should be trained in probability models. The leader's responsibility is to make sure that the investigation is carried out thoroughly and to provide content expertise.
2. When a sentinel event is reported, the employees closest to the incident are asked to record facts (not accusations) about the event, including what happened, who was present, where the event

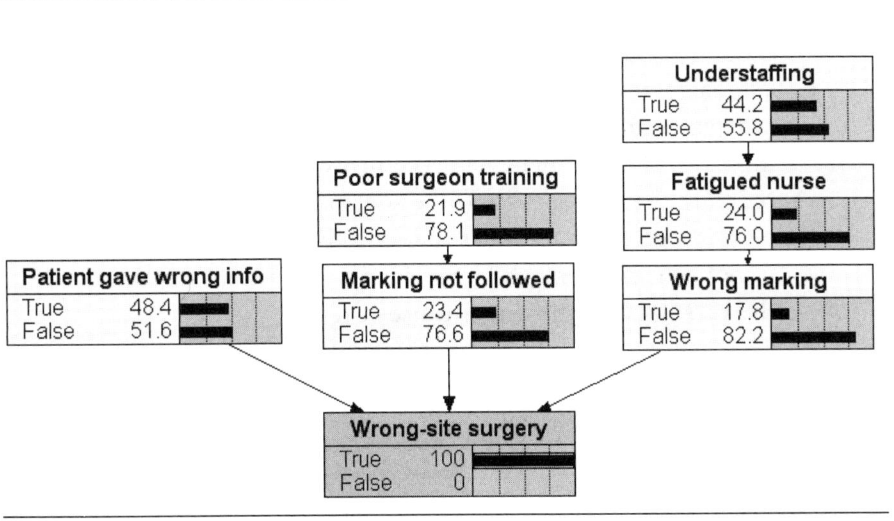

FIGURE 7.10 Prevalence of Understaffing Among Wrong-Site Surgery

occurred, when it occurred, and what the time sequence of the events that preceded the sentinel event was.

3. The investigative team meets and brainstorms the following: (1) potential causes for the incidence and (2) key constraints that would have prevented the incidence if they had been in place. Two steps are taken to make sure the listing is comprehensive. First, the framing bias is reduced by using alternative prompts. Because constraints can be thought of as reverse causes, the team should be asked to list both the constraints and causes. Furthermore, because the team is focused on conditions that led to the sentinel event, they should also be asked to examine conditions that prevented sentinel events on other occasions.
4. The facilitator interviews the investigative team or uses existing data to assign a probability to each cause and a conditional probability for each effect following the cause.
5. The facilitator checks the accuracy of the causal model and asks the investigative team to revise their model. The following steps allows one to check the accuracy or consistency of the causal model:
    a. The facilitator uses the model to predict the probability of the sentinel event. If this probability is several magnitudes higher than historical patterns or investigative team's intuitions, the facilitator seeks additional constraints that would reduce the probability of the sentinel event. If the probability is lower than historical experience or the investigative team's intuitions, the team is asked to describe additional mechanisms and causes that may lead to the sentinel event.
    b. The facilitator uses the model to calculate the prevalence of the causes among sentinel events. These data are checked against the investigative team's intuitions as well as against observed industry rates published by JCAHO.
    c. The facilitator checks that claimed root causes are conditionally independent from the sentinel event. If a root cause is directly linked to the sentinel event, the investigative team is asked to redefine the direct cause to be specific to the mechanism used by the root cause to affect the sentinel event. If few root causes have been specified, the investigative team is asked to rethink the reasons why the direct causes occur.
    d. The facilitator checks the marginal probabilities against objective data. If the probabilities do not match, the facilitator should use the objective probabilities whenever available.
6. The findings are documented. A flowchart shows the nodes for the root causes, direct causes, and sentinel events connecting to each

other with arrows. Arrows are drawn from root causes to direct causes and from direct causes to sentinel events.

Summary

Investigative teams often rely on their own intuitions for listing the root causes of a sentinel event. They rarely check the validity of their analysis. Bayesian networks can be applied to root-cause analyses to test the validity or consistency of the analyses. Real analysis should be a careful examination of facts and not a cover for wishful speculation. By creating a Bayesian network and estimating the probabilities of various events, one can scrutinize assumptions made in a root-cause analysis. In particular, one can check if important root causes have been missed, if the analysis is focused on root causes or direct causes, if the frequency of the sentinel event corresponds to expectations and experienced rates, if the prevalence of the causes of sentinel events corresponds to known rates, and if the assumptions of dependence or independence are wrong. These are not exact ways of checking the accuracy of the analysis, but these methods allow one to check the intuition of investigative teams and help them think through the implication of their analysis.

Review What You Know

1. When *A* causes *B*, *B* causes *C*, and there are no other causal relationships, what implication do these relationships have for the conditional probabilities?
2. What are the steps in conducting a root-cause analysis?
3. How can you validate the root-cause analysis? List specific ways that assumptions in root-cause analysis can be verified.
4. If a root-cause analysis of wrong-site surgery exceeds by several folds the observed frequency of wrong-site surgery, what implication does this have for the analysis?
5. What are serial, diverging, and converging structures, and which ones imply conditional independence?
6. What is meant by reverse prediction, and why is that more useful than directly predicting a rare accident?
7. In the root-cause analysis of wrong-site surgery, what is the probability of finding that the patient was responsible? If in the past you have reviewed 100 wrong-site surgeries and found that 5 percent of them were because of patient misinformation, what is the implication of this finding for the root-cause analysis?

Rapid-Analysis Exercises

1. Interview a colleague at work to analyze root causes of an adverse outcome (not necessarily a sentinel event). Make sure that you list at least three direct causes or constraints and that you include the categories suggested by JCAHO. Draw a flowchart.
2. Indicate the direct and root causes of the sentinel event in your model.
3. Give an example question that can check the conditional independence assumption associated with root causes. Make sure the question is not awkward.
4. Verify all assumptions of conditional independence in your model by interacting with your expert. Show what assumptions were checked and what assumptions were violated.
5. Estimate marginal and conditional probabilities by interviewing your expert.
6. Use Netica to estimate the probability of the sentinel event.
7. Use Netica to calculate the probability of sentinel event in at least three different scenarios (i.e., combination of causes occurring or not occurring).
8. Ask your expert if the various estimates in questions 6 through 7 are within your expert's expectations.
9. Calculate the prevalence of root causes for the sentinel event in your analysis. Compare these data to JCAHO's reports on prevalence of causes of sentinel events. Report the difference between your model assumptions and JCAHO's data.
10. Suggest how you would change the causal model to better accommodate your expert's insights. Show how your root-cause analysis changed as a consequence of the data you examined.
11. Bring your work to class.

Audio/Visual Chapter Aids

To help you understand the concepts of root-cause analysis, visit this book's companion web site at ache.org/DecisionAnalysis, go to Chapter 7, and view the audio/visual chapter aids.

References

Boxwala, A. A., M. Dierks, M. Keenan, S. Jackson, R. Hanscom, D. W. Bates, and L. Sato. 2004. "Organization and Representation of Patient Safety Data: Current Status and Issues Around Generalizability and Scalability." *Journal of the American Medical Informatics Association* 11 (6): 468–78.

Joint Commission on Accreditation of Healthcare Organizations (JCAHO). 2005. "Glossary of Terms." [Online information; retrieved 06/16/05.] http://www.jcaho.org/accredited+organizations/sentinel+event/glossary.htm.

Ludke, R. L., F. F. Stauss, and D. H. Gustafson. 1977. "Comparison of Five Methods for Estimating Subjective Probability Distributions. *Organizational Behavior and Human Performance* 19 (1): 162–79.

Spizzichino, F. 2001. *Subjective Probability Models for Lifetimes.* Boca Raton, FL: Chapman and Hall.

CHAPTER

8

COST-EFFECTIVENESS OF CLINICS

Farrokh Alemi

This chapter demonstrates the application of decision trees to the analyses of the cost-effectiveness of clinics. Healthcare managers often start clinics and programs. They need to understand how much to charge for the services offered through their new investment. They need to justify the effectiveness of clinics to various funding agencies. They need to identify weak and money-losing operations and work on improving them. Unfortunately, the cost-ffectiveness of clinics is not always clear because it is difficult to distinguish program costs from other expenditures in the organization. Many clinicians have multiple roles within the organization, and it is not clear how much of their time and effort are going into the new program versus other activities within the organization. It is difficult to understand how management personnel and other indirect costs affect the viability of the new clinic. To make things more confusing, new clinics share facilities with existing programs, making it difficult to charge them rent or allocate a portion of capital expenditures to these clinics. A rational approach would require one to isolate the cost of the program from other costs and to decide how much of the overhead should be carried by the program.

In addition, a program's cost is just part of the picture. Any program or clinic not only has its own services but also affects the services offered by other units. For example, offering a new program in cardiology might help identify patients for the existing home health care service of the organization. If the new clinic is more modern and advanced than existing operations (e.g., it uses electronic medical records or new surgical equipment), then it might change the image of the entire organization and affect the referral to all existing clinics. The new clinic might be the loss leader that attracts patients to other parts of the organization. In short, any new investment may have many consequences. If you are evaluating the cost-effectiveness of a new clinic, it is important to go beyond a program's operations and costs and look at its affect on other services too. This chapter shows how healthcare managers can isolate the cost of a clinic or program and trace the consequences of offering a service by using decision analytic tools.

Managers who have to justify the operations of a clinic to outside planning offices or insurance companies might be interested to look at the

This book has a companion web site that features narrated presentations, animated examples, PowerPoint slides, online tools, web links, additional readings, and examples of students' work. To access this chapter's learning tools, go to ache.org/DecisionAnalysis and select Chapter 8.

broad consequences of the clinic. Instead of just looking at how the clinic affects their existing services, they might want to look at the effect of the clinic on payers. They might not want to limit the analysis to specific internal components but also include utilization of services outside the organization. This chapter will show how such a broad analysis of the consequences of opening a clinic can be carried out.

These ideas will be demonstrated by an example that applies them to an evaluation of the cost-effectiveness of locating a substance abuse treatment clinic within a probation agency (Alemi et al. 2006). More than four million adults are on probation or parole supervision. Supervision failures, often linked to a return to drug use, create a cycle back into prison and jail. If supervision can be enhanced with treatment, then perhaps the cycle can be broken and offenders can return to the community, not only restoring their lives but also perhaps saving money associated with crime and multiple returns to prison. In recent years, a number of studies have examined the cost-effectiveness of substance abuse treatment (Shepard and Reif 2004; Kunz, French, and Bazargan-Hejazi 2004; Kedia and Perry 2003; Kaskutas, Witbrodt, and French 2004; Jofre-Bonet et al. 2004; French et al. 2002; Doran et al. 2004; Dismuke et al. 2004; Dennis et al. 2004; Daley et al. 2004; Caulkins et al. 2004; Berger 2002) and ways to reduce recidivism (McCollister et al. 2004, 2003; Logan et al. 2004; Fass and Pi 2002; Aos 2002, 2003; Aos and Barnoski 2003; Aos et al. 2001, 2004). For ease of reference, the model of coordinating the clinic with the probation agency is referred to as "seamless probation" and is compared to the traditional model of providing probation and substance abuse treatment services independently.

Perspective

In any analysis, the perspective of the analysis dictates whose costs are included. If one is analyzing cost to the patient, then cost to the hospital is not included. If one is analyzing cost to the organization only, then cost to external agencies are not included. A societal perspective may include costs incurred to caregivers and other social components of care. If the analysis is done for payers, then costs to these organizations are included, and other costs are ignored.

In the seamless probation study, the focus of the analysis was costs and benefits to the government agencies that were expected to fund the clinic.

Time Frame

Many of the benefits of new procedures may occur several years later (e.g., reduced hospitalizations), while the cost may occur during the clinic visits. It is therefore important to precisely define the time frame for the cost-benefit analysis and to discount future returns to current values. For example, the benefit of seamless probation is observed years later in the form of reduced crime. To capture these future outcomes, a sufficiently long perspective is needed. The study on seamless probation examined the effect of the substance abuse clinic for two to three years after enrollment in the study. This was long enough to see the effect of short-term events but not long enough to capture lifetime events.

Steps in the Analysis

The analysis of the cost-effectiveness of a clinic requires the estimation of a number of related concepts, including the following:

1. Create a decision analytic model that includes clinic utilization, clinic operating costs, and the effect of the clinic on other costs.
2. Estimate probabilities of daily clinic utilization and various consequences.
3. Estimate the daily cost of the clinic's operation from the clinic's budget.
4. Estimate the daily cost of various consequences from the literature.
5. Calculate the expected cost of the clinic.
6. Conduct a sensitivity analysis.

Each of these steps is further explained in the remainder of this chapter.

Step 1: Create a Decision Analytic Model

Decision models have been used to model costs and benefits of a wide array of services (Varghese, Peterman, and Holtgrave 1999; Marley 1990; Davis 1989; McNeil 2000; Carlos et al. 2001; Palmer et al. 2002; Post, Kievit, and Van Bockel 2004; Kocher and Henley 2003; Inadomi 2004; Sonnenberg 2004; You et al. 2004; Targownik et al. 2004; Culligan et al. 2005; Lejeune et al. 2005; Jordan et al. 1991; Malow, West, and Sutker 1989). The

FIGURE 8.1 A Decision Trees for Evaluaing Cost-Effectiveness in New Clinics

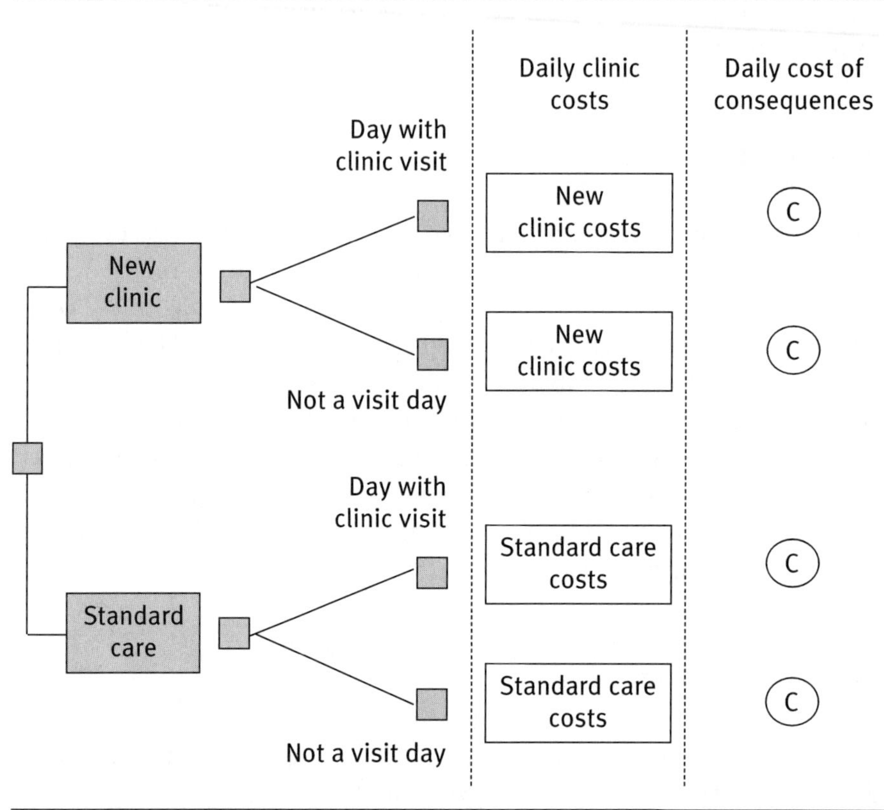

typical analysis, as shown in Figure 8.1, starts with a decision node that contrasts joining the new clinic against the standard care alternative. Then, the various events within the program are indicated (e.g., visits). Because the analysis is done per day, these events are shown as days in which a visit has occurred. Next, two costs are reported: the daily cost of the clinic and the daily cost of the clinic's consequences. The daily cost of the clinic includes the personnel, material, information system, building, and other capital and operating costs of delivering the program. The cost of the clinic's consequences is itself a separate decision tree. In Figure 8.1, cost of the consequences is shown as node "C." This node is broken into a more detailed decision tree in Figure 8.2, which shows the daily probability of various consequences and the daily cost associated with each.

Note that, in the analysis, all probabilities and costs are calculated per day. Thus, cost is discussed in terms of the daily probability of initiating treatment and the daily probability of retaining a client. Consequences are discussed in terms of the daily probability of needing a service and the daily cost of various services. In this fashion, a consistent unit of analysis is kept throughout the analysis.

Figure 8.2 assumes that the patient may have a day of hospitalization or a day in which a clinic visit occurs. In addition, the figure has a

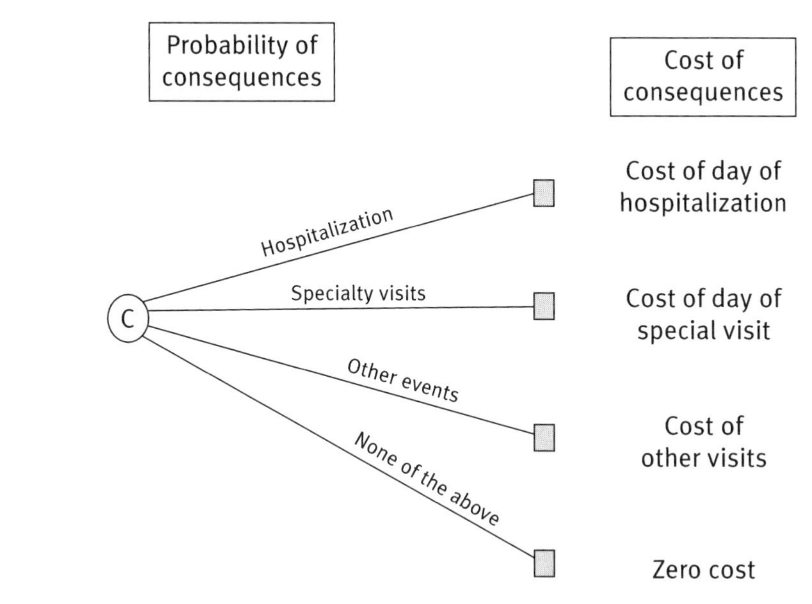

FIGURE 8.2 An Example of a Decision Tree for Costs of Consequences

placeholder for other major events that might occur as a consequence of the clinic visit. Finally, to make the list of possible events complete, one needs to also include the situation in which none of the major events imagined will happen. Strictly speaking, the events depicted must be mutually exclusive and exhaustive. Some events—for example, visiting a specialist and being hospitalized—may occur on the same day and thus may not be mutually exclusive. If this is not occurring often, the analysis depicted in Figure 8.2 may continue as is and be considered an approximation of the reality.

One advantage of a decision tree is that it separates the probability of an event from its unit cost. For example, in Figure 8.2, the probability of a day of hospitalization is separated from the cost of a day of hospitalization. Unit costs of services are unlikely to change under different alternatives. Therefore, the analyst does not need to estimate the unit cost for each alternative. For example, although the new clinic is expected to affect the probabilities of hospitalization, it is not expected to affect the unit cost of a day of hospital care. Because the unit cost is the same under each alternative, changes to the unit cost are unlikely to affect the analysis in significant ways. Therefore, the analyst can use national estimates for unit costs and does not need to collect data to assess these costs within the organization. Decision analysis makes data collection easier and perhaps more accurate by reducing the number of estimates needed and by using national estimates for components that do not change under various alternatives.

Figure 8.3 shows the overall structure of the analysis for seamless and traditional probation. The left section of the decision tree depicts the decision. Immediately after this node, the probability of receiving one day

FIGURE 8.3 Decision Tree for Seamless and Traditional Probation

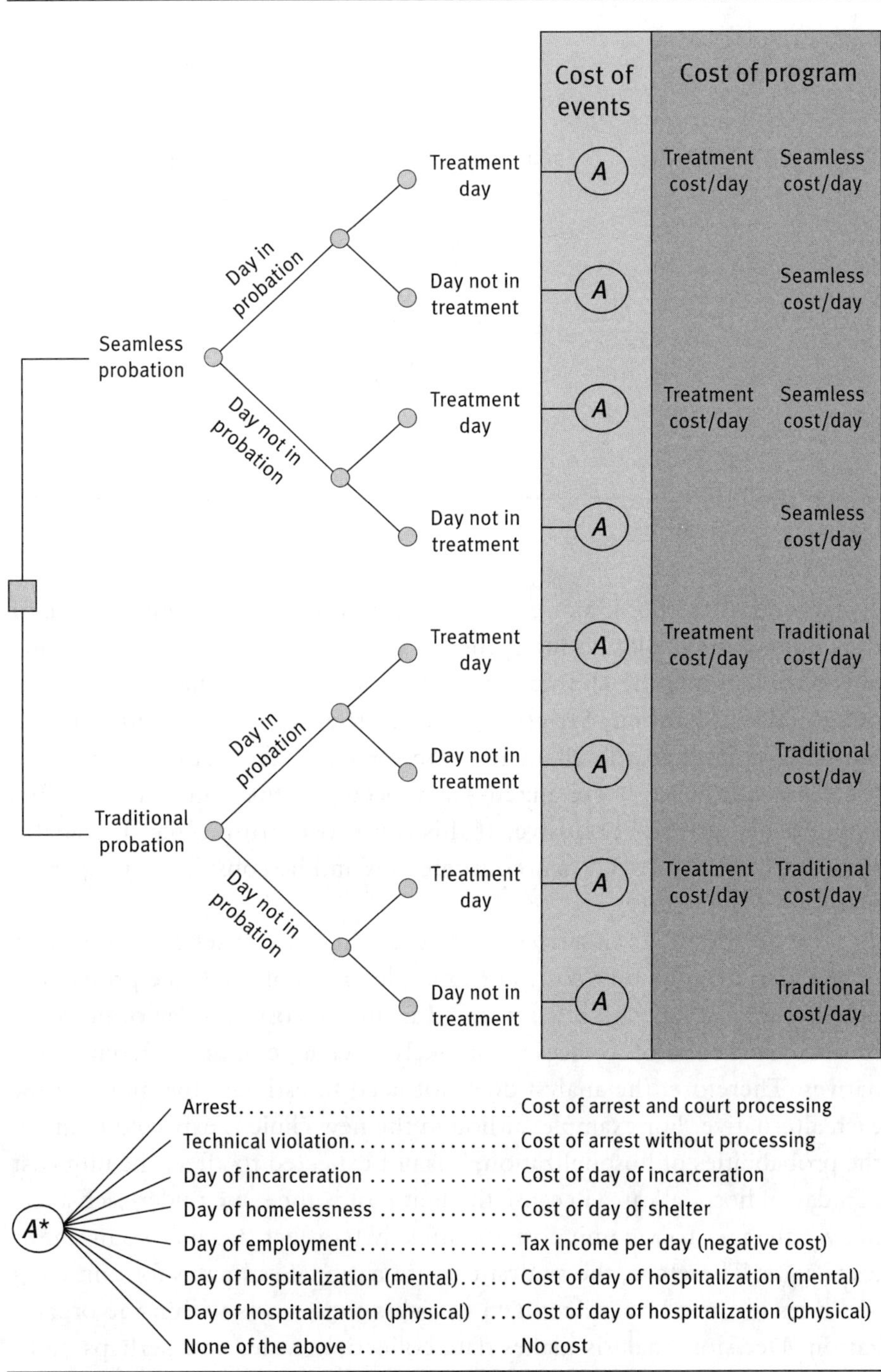

of probation or one day of treatment is shown. These branches indicate the utilization of services. The middle section of the decision tree depicts treatment and probation outcomes—previously referred to as the consequences of clinic visits. Next, the decision tree assumes that the probabilities for a day of homelessness, a day of unemployment, a day of foster care for children, a day of hospitalization, and a day in prison will vary with client's probation and treatment status. The right section of the decision tree depicts the cost associated with each path in the tree, measured per client per day.

Step 2: Estimate Probabilities

This section discusses how the probabilities needed for the analysis are calculated. There are four ways to assess these probabilities, as shown in see Table 8.1.

The first method is to monitor a large cohort of patients (preferably randomly assigned to various alternative arrangements) over time and count the frequency of the events. This method is objective and requires considerable follow-up time and access to a large number of patients. For example, one might follow up 100 patients in the clinic and report the frequency with which they are hospitalized.

The second method is to examine the time between reoccurrences of events in the decision tree. If you can assume that the daily probability of the event has a binomial distribution, then the time between the occurrences of the event has a geometric distribution, and the daily probability can be calculated by number of days in between the reoccurrence:

$$\text{Daily probability of event} = \frac{1}{1 + \text{Number of days to reoccurrence of the event}}.$$

TABLE 8.1 Four Ways of Assessing Probabilities

	Time to Event	*Frequency Counts*
Objective	Number of days to event is measured and transferred by formula to daily probabilities of the event.	A large cohort of patients is followed up and frequencies of various events are calculated.
Subjective	Experts are asked to estimate the number of days to the event, and daily probabilities are calculated from these estimates.	Experts are asked to estimate the frequency of events.

This method is objective but requires a shorter follow-up time than the first method, especially if the probabilities being assessed are relatively small. For example, the daily probability of hospitalization might be calculated as the number of days before the patient is hospitalized. If a patient is hospitalized after 80 days, then the daily probability of hospitalization is 1/81.

The third and fourth methods are the same as the first two but are based on experts' opinions rather than objective data. You might ask experts about days to the event or the frequency of the event. You might ask a clinician to estimate how many days before a patient is hospitalized; or you might ask an expert about the patient's prognosis by asking him to specify the likelihood that the patient might be hospitalized within 30 days.

In the seamless probation example, the first method was used. The researchers recruited 272 offenders with extensive criminal justice histories and randomly assigned them to seamless and traditional probation. Offenders were interviewed at baseline and at three 12-month follow-up periods to examine their utilization of various services. Of the clients, 78 percent of those on traditional probation and 77 percent of those in the seamless group were available for follow-up interviews.

When assessing objective frequencies, it is important to keep in mind that the decision tree requires the calculation of the daily probability of various events. These probabilities are calculated by dividing the length of time that an event occurs (e.g., days of hospitalization) by the total number of follow-up days. When calculated in this fashion, the probability of one day of an event is affected by the duration of the event. For example, the client's length of stay in treatment alters the probability of a day of treatment. The longer the treatment program, the larger the daily probability. A client who is in treatment for one year will have a daily probability of 1 percent. A client in treatment for one month in a year will have a daily probability of 8 percent. As clients stop and restart treatment, the daily probability changes. The proposed method of calculating the probability of the event takes into account multiple returns to treatment. Table 8.2 provides the average length of various events for the clients who were followed up in the study, and Table 8.3 turns these durations into daily probabilities.

Table 8.2 shows that the clients in the seamless group had more treatment, more probation time, and lower arrest rates but also more technical violations (instances in which a probation officer jails the client while he is waiting to appear in front of the judge). The clients in the seamless group also spent more days in prison/jail—despite the fact that they were arrested less often—in part because they had more technical violations.

TABLE 8.2 Average Duration of Various Events per Client

	Traditional		*Seamless*	
	Average for 100 Clients	*Standard Deviation*	*Average for 101 Clients*	*Standard Deviation*
Follow-up days	1,001.20	308.60	1,006.21	339.03
Treatment days	114.78	212.21	200.00	215.00
Probation days	410.12	195.54	456.81	213.52
Arrests in first year	1.00	1.40	0.86	1.09
Technical violation of probation	0.35	0.48	0.40	0.49
Days in prison	112.15	193.46	140.23	213.38
Days employed	378.65	390.59	391.32	439.38
Days in hospital (mental illness)	0.30	1.49	1.65	12.31
Days in hospital (physical illness)	0.25	1.70	0.12	1.19
Days in homeless shelter	1.22	8.96	6.51	40.44

SOURCE: Alemi et al. (2006). Used with permission.

Table 8.3 shows the probability of events in each pathway of the decision tree in Figure 8.3. The probability of each consequence for each pathway in the decision tree is calculated by dividing the duration of the events (e.g., length of stay) observed for patients in the pathway by the number of days these patients were followed up. With the exception of arrest and technical violations, these probabilities reflect both the incidence of the event and the duration of the event.

The decision tree in Figure 8.3 depicts eight pathways. By convention, the probabilities of events in a pathway are conditioned on the events preceding them. In the decision tree, treatment occurs after participation in probation; therefore, the analyst needs to show the conditional probability of treatment given probation. Conditional probabilities, as discussed in Chapter 3, are calculated by restricting the universe of possible events to the condition and then examining the joint frequency of the condition and the event. In this case, the conditional probability of probation and treatment is calculated by dividing the joint probability of these two events with the marginal probability of being in probation. For example, using Table 8.4, the conditional probability of clients in seamless probation seeking treatment while they are in probation was $0.14 \div 0.45 = 0.31$. In contrast, the same conditional probability for clients who were in a traditional probation was $0.05 \div 0.41 = 0.12$.

TABLE 8.3
Conditional Probabilitiy of Consequences of Lack of Treatment and Probation

Conditions			Probability of Event Given Probation and Treatment Conditions						
Type of Probation	*Probation Day*	*Treatment Day*	*Technical Violation*	*Arrest**	*Hospital Day (Mental)*	*Hospital Day (Physical)*	*Day in Prison*	*Day Employed*	*Day Homeless*
Traditional	No	No	.0001	.0005	.0004	.0003	.1221	.4430	.0016
Traditional	No	Yes	.0010	.0007	.0000	.0000	.3725	.1250	.0000
Traditional	Yes	No	.0011	.0020	.0000	.0001	.0800	.3432	.0000
Traditional	Yes	Yes	.0003	.0005	.0000	.0000	.0990	.1663	.0000
Seamless	No	No	.0001	.0001	.0036	.0002	.1850	.4631	.0061
Seamless	No	Yes	.0000	.0000	.0599	.0000	.3069	.2873	.0208
Seamless	Yes	No	.0011	.0016	.0073	.0000	.1029	.2629	.0005
Seamless	Yes	Yes	.0034	.0012	.0296	.0000	.0898	.2787	.0147
Total for traditional probation			.0003	.0027	.0003	.0002	.1075	.3993	.0009
Total for seamless probation			.0004	.0024	.0021	.0001	.1405	.3824	.0075

* Probability of arrest was calculated for 1 year; all other rates were calculated for 2.75 years.

SOURCE: Alemi et al. (2006). Used with permission.

TABLE 8.4 Probability of Successfully Completing a Day of Probation and Treatment

	Traditional Clients (n = 100)			*Seamless Clients (n =101)*		
	Not a Probation Day	*Probation Day*	*Total*	*Not a Probation Day*	*Probation Day*	*Total*
Not a treatment day	0.53	0.36	0.89	0.48	0.32	0.80
Treatment day	0.06	0.05	0.11	0.06	0.14	0.20
Total	0.59	0.41	1.00	0.55	0.45	1.00

SOURCE: Alemi et al. (2006) Used with permission.

Step 3: Estimate the Daily Cost of the Clinic

The daily cost of a clinic or program is calculated by dividing the total cost of a program (including operating and fixed costs) by the number of days clients were enrolled in the program during the previous year (program census). Total program costs are estimated from the organization's budget. Typically, the budget provides cost of personnel, supplies, equipment, buildings, and information services.

Not everything shows in the organization's budget, however. To the costs available in budgets, one adds the market value of buildings, volunteer services, and unaccounted retirement costs. Economic cost of a clinic differs from accounting cost because it includes the value of assets or personal services donated to the program. For example, accounting procedures usually depreciate building costs. This distorts the real market value of the asset. To correct for these inaccuracies within the budget, whenever possible the analysis should rely on the lease value of major assets such as buildings, office space, or information technology.

When a picture of true economic costs is established, the costs are allocated to various programs within the organization. Sometimes these allocations are clear, as when the budget of the clinic is separate from that of other operations. At other times, costs of various programs and clinics are mixed together in the same budget and an allocation scheme must be decided upon. Table 8.5 provides an allocation scheme for various component of the budget.

The costs of many budget categories are allocated to the program using the activity of employees by the following formula:

$$C_{p,c} = \frac{(C_{b,c} + C_{m,c})\, E_p}{E_b},$$

where

- $C_{p,c}$ is the program cost in budget category c;
- $C_{b,c}$ is the cost to the entire organization in budget category c, estimated from the budget;
- $C_{m,c}$ is the market value of donated services or unreported capital resources in budget category c;
- E_p is the number of full-time equivalent personnel working in the program; and
- E_b is the number of full-time equivalent personnel working in the entire organization.

The key for allocating the organization's budget to program costs is determining personnel activities. Clearly, some personnel will have dual roles, and it is important to ask them the percent of time they work on different activities. This is typically done by a survey of employee activities. Because of the focus on employee activities, the approach described above is often called *activity-based costing*.

In the seamless probation, two new operations were introduced: a new clinic for providing substance abuse treatment and a new way of doing probation. The study estimated the daily costs of both operations. The daily cost of providing the probation was calculated from the budget of the probation agency and the market value of items not in the budget. Building costs were based on the lease value of equivalent office space. The cost of information services provided by other state agencies, which were not directly on the budget of the probation agency, was added in. Table 8.6 shows the

TABLE 8.5 Allocation Schemes for Calculating Program Cost from Budget

Budget Category	*Allocation Scheme for Shared Items*
Clinical and support personnel	Distribution of personnel's time
Management personnel	Distribution of clinic and support personnel
Information services	Frequency of requests to the service
Equipment cost	Frequency of use and age of equipment
Building	Square footage based on patient census
Supplies	Personnel if supplies are used by employee; otherwise proportional to census if supplies are used by patients
Utilities and other overheads	Total cost of clinic and other operations (after above allocations)

TABLE 8.6
Cost of Probation per Day and per Client

		Costs (June 30, 2000 to July, 2001)		
	Agency Costs	*Investigative Reporting**	*Seamless Supervision**	*Traditional Supervision**
Personnel services	$1,191,362	$163,182	$79,320	$948,859
Contractual services	$11,984	$1,641	$798	$9,544
Supplies and materials	$9,436	$1,293	$628	$7,516
Building rental	$206,144	$28,236	$13,725	$164,183
Equipment rentals+	$122,083	$16,722	$8,128	$97,233
Information services++	$148,621	$20,357	$9,895	$118,369
Economic cost of volunteers	$5,013	$687	$334	$3,993
Total	$1,694,643	$232,117	$112,828	$1,349,697
Cost per work day	$6,009	$823	$400	$4,786
Number of client days		15,792	9,588	206,424
Cost per day per client		$15	$12	$7

* Personnel, contractual, supplies, building, equipment, information services, and volunteer costs were allocated proportional to activities of probation officers involved in investigative reporting, seamless supervision, and traditional supervision.
+ Estimated from market lease value.
++ Estimated from state and city operating budgets.

SOURCE: Alemi, F., F. Taxman, V. Doyon, M. Thanner, and H. Baghi. 2004. "Activity Based Costing of Probation With and Without Substance Abuse Treatment: A Case Study." *Journal of Mental Health Policy and Economics* 7 (2): 51–57. Used with permission.

total agency budget and allocation of these costs to various activities: investigative reporting, seamless supervision, and traditional supervision.

A similar procedure was followed for the cost of the substance abuse treatment clinic. Table 8.7 shows the total budget of the clinic and its allocation to three programs within the clinic. Like before, items that did not show in the budget of the clinic (e.g., centralized management costs) were added to the accounting costs.

Program Census

A key factor in estimating cost per day of service is estimating the number of days of enrollment, or *program census*. Errors in calculating program census could lead to surprising results. Very expensive programs may show a low daily cost if one overestimates the program's census. Likewise, inexpensive programs may have a high daily costs if the census is estimated to be too low. Given the importance of census in calculating daily costs, it is important to have an accurate estimate of this factor.

Note that the number of days clients are enrolled in the program is not the same as the number of visits. Clients stay in a service even when they do not visit the clinic. There are three methods for estimating enrollment days. First, if admission and discharge dates are available, enrollment can be measured from the difference. Sometimes these data are not readily available. In the second method, the clinicians can be asked to

TABLE 8.7 Cost of a Day of Treatment

Category	*Total*	*CROP Program*	*Outpatient Program*	*Methadone Program*
Personnel	$1,266,651	$64,425	$732,452	$469,774
Building lease value	$75,435	$5,372	$48,275	$21,788
Equipment lease value	$65,420	$2,456	$26,773	$36,191
Operations	$47,425	$1,259	$15,888	$30,278
Centralized management	$397,259	$15,814	$240,449	$140,996
Total costs	$1,852,189	$89,325	$1,063,836	$699,027
Enrollment days based on counselor's estimated panel size		$9,490	$89,790	$40,150
Enrollment days based on time between most recent discharge and admission dates		$11,043	$44,860	$57,945
Cost per enrollment day		$8.70	$15.80	$14.25

SOURCE: Alemi, F., and T. Sullivan. "A Example of Activity Based Costing of Treatment Programs Using Time Between Discharges." Working paper. Used with permission.

estimate their average panel size during the previous month. Then enrollment days are calculated as 365 days × the average panel size. The third method is to look at the time between the most recent discharge and the admission dates for the clinician. All three methods are subject to errors, because clinicians may overestimate their panel size, and historical discharge and admission dates may not reflect recent patterns. To make a more stable estimate, the enrollment days estimated from the various methods can be averaged. In addition, the range of the estimates can be used to guide the sensitivity analysis.

Table 8.7 shows the estimates of the enrollment days using different methods. The estimates vary a great deal. In two programs, the two estimates are close to each other, but for the outpatient program the two estimates are considerably different.

Step 4: Estimate the Cost of Consequences

Typically, the daily cost of consequences (e.g., day of hospitalization) does not change across alternatives. The clinic and the standard care alternative will differ in the frequency of occurrences of various consequences but not in the daily cost of each occurrence. Therefore, these daily costs can be estimated from national or regional values available through the literature.

For example, the decision tree in Figure 8.3 separates the probability of arrest from its cost. Because cost of arrest is unlikely to change with the use of the seamless probation program, national estimates were used for these costs. Table 8.8 shows the estimated cost of arrest and court processing using 2001 and 2004 values.

Table 8.9 shows the daily cost of various consequences as estimated from published national or regional data. The cost of a day of employment

TABLE 8.8
Cost of Arrest and Court Processing*

	Number of Cases in Millions	*Expenditure in 2001 in Millions*	*Cost per Case in 2001*	*Cost per Case Inflated to 2004 Prices*
Police arrests	13.7	$72,406	$5,285.11	$6,330.35
Adult judicial cases	92.8	$37,751	$406.80	$487.25

* Includes local, state, and federal costs.

SOURCE: Bauer, L., and S. D. Owens. 2004. "Justice Expenditure and Employment in the United States 2001." *Bureau of Justice Statistics Bulletin*, May.

TABLE 8.9 Cost per Occasion or per Day of a Consequence

	Technical Violation	*Arrest*	*Hospital Day (Mental)*	*Hospital Day (Physical)*	*Day in Prison*	*Day Employed*	*Day of Shelter*
Cost of consequences	$487	$6,818	$1,164	$1,868	$74	($1.50)	$30

was the exception to the rule. This cost was estimated by the tax paid by offenders on legal income they had during probation.

The cost of various consequences can be calculated by multiplying the daily probability of the consequence by its daily cost. Table 8.10 provides the expected cost for the eight pathways in the decision tree in Figure 8.3.

Step 5: Calculate the Expected Cost

As mentioned in Chapter 4, expected cost can be calculated by folding back a decision tree so that each node is replaced by its expected value, starting from the right side of the tree. Another way of calculating the expected cost, a method that is easily implemented within Excel, is to calculate the joint probability of events within each pathway and multiply this probability by the total costs incurred during the pathway. For example, in Figure 8.1 there are four pathways, each with a probability of occurring and corresponding program and consequence costs. The expected value of this decision tree can be calculated by first calculating the expected cost of consequences by multiplying the cost of each consequence by its probability and then summing across all consequences. Next, the expected cost for each pathway is calculated by multiplying the probability of the path by its total costs (sum of the program's cost and expected cost of consequences). The expected cost of each alternative is calculated by summing the expected cost of each pathway that emerges from the alternative.

The expected cost for seamless and traditional probation was calculated in the three steps. First, the expected cost of the consequence was calculated by multiplying its probability by its cost. This is shown in columns four through ten in Table 8.10. Next, the expected cost of each pathway was calculated. This was done by summing the expected cost of consequences (all rows in Table 8.10) and multiplying the total by the joint probability of events in the pathway. Finally, the expected cost of seamless probation was calculated by summing the costs of the pathways that followed from joining seamless probation (rows five through eight in Table

TABLE 8.10
Expected Cost in Different Decision Tree Paths

Condition			*Cost of Consequences*							*Cost of Programs*	
Type of Probation	*Probation Day*	*Treatment Day*	*Technical Violation*	*Arrest*	*Hospital Day (Mental Illness)*	*Hospital Day (Physical Illness)*	*Day in Prison*	*Day Employed*	*Day of Shelter*	*Cost of Probation*	*Cost of Treatment*
Traditional	No	No	0.03	3.27	0.45	0.58	9.04	(0.66)	0.05	$0	$0
Traditional	No	Yes	0.51	4.53	0.00	0.00	27.56	(0.19)	0.00	$0	$15.8
Traditional	Yes	No	0.54	13.70	0.05	0.18	5.92	(0.51)	0.00	$7	$0
Traditional	Yes	Yes	0.16	3.74	0.00	0.00	7.33	(0.25)	0.00	$7	$15.8
Seamless	No	No	0.04	0.64	4.20	0.33	13.69	(0.69)	0.18	$0	$0
Seamless	No	Yes	0.00	0.00	69.77	0.00	22.71	(0.43)	0.63	$0	$15.8
Seamless	Yes	No	0.56	10.96	8.50	0.00	7.61	(0.39)	0.01	$12	$0
Seamless	Yes	Yes	1.68	8.24	34.49	0.00	6.64	(0.42)	0.45	$12	$15.8
Cost per day or occasion			$487	$6,818	$1,164	$1,868	$74	($1.50)	$30	—	—
Difference of seamless and traditional expected costs			$0.17	($2.31)	$13.50	($0.20)	$2.08	$0.01	$0.17	$2.58	$1.24

SOURCE: Alemi et al. (2006). Used with permission.

8.10). The expected cost of traditional probation was calculated by summing the costs associated with the pathways that followed traditional probation (rows one through four in Table 8.10). The expected cost for seamless probation was $38.84 and for traditional probation was $21.60 per follow-up day per client. The net difference was $6,293 per client per year. Seamless probation had led to reduced arrest rates ($2.31 reduction in expected cost per client per follow-up day), but this savings was not enough to compensate for the increased cost of mental hospitalization ($13.50 per client per follow-up day), increased cost for delivery of seamless probation ($2.58 per client per follow-up day), additional cost because of the use of prison/jail ($2.08 per client per follow-up day), and increased cost of providing treatment ($1.24 per client per follow-up day). Therefore, locating the clinic within probation agency had not led to savings.

Step 6: Conduct a Sensitivity Analysis

In any analysis, numerous assumptions are made. Sometimes assumptions can be wrong without changing the conclusions of the analysis. At other times, parameters need to be estimated precisely because small variations in estimates could reverse the conclusion. A sensitivity analysis can establish whether assumptions are significant enough to change the conclusions. For each parameter in the decision tree, a break-even point is found by changing the parameter until the conclusion is reversed. The percent of change to reach the break-even point is reported. In addition, where alternative estimates are available, the other estimates are used to see if conclusions change.

Decision makers are often concerned with how much confidence they should put in an analysis. Statisticians answer these concerns by measuring statistical significance of differences between the new clinic and the standard care alternative. In a decision analysis, one way to help decision makers gain confidence in the analysis is to conduct a sensitivity analysis. First, single parameters are changed. Then, two parameters are changed at the same time; finally, multiple parameters are changed. If conclusions are insensitive to reasonable changes in the parameters, then decision makers will gain confidence in the analysis.

Table 8.11 shows the sensitivity of the conclusion in the seamless probation case to changes in rates of any one of the consequences. There was no change in rates of any adverse outcome that could make seamless probation more cost-effective than traditional probation (e.g., even when the arrest rate of the seamless population was set to zero, the traditional probation was still more cost-effective). The break-even points were examined for simultaneous changes in several variables. A 54 percent reduction

TABLE 8.11 Sensitivity of Conclusion to Changes in One Estimate

	Initial Rate	*Break-even Rate*	*Percent of Initial Rate*
Changes in estimates for seamless probation			
Technical violation	0.0004	None	—
Arrest rate	0.0010	None	—
Hospitalization (mental illness)	0.0021	None	—
Hospitalization (physical illness)	0.0001	None	—
Incarceration	0.1405	None	—
Employment	0.3824	None	—
Homeless	0.0075	None	—
All adverse outcome rates	1	0.4609	46%
Arrest rates, hospitalization for mental illness, and incarceration rates	1	0.4255	43%
Arrest and mental hospitalization rates	1	None	—
Hospitalization for mental illness and incarceration rates	1	0.3130	31%
Changes in estimates for traditional probation			
Technical violation	0.0003	None	—
Arrest rate	0.0027	0.0093	339%
Hospitalization (mental illness)	0.0003	0.0193	7,042%
Hospitalization (physical illness)	0.0074	0.0925	1,245%
Incarceration	0.1075	0.3145	293%
Employment	0.3993	None	—
Homeless	0.0009	0.6597	69,877%
Cost of arrest	$6,818	$57,721	847%
Cost of seamless probation	12	None	—

in all adverse outcome rates would have made seamless probation more cost-effective than traditional probation. The analysis was most sensitive to reductions in arrest rates, hospitalization for mental illness, and incarceration rates. A 57 percent reduction in these three rates would have made seamless probation more cost-effective.

The sensitivity of conclusions to changes in any one of the estimated daily costs was examined. Note that both the traditional and seamless probation have the same daily cost for all adverse events, and therefore small changes in these estimates are unlikely to affect the difference between the two groups. For example, the daily cost of arrest is the same for both seamless and traditional probations. The cost of arrest had to increase by nearly eightfold (from $6,818 to $57,721) before the conclusion that traditional probation is more cost-effective is reversed. This analysis suggests that small variations in daily cost estimates of adverse outcomes were unlikely to affect the conclusion.

Summary

This chapter has shown how the cost-effectiveness of a clinic can be examined. A decision tree allows the calculation of cost-effectiveness to be broken down into several estimates: daily probability of enrolling in clinic services, daily probability of facing various consequences, daily cost of clinic operations, and daily cost of various consequences. The latter is available through the literature, and the former variables can be measured through tracking a large cohort of patients through subjective estimates of experts familiar with the clinic operations.

The advantage of decision analytic evaluation of a clinic is that it reduces the number of estimates needed as the daily cost of consequences can be obtained from the literature. In addition, a sensitivity analysis could be used to understand how conclusions might depend on various estimates. When conclusions are sensitive to the estimated model parameters, then additional data should be collected to improve the precision of the estimates.

These concepts were applied to the measurement of the cost-effectiveness of substance abuse clinic coordinated with traditional probation or seamless probation. The total cost of seamless probation exceeded the total cost for traditional probation by $6,293 per client per year. Sensitivity analysis suggested that the analysis was not sensitive to small changes in the estimated parameters.

Review What You Know

1. What is the meant by the terms *activity-based costing*, *economic cost* (distinct from accounting cost), *break-even point*, and *program census*?
2. Which of the following are used for calculating the cost of delivering a new clinic?
   a. Published changes for a day of service
   b. Accounting expenditures within the new clinic
   c. Market value of buildings and information technology used by the new clinic
3. Describe three ways of calculating a program census.
4. Describe two ways of analyzing a decision tree to obtain an expected value for each alternative in the tree.

5. What is the purpose of sensitivity analysis, and in what way is it similar to the concept of confidence intervals?
6. When comparing decision analysis and cost-benefit analysis, how does decision analysis reduce the number of estimates needed?
7. Using Excel and the data provided in Tables 8.3, 8.4 and 8.10, calculate the expected cost of consequences associated with days clients are in probation but not in treatment. This is done by first reading the data on cost and probabilities into Excel and setting the probability of null events relative to the probability of all events. Then, multiply the probability of incurring a cost by its amount and sum over all possible consequences. Make sure that all calculations are done using relative cell values and not by entering the results by hand. Check that your answers correspond roughly with the answers in Table 8.10 to make sure that formulas lead to same answers as the reading.
8. Using Excel and the data provided in Tables 8.3, 8.4, and 8.10, calculate the expected cost of seamless probation and traditional probation per client per day. These three tables show either the probability or the cost. The expected cost can be calculated as the sum of probability of incurring a cost times the dollar amount of the cost. For seamless and traditional probations, this is done by multiplying the probability of four situations—in probation and in treatment, in probation but not in treatment, not in probation but in treatment, and not in probation and not in treatment—by the cost at each of these situations. The cost at any of these situations is calculated as the cost of consequences plus the cost of the program (probation or treatment). Make sure that all calculations are done using relative cell values and not by entering the results by hand. The expected value should be calculated as the probability of the combination of probation and treatment times the cost of that combination. Check that your answers correspond roughly with the answers in the reading.
9. Conduct a sensitivity analysis on the data by making single parameter changes in the decision tree in the section on seamless probation. Before doing so, make sure that the probability of opposite events are calculated as 1 – the probability of the event. For example, make sure that the probability of not being a probation day is calculated as one minus the probability of a probation day. In this manner, if the values of a probation day change in the sensitivity analysis, all related values will change too. Report the breakeven points for the parameters in Table 8.12.
10. Draw a chart showing the sensitivity of conclusions of the analysis to changes in the probability of arrest in traditional probation. Put the

TABLE 8.12 Worksheet for Reporting Sensitivity of Conclusions

Name of Parameter Changed	*Current Value*	*Value at Break-even Point*	*Percent of Change to Reach Break-even Point*
1. Probability of a seamless probation day	______	______	______
2. Probability of treatment day given seamless probation	______	______	______
3. Probability of technical violation given seamless probation and treatment day	______	______	______
4. Probability of arrest given seamless probation and treatment day	______	______	______
5. Probability of technical violation given seamless probation day and no treatment	______	______	______
6. Probability of hospitalization (mental illness) given traditional probation and treatment days	______	______	______
7. Probability of employment given traditional probation and treatment days	______	______	______
8 Cost of treatment	______	______	______
9 Cost of seamless probation	______	______	______
10. Cost of arrest	______	______	______

probability of arrest on the x-axis. On the y-axis, put the expected cost. Draw two lines, one showing how the expected cost of seamless probation changes when the probability of arrest in the seamless probation changes from 0 to 1. Draw another line showing how the expected cost for traditional probation changes when the cost of arrest in the seamless probation changes from 0 to 1. Note the point when the two lines meet. This is the point at which the conclusion regarding which program is preferred is reversed.

11. Conduct a multi-parameter sensitivity analysis by simultaneously allowing following changes:
    a. A 30 percent increase in the cost of arrest (from \$6,818 to \$8,863)
    b. Any change in the probability of arrest in the seamless probation and treatment group (from 0 to 1)

c. Any change in the probability of arrest in the traditional probation and treatment group (from 0 to 1)

Report what parameters need to change to arrive at a break-even point, where current conclusions are reversed. To accomplish this assignment, instruct the Excel program to set the difference between the expected cost for traditional and seamless probations to zero subject to several constraints. Include at least the following constraints:

a. Cost of arrest < $8,863.
b. Cost of arrest > $6,818. \
c. Probability of arrest in seamless probation and treatment group > 0.
d. Probability of arrest in seamless probation and treatment group < 1.
e. Probability of arrest in traditional probation and treatment group > 0.
f. Probability of arrest in traditional probation and treatment group > 0.

Report if there is a combination of changes in these estimates that would set the difference of expected value of seamless and traditional probation equal to zero. Alternatively, you can complete this assignment by creating best- and worst-case scenarios. For each of the constraints, calculate the expected value under the worst scenario and repeat under the best scenario. If the conclusion is reversed, then the analysis is sensitive to the range of changes in the parameters.

Rapid-Analysis Exercises

1. Estimate the daily and per-visit cost of a clinic operation. The purpose of this assignment is to use the steps described here to analyze the cost of operating a clinic. To accomplish this task, use your own familiarity with the clinic operations to estimate the following:
   a. Proportion of employees working in the clinic
   b. Proportion of volunteers to employees within the clinic
   c. Proportion of patients cared for in the clinic
   d. Square footage used by the clinic based on your estimate of the square footage used by the clinic exclusively and the square footage shared among clinics
   e. Number of clients served in the organization and in the clinic in the last year or last month

f. Panel size of clinicians working in the clinic
g. Time between visits per client

2. Follow these steps to accomplish the cost analysis:
   a. Select a publicly available operating budget of a healthcare organization, preferably one in which you work or one in which you have a friend who is interested in your help in analyzing their costs.
   b. Identify the various clinics within the organization and, based on the proportion of employees who work in the clinic, allocate the operating budget to the cost of the clinic. Divide the operating budget into personnel and other operating costs. Increase the personnel expenses of the clinic proportional to the ratio of volunteers to employees within the clinic.
   c. Add the building capital costs to the clinic cost. Estimate this based on your estimated square footage used by the clinic times the market value of medical office space in the zip code of the clinic. Collect this information from real estate agents in your community or through the Internet.
   d. If the clinic relies on information systems or medical records provided by other units of the organization that are not part of the operating budget you have analyzed, add this cost into the total expense proportional to the number of clients served in the clinic.
   e. Estimate the daily clinic census from the panel size of clinicians.
   f. Estimate the number of visits of an average client (estimate this as 1 / 1 + time between visits for an average client).
   g. Estimate the total number of visits during the previous year by multiplying the number of visits of the average client by the number of clients.
   h. Report the daily cost of operating the clinic and cost per visit.
   i. Report which source of data in your analysis needs additional precision and what steps you can take to collect this information. Include estimate of how much time would be needed to collect this information.
3. Analyze the consequences of purchasing a physician primary care practice on a tertiary hospital system. Select a clinic and tertiary clinical service group, preferably settings you are familiar with or settings where you have access to someone who is familiar with the operations. Estimate the variables needed based on your knowledge of these organizations and publicly available data. Follow these steps:
   a. Create a decision model that has as its first decision node whether the to purchase or not to purchase the primary care office. The chance node should indicate the frequency of visits to the primary

care setting, the frequency of visits to specialists, and the probability of hospitalization at tertiary hospital after visit to a specialist.

b. Estimate the probabilities for the model and use publicly available estimates of the cost of clinic visits and hospital visits. Adjust the cost of hospitalization based on your estimate of differences in case mix in the tertiary hospital and the types of patients needing hospitalization in the primary care setting.
c. Report the expected increase in revenues if the office is purchased.
d. Conduct a single-variable sensitivity analysis to see which estimate is most likely to affect the expected increase in revenues. Indicate how much of the additional revenue comes from direct primary care visits and how much from subsequent referrals.
e. Report on the availability of the data needed to conduct the analysis, where you would look for each data item, and how long you think collection of the data would take.

Audio/Visual Chapter Aids

To help you understand the concepts of cost-effectiveness of clinics, visit this book's companion web site at ache.org/DecisionAnalysis, go to Chapter 8, and view the audio/visual chapter aids.

References

Alemi, F., F. Taxman, H. Baghi, J. Vang, M. Thanner, and V. Doyon. 2006. "Costs and Benefits of Combining Probation and Substance Abuse Treatment." *Journal of Mental Health Policy and Economics* 9: 57–70.

Aos, S. 2002. *The Juvenile Justice System in Washington State: Recommendations to Improve Cost-Effectiveness.* Olympia, WA: Washington State Institute for Public Policy.

Aos, S. 2003. *The Criminal Justice System in Washington State: Incarceration Rates, Taxpayer Costs, Crime Rates, and Prison Economics.* Olympia, WA: Washington State Institute for Public Policy.

Aos, S., and R. Barnoski. 2003. *Washington State's Drug Courts for Adult Defendants: Outcome Evaluation and Cost-Benefit Analysis.* Olympia, WA: Washington State Institute for Public Policy.

Aos, S., R. Lieb, J. Mayfield, M. Miller, and A. Pennucci. 2004. *Benefits And Costs of Prevention and Early Intervention Programs for Youth.* Olympia, WA: Washington State Institute for Public Policy.

Aos, S., P. Phipps, R. Barnoski, and R. Lieb. 2001. *The Comparative Costs and Benefits of Programs to Reduce Crime, Version 4.0*. Olympia, WA: Washington State Institute for Public Policy.

Berger, L. M. 2002. "Estimating the Benefits and Costs of a Universal Substance Abuse Screening and Treatment Referral Policy for Pregnant Women." *Journal of Social Service Research* 29 (1): 57–84.

Carlos, R. C., R. L. Bree, P. H. Abrahamse, and A. M. Fendrick. 2001. "Cost-Effectiveness of Saline-Assisted Hysterosonography and Office Hysteroscopy in the Evaluation of Postmenopausal Bleeding: A Decision Analysis." *Academic Radiology* 8 (9): 835–44.

Caulkins, J. P., R. L. Pacula, S. Paddock, and J. Chiesa. 2004. "What We Can—and Cannot—Expect from School-Based Drug Prevention." *Drug and Alcohol Review* 23 (1): 79–87.

Culligan, P. J., J. A. Myers, R. P. Goldberg, L. Blackwell, S. F. Gohmann, and T. D. Abell. 2005. "Elective Cesarean Section to Prevent Anal Incontinence and Brachial Plexus Injuries Associated with Macrosomia—A Decision Analysis." *International Urogynecology Journal and Pelvic Floor Dysfunction* 16 (1) 19–28.

Daley, M., C. T. Love, D. S. Shepard, C. B. Peterson, K. L. White, and F. B. Hall. 2004. "Cost-Effectiveness of Connecticut's In-Prison Substance Abuse Treatment." *Journal of Offender Rehabilitation* 39 (3): 69–92.

Davis, J. E. 1989. "Decision Analysis: A Prescriptive Method for Decision and Cost-Effectiveness Research." *Journal of Family Practice* 29 (4): 367–9.

Dennis, M., S. H. Godley, G. Diamond, F. M. Tims, T. Babor, J. Donaldson, H. Liddle, J. C. Titus, Y. Kaminer, C. Webb, N. Hamilton, and R. Funk. 2004. "The Cannabis Youth Treatment (CYT) Study: Main Findings from Two Randomized Trials." *Journal of Substance Abuse Treatment* 27 (3) 197–213.

Dismuke, C. E., M. T. French, H. J. Salome, M. A. Foss, C. K. Scott, and M. L. Dennis. 2004. "Out of Touch or on the Money: Do the Clinical Objectives of Addiction Treatment Coincide with Economic Evaluation Results?" *Journal of Substance Abuse Treatment* 27 (3): 253–63.

Doran, C. M., M. Shanahan, J. Bell, and A. Gibson. 2004. "A Cost-Effectiveness Analysis of Buprenorphine-Assisted Heroin Withdrawal." *Drug and Alcohol Review* 23 (2) 171–5.

Fass, S. M., and C. R. Pi. 2002. "Getting Tough on Juvenile Crime: An Analysis of Costs and Benefits." *Journal of Research in Crime and Delinquency* 39 (4): 363–99.

French, M. T., M. C. Roebuck, M. L. Dennis, G. Diamond, S. H. Godley, F. Tims, C. Webb, and J. M. Herrell. 2002. "The Economic Cost of Outpatient Marijuana Treatment for Adolescents: Findings from a Multi-Site Field Experiment." *Addiction* 97 (Suppl. 1): 84–97.

Jofre-Bonet, M., J. L. Sindelar, I. L. Petrakis, C. Nich, T. Frankforter, B. J. Rounsaville, and K. M. Carroll. 2004. "Cost Effectiveness of Disulfiram: Treating Cocaine Use in Methadone-Maintained Patients." *Journal of Substance Abuse Treatment* 26 (3): 225–32.

Jordan, T. J., E. M. Lewit, R. L. Montgomery, and L. B. Reichman. 1991. "Isoniazid as Preventive Therapy in HIV-Infected Intravenous Drug Abusers. A Decision Analysis." *JAMA* 265 (22): 2987–91.

Inadomi, J. M. 2004. "Decision Analysis and Economic Modelling: A Primer." *European Journal of Gastroenterology and Hepatology* 16 (6): 535–42. Review.

Kaskutas, L. A., J. Witbrodt, and M. T. French. 2004. "Outcomes and Costs of Day Hospital Treatment and Nonmedical Day Treatment for Chemical Dependency." *Journal of Studies on Alcohol* 65 (3): 371–82.

Kedia, S., and S. W. Perry. 2003. "Substance Abuse Treatment Effectiveness of Publicly Funded Clients in Tennessee." *Journal of the National Medical Association* 95 (4): 270–77.

Kocher, M. S., and M. B. Henley. 2003. "It Is Money that Matters: Decision Analysis and Cost-Effectiveness Analysis." *Clinical Orthopaedics and Related Research* 413: 106–16.

Kunz, F. M., M. T. French, and S. Bazargan-Hejazi. 2004. "Cost-Effectiveness Analysis of a Brief Intervention Delivered to Problem Drinkers Presenting at an Inner-City Hospital Emergency Department." *Journal of Studies on Alcohol* 65 (3): 363–70.

Lejeune, C., K. Al Zahouri, M. C. Woronoff-Lemsi, P. Arveux, A. Bernard, C. Binquet, and F. Guillemin. 2005. "Use of a Decision Analysis Model to Assess the Medicoeconomic Implications of FDG PET Imaging in Diagnosing a Solitary Pulmonary Nodule." *European Journal of Health Economics* 6 (3): 203–14.

Logan, T. K., W. H. Hoyt, K. E. McCollister, M. T. French, C. Leukefeld, and L. Minton. 2004. "Economic Evaluation of Drug Court: Methodology, Results, and Policy Implications." *Evaluation and Program Planning* 27: 381–96.

Marley, D. S. 1990. "Decision and Cost-Effectiveness Analysis." *Journal of Family Practice* 30 (2): 233, 236.

Malow, R. M., J. A. West, and P. B. Sutker. 1989. "Anxiety and Pain Response Changes Across Treatment: Sensory Decision Analysis." *Pain* 38 (1): 35–44.

McCollister, K. E., M. T. French, J. A. Inciardi, C. A. Butzin, S. S. Martin, and R. M. Hooper. 2003. "Post-Release Substance Abuse Treatment for Criminal Offenders: A Cost-Effectiveness Analysis." *Journal of Quantitative Criminology* 19 (4): 389–407.

McCollister, K. E., M. T. French, M. L. Prendergast, E. Hall, and S. Sacks. 2004. "Long-Term Cost Effectiveness of Addiction Treatment for Criminal Offenders." *Justice Quarterly*, 21 (3): 659–79.

McNeil, B. J. 2000. "Changing Roles of Decision Analysis and Cost-Effectiveness Analyses in Medicine and Radiology." *European Radiology* 10 (Suppl. 3): S340–3.

Palmer, C. S., E. Brunner, L. G. Ruiz-Flores, F. Paez-Agraz, and D. A. Revicki. 2002. "A Cost-Effectiveness Clinical Decision Analysis Model for Treatment of Schizophrenia." *Archives of Medical Research* 33 (6): 572–80.

Post, P. N., J. Kievit, and J. H. Van Bockel. 2004. "Optimal Follow-Up Strategies after Aortoiliac Prosthetic Reconstruction: A Decision Analysis and Cost-Effectiveness Analysis." *European Journal of Vascular and Endovascular Surgery* 28 (3): 287–95.

Shepard, D.S., and S. Reif. 2004. "The Value of Vocational Rehabilitation in Substance User Treatment: A Cost-Effectiveness Framework." *Substance Use and Misuse* 39 (13–14): 2581–609.

Sonnenberg, A. 2004. "Decision Analysis in Clinical Gastroenterology." *American Journal of Gastroenterology* 9 (1): 163–9. Erratum in *American Journal of Gastroenterology* 9 (2): following 398.

Targownik, L. E., B. M. Spiegel, J. Sack, O. J. Hines, G. S. Dulai, I. M. Gralnek, and J. J. Farrell. 2004. "Colonic Stent vs. Emergency Surgery for Management of Acute Left-Sided Malignant Colonic Obstruction: A Decision Analysis." *Gastrointestinal Endoscopy* 60 (6): 865–74.

You, J.H., F. W. Chan, R. S. Wong, and G. Cheng G. 2004. "The Potential Clinical and Economic Outcomes of Pharmacogenetics-Oriented Management of Warfarin Therapy—A Decision Analysis." *Thrombosis and Haemostasis* 92 (3): 590–7.

Varghese, B., T. A. Peterman, and D. R. Holtgrave. 1999. "Cost-Effectiveness of Counseling and Testing and Partner Notification: A Decision Analysis." *AIDS* 13 (13): 1745–51.

CHAPTER

9

SECURITY-RISK ANALYSIS[1]

Farrokh Alemi and Jennifer Sinkule

These days, there is a palpable frustration with risk analysis and vulnerability assessments because critics believe they have misdirected security and recovery efforts. Some think these tools are misinforming people and causing an epidemic of fear (Siegel 2005). Organizations may misunderstand small probabilities of rare events and may seek remedies that cause more harm than the original threat would have (Gray and Ropeik 2002).

Other critics point out that the real problem is not miscommunication about the risk but faulty analysis leading to wrong priorities (Siegel 2005). Organizations may protect against long lists of security threats that are not likely to happen and fail to safeguard against prevalent risks. For example, such reviews may put an anthrax terrorism attack (Leask, Delpech, and McAnulty 2003) at a higher risk level than a hurricane as devastating as Katrina; obviously, the hurricane has more devastating impact. People using risk analysis need to be more accurate in the way they set priorities for action and ranks potential threats.

Let's start with a few obvious principles and assumptions. Risk analysis does not help when the outcome is a recommendation that all security steps are equally important and should be pursued. To be helpful, risk analysis must help organizations set priorities. To set priorities, there must be a process that could establish that the risk of one event is higher than another. To help groups understand differential risks, risk analysis must be based an objective, defensible fact; relying on consensus is not enough unless one can show that the consensus is based on actual events. This chapter shows how the accuracy of risk analysis could be improved by shifting away from consensus and comprehensive vulnerability assessments to more a focused, probabilistic, and objective analysis.

There are three possible objections to probabilistic and focused (not comprehensive) security analysis. The first is that terrorism and major catastrophic events are rare, and therefore it is not possible to measure their frequency (Kollar et al. 2002). Second, the approach is not practical; a probabilistic risk assessment is too time consuming and cumbersome. Finally, the approach should not be done because objective risk

This book has a companion web site that features narrated presentations, animated examples, PowerPoint slides, online tools, web links, additional readings, and examples of students' work. To access this chapter's learning tools, go to ache.org/DecisionAnalysis and select Chapter 9.

analysis focuses on historical precedents and leaves organizations vulnerable to new and emerging threats. These are important criticisms of probabilistic risk analysis, and they are addressed in this chapter. In particular, examples are used to show that a focused analysis is surprisingly more practical than a comprehensive analysis. A focused analysis may be done in less time, even though it relies on objective data. Also, by using new probability tools, it is possible to estimate the chances that very rare events will occur. Although these estimates are not precise to the last digit, they are accurate in magnitude and provide a consistent method of tracking the probabilities of many rare events. Furthermore, the methodology can be extended to anticipate emerging threats, starting from a kernal of truth (a fact about an event that has happened) and extending scenarios of how similar events might happen elsewhere.

Definitions

Before proceeding, it is important to define various terms. *Risk analysis* assesses the probability of an adverse outcome—in this case, security violations. Included in this broad definition are terrorism, cyber attacks, and physical attacks. Risk analysis is not the same as threat analysis, however, in which the environment is scanned for credible attacks against the organization. Figure 9.1 shows the relationship between environmental threats, organization vulnerabilities, and security violations.

Organization vulnerability is an internal weakness that could, but does not always, lead to security violations. *Security controls* are business process changes and information technology steps that organizations can take to reduce their vulnerability or to mitigate the consequences of security violations. To conduct a *vulnerability assessment*, one needs to step back from actual security violations and look for causes of security violations. When a *security violation* occurs, there are often multiple causes for it. For example, a hacker or a cyber terrorist might be able to gain access to the organization's network through a disgruntled employee. Using this definition, penetration into the network is considered a security violation, the

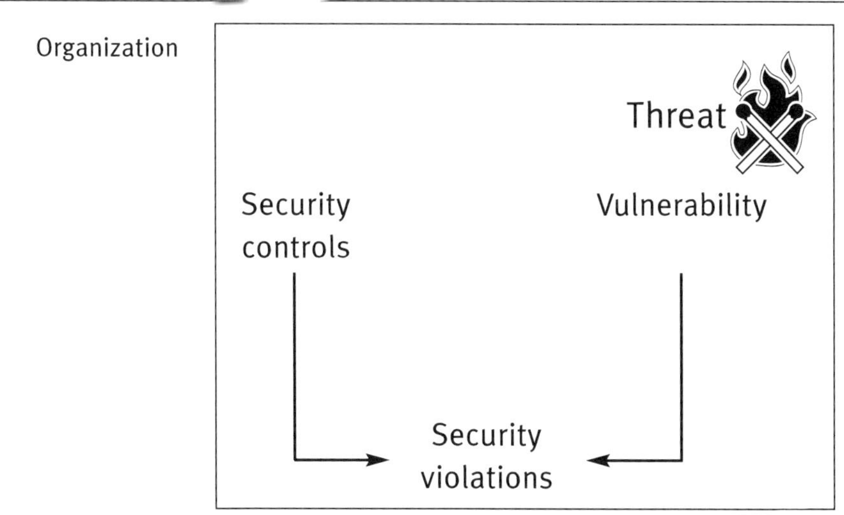

FIGURE 9.1 Threats, Vulnerability, and Security Violations

disgruntled employee is a vulnerability, and the hacker is the outside threat. In this sense, the risk analysis of security violations assesses the joint effect of threats, vulnerabilities, and security controls.

This chapter repeatedly refers to *security incidents*. A security incident is defined as "any action or event that takes place, whether accidental or purposeful, that has the potential to destabilize, violate, or damage the resources, services, policies, or data of the organization or individual members of the organization" (Rezmierski et al. 2005).

Analysis is the process of enumerating a set of scenarios for security violations (Kaplan and Garrick 1981). A focused risk analysis starts with objective data about security incidents and builds the scenarios around these incidents. Because it starts with actual incidents, the approach is also referred to as *objective risk analysis*. A *scenario* consists of one or more vulnerabilities that can lead to security violations. Examples of vulnerabilities include, but are not limited to, (1) discharging an employee without turning off access codes, (2) theft of computers, (3) attempted worm attacks, or (4) spy software on desktops. A *cyber security violation* is defined as network or desktop penetration by an outside agent independent of the intention.

History

In recent years, there have been many occasions in which risks for rare events have been assessed and subsequent events have helped confirm the accuracy of the risk analysis or improve aspects of the analysis. Probabilistic risk analysis originated in the aerospace industry. One of the earliest comprehensive studies was started after the loss of life because of a fire in Apollo flight AS-204 in 1967. In 1969, the Space Shuttle Task Group in the Office of Manned Space Flight of NASA suggested that the probability of the loss of life should be less than 1 percent. Colglazier and Weatherwax (1986) conducted a probabilistic risk analysis of shuttle flights. But over time, NASA administrators abandoned the numerical forecast of risks because the projected risks were so high that they undermined the viability of the entire operation. Cooke (1991) and Bell and Esch (1989) report that NASA administrators "felt that the numbers could do irreparable harm" (Bell and Esch 1989). But subsequent shuttle accidents returned the emphasis on probabilistic risk analysis. Today, almost all components of space shuttles go through an independent risk analysis (Safie 1991, 1992, 1994; Planning Research Corporation 1989; Science Applications International Corporation 1995). A good example of such a risk analysis can be found in the work of Pate-Cornell and Fischbeck (1993, 1994); in this award-winning study, the authors link management practices to the risk that tiles on the shuttle will break away.

Probabilistic risk analysis has also been utilized to determine nuclear safety. Several studies have focused on reactor safety. The first such study was the reactor safety study conducted by the U.S. Nuclear Regulatory Commission (1975). The study was followed by a series of critical reviews (Environmental Protection Agency 1976; Union of Concerned Scientists 1977; Lewis et al. 1975), including a 1997 Congressional bill to mandate a review panel to examine the limitations of the study. The near failure of the reactor core at Three Mile Island, however, proved that the scenarios anticipated in the study were indeed correct, although the probability of human failures was underestimated. Not surprisingly, reviews of Three Mile Island emphasized the need for conducting a probabilistic risk analysis (Rogovin and Frampton 1980; Kemeny 1979). Kaplan and Garrick (1981) conducted a study of the probability of a reactor meltdown. The U.S. Nuclear Regulation Commission (1983) issued a manual for how to conduct a probabilistic risk analysis for the nuclear industry. Probabilistic risk analysis has also been used by energy firms that focus on sources of power other than nuclear power to predict catastrophic events (Cooke and Jager 1998; Rasmussen 1981; Ortwin 1998).

In addition to its use in the aerospace and nuclear industries, probabilistic risk analysis has also been applied to the prediction of a variety of natural disasters, including earthquakes (Chang, Shinozuka, and Moore 2000) and floods, as well as to the informed planning of coastal designs

(Voortman, van Gelder, and Vrijling 2002; Mai and Zimmerman 2003; Kaczmarek 2003). Probabilistic risk analysis has also been used to predict environmental pollution (Slob and Pieters 1998; Moore et al. 1999). A large number of studies have used probabilistic risk analysis to access waste disposal and environmental health (Ewing, Palenik, and Konikow 2004; Sadiq et al. 2003; Cohen 2003; Garrick and Kaplan 1999).

Probabilistic risk analyses are becoming increasingly utilized in healthcare organizations. In healthcare, probabilistic risk analyses have focused on root causes of sentinel adverse events, such as wrong-site surgery or failure mode and effect analysis of near catastrophic events (Bonnabry et al. 2005). Amgen Pharmaceutical has also used the procedure for making decisions regarding new product development (Keefer 2001). One difficulty in using probabilistic risk analyses for healthcare systems is the fact that in identifying and protecting against risks, organizations often rely on a rank orders and ignore the magnitude of the probability for a given adverse event (DeRosier et al. 2002).

New applications of probabilistic risk analyses are being used with respect to terrorism. Taylor, Krings, and Alves-Foss (2002) have applied a probabilistic risk analysis to assessing cyber terrorism risks. Others have suggested using these techniques in assessing other types of terrorism (Apostolakis and Lemon 2005; Haimes and Longstaff 2002).

Procedures for Conducting a Focused Risk Analysis

Step 1: Specify Decisions to Be Made

Before analyzing risks, an organization needs to clarify how the risk assessment will be used. For example, an organization might want to use the risk assessment to allocate the budget for security controls. If the assessment finds that the organization is most vulnerable to a cyber attack, then money can be spent on improving the security of its computers. If the organization finds that employees' departures from the organization are leading to many security violations, then more money may be spent on improving this process. The point is that it should be clear what choices are available to the chief security officer. It should also be clear how security assessments can lead to corrective action.

Step 2: Organize an Incident Database

A focused risk analysis starts with historical precedence and adds to this list additional information about emerging threats. It assumes that history repeats itself and that the first place to anticipate the future is by examining the recent past. This is done by organizing a *security incident database.* An incident database lists the security violation, its date of occurrence, and the risk factors or vulnerabilities that led to it.

An incident database of security violations is used to collect data from one participant and report it to all others. In this fashion, participants have access to patterns of violations across the industry. First, participants register and sign a consent form. Then, participants are asked to report the security violations within their organization, including the date of the violation.

In this fashion, as more participants contribute data to the incident database, a list of types of security violations and their contributing causes emerges. In focused risk analyses, an incident database is used in two ways. First, it is used to focus the investigation on the types of violations and vulnerabilities listed in the database. Because this list is by definition more limited than comprehensive lists of what could possibly lead to security violations, focused analysis radically reduces the effort needed for conducting a risk analysis. The incident database is also used to assess the frequency of security violations, as well as the relationship between the security violation and various vulnerabilities.

Examples of incident databases abound. The Symantec Corporation collects and reports the largest database of cyber attacks.[2] This database of incidents can be used to assess the conditional probability of a security violation given specific cyber vulnerabilities. Another example is the National Vulnerability Database, which also maintains a listing of incidents of cyber security vulnerabilities.[3]

A broad example of security violations can be found in voluntary databases maintained by associations. For example, the Joint Commission on Accreditation of Healthcare Organizations (JCAHO) has created a database for voluntarily reported incidents of sentinel events (e.g., medication errors or wrong-site surgery). If JCAHO would consider security violations to be sentinel events, then its database could serve as the repository for this proposed incident database.

Incident databases can be constructed from publicly available data. For example, Alemi and Arya (2005) needed an incident database for unauthorized disclosures. They identified publicly available reports of unauthorized disclosures from (1) reviews of complaints to the U.S. Department of Health and Human Services regarding privacy issues, and (2) legal and news databases for reports of unauthorized disclosures. Table 9.1 shows the terms used to search for unauthorized disclosures and the number of unique cases found.

It is possible, and perhaps likely, that there exist other cases in which unauthorized disclosures have occurred. Public sources do not include

TABLE 9.1
Frequency of Publicly Reported Incidents of Unauthorized Disclosures

Terms Searched	*Databases Searched*	*Records Found*	*Number of Unauthorized Disclosures*	*Dates*	*Probability of Unauthorized Disclosure*
Patient confidentiality [keyword]; OR confidential medical records [keyword]; OR privacy [keyword]; medical records [additional terms]; OR privacy [keyword]; medical records [additional terms]; unauthorized disclosure [focus]	LexisNexis Academic	47	2	01/01/03–12/31/03	.005
Privacy of [subject] cases [subdivision]; OR medical records [subject] cases [subdivision]; OR medical records [subject] laws, regulations, and rules [subdivision]; OR hospital information systems [subject] safety and security measures [subdivision]	Health Reference Center-Academic Infotrac	141*	8	01/01/90–12/31/03	.022
U.S. Department of Health and Human Services; HIPAA complaints	DHHS reports	22	16	01/01/03–12/31/03	.044
Direct reports		3	3	01/01/03–12/31/03	.008
Total:		213	29	01/01/90–12/31/03	.079

* Also includes additional journal reports of unauthorized disclosure.

many of the private incidents. Therefore, their list of security violations and related risk factors might be incomplete. But no matter how many cases are reviewed, the number of risk factors will be relatively small because many risks can be imagined but few actually occur. Because relying on case histories reduces the number of risk factors, it reduces the time it takes to conduct a risk analysis.

In some industries, public incident databases are not available. If an incident database does not exist, it is possible to collect one through industry contacts. A handful of organizations can collaborate and share security violations across their organizations and thus start a small incidence database. This certainly would not be a complete list of violations, but it is better than having no data at all. Obviously, any incident database becomes more accurate as a larger percentage of security violations are reported. The more data, the more the security assessment is grounded in reality.

Step 3: Estimate the Probability of Security Violations

There are two ways to estimate probability of future security violations: direct and indirect methods. The latter method estimates probability of security violations from various vulnerabilities and risk factors within the organization. The former method estimates it from past patterns of violations. Both methods are described below in more detail.

Direct Method

The next step is to use the incident database to estimate the probability of various types of security violations. Security violations are often rare, and the incident database may contain only one or two examples of such violations. Furthermore, the probability of the violations cannot be estimated from experts' or employees' recall because, when it comes to describing rare events, people have a hard time talking about or keeping track of small probabilities.

Psychological research has shown that people often exhibit selective memory bias for events that are personally relevant (Ellwart, Rinck, and Becker 2003; Becker, Roth, and Andrich 1999; Gardner, Pickett, and Brewer 2000). In addition, emotionally arousing events often cause individuals to recall the event with greater detail and specificity (Schmidt 2004; Cahill and McGaugh 1998). Often, rare security events are personally relevant to many and are of an emotionally arousing nature. A situation in which a hospital is attacked by terrorists who kill hundreds of helpless patients is very personally relevant, even to those unaffected directly by the attack, because such an event exposes everyone's vulnerability. By the same token, witnessing such an event, either firsthand or through news coverage, causes extreme feelings of sorrow, fear, and anger. These factors will cause such events to stick out in people's minds and distort their understanding of the probability of such an attack. Memories of such events will be more salient and vivid than for other events. In sum, people are bad at accurately estimating the probability of rare security events.

Surprisingly, experts can describe with considerable confidence the time to the event. For example, many have difficulty referring to or imagining the probability of 0.000274, but they may easily make statements such as "this event has occurred once in the last decade." Because experts and employees have an easier time thinking of rare events in terms of the time to the event as opposed to a frequency count, one way to estimate probability of rare security events is through the time to the event.

If one assumes that an event has a Bernoulli distribution (i.e., the event either happens or does not happen; it has a constant daily probability of occurrence; and the probability of the event does not depend on prior occurrences of the event), then the time to the next occurrence of the event has a geometric distribution. In a geometric distribution, the probability of a rare event, P, can be estimated from the average time to the occurrence of the event, T, using the following formula:

$$P = \frac{1}{1 + T}.$$

In this approach, the frequency of an event is first estimated by calculating the time to reoccurrence of the event. For example, investigators often assume an event happens daily, weekly, monthly, once a year, once every two years, once every five years, or once a decade. This time to the event can be transferred to a frequency count using the above formula (see Table 9.2).

Some security violations are so rare that they may not occur during the observation period at all, or they may occur only once. In these

TABLE 9.2 Calculated Probabilities for Various Terms

Word Assignment	*Frequency of Event*	*Calculated Probability*
Negligible	Unlikely to occur*	0.0003
Very low	2–3 times every 5 years	10.0014
Low	≤ once per year	0.0027
Medium	≤ once every 6 months	30.0056
High	≤ once per month	0.0055
Very high	> once per month**	0.1429
Extreme	> one per day	1.0000

* Assumes less than once every 10 years
** Assumes once per week

circumstances, the length of the observation period can be used as a surrogate for the time between reoccurrences. This assumes that the security violation would occur the day after the end of the observation period, and thus it provides an upper limit for the prevalence of the security event. For an example of the use of the formula, consider that you want to assess the prevalence of physical theft of a computer. Suppose your records show that such theft occurs once every three months; then the time between two thefts is 90 days, and the probability of a theft for any day is calculated as

$$P(\text{Physical theft of a computer}) = \frac{1}{1+91} = 0.01.$$

Another method of improving the accuracy of estimates of rare events is to purposefully examine the event in artificially constructed samples where the event is not rare (Heidelberger 1995). Then the frequency of the event in the sample can be extrapolated to the remaining situation proportional to how narrowly the sample was drawn. The procedure is generally known as "importance sampling" and involves sampling data from situations where one expects to find the rare event. Assume that you have taken m narrowly defined samples, and sample i represents W_i cases in the population of interest. If P_i is the probability of the event in the narrowly defined sample, then the probability of the rare event, P, can be calculated as

$$P = \frac{\sum_{i=1,\ldots,m} W_i \times P_i}{\sum_{i=1,\ldots,m} W_i}.$$

An example may demonstrate this concept. Suppose you want to estimate the probability that electronic data could be stolen by someone overcoming the password protection in a computer. For most organizations, such an attack is rare, but the attack is more likely to be seen in computers that are infected by a virus. Suppose that in an organization, one in 100 computers has a major virus. Also suppose that the examination of data trails in these infected computers shows that 0.3 percent involve a loss of data. What is the probability of the loss of data anywhere in the organization? This probability is calculated by weighting the narrow sample of infected computers to reflect the proportion of these computers inside the organization:

$$P = \frac{1}{100} \times 0.003 + \frac{99}{100} \times 0.$$

Note that in this calculation it is assumed that a loss of data does not occur in computers without a virus infection. This may be wrong but, as a first approximation, may be reasonable, because it is anticipated that most data loss occurs among infected computers. The importance weighting procedure requires one to know a priori, with a high level of certainty, both the conditions under which the rare event are more likely to occur and the prevalence of the conditions.

Indirect Method

In the indirect approach, the probability of security violations is estimated from the presence of various vulnerabilities and risk factors within the organization. A survey is constructed based on the risk factors identified across the industry through the incident database. Then, the organization's employees are surveyed regarding practice patterns in their midst, and data from the survey and incident database are used to estimate the probability of future security violations using the following formula:

$$P(V | R_1, \ldots, R_n) = \sum_{i=1,\ldots,n} P(V | R_i) \times P(R_i).$$

where

- n is the number of hazards;
- R_i is the risk factor i;
- $P(V | R_1, \ldots, R_n)$ is the probability of security violations given various risk factors (vulnerabilities) in the organization;
- $P(V | R_i)$ is the conditional probability of security violations given the presence of a risk factor in the organization. This variable is calculated using the Bayes's theorem presented below; and
- $P(R_i)$ is the prevalence of the risk factor in the organization. This variable is calculated from the time to occurrence of the events (see below).

This formula is known as the *law of total probability*, and it states that the probability of a security violation is the sum of all the ways in which a security violation can happen from different risk factors (see Chapter 3).

The frequency of risk factors within an organization, $P(R_i)$, is estimated by surveying key informants within the organization. As risk factors can also be rare, one should assess the probability of their presence from the average time between reported occurrences of the risk factor. As before, use of this formula assumes that the risk factor has a binomial distribution of occurrence, in which the probability of the risk factor is relatively rare but is constant and independent from future occurrences. These assumptions may not be reasonable. For example, when organizations actively improve their security, the assumption of constant probability is violated. If the assumptions of binomial distribution are met or are acceptable as a first approximation, then the time between the presence of risk factors has a geometric distribution, and the formula presented earlier can be used.

Bayes's theorem is used to calculate the probability of unauthorized disclosure after the occurrence of a risk factor:

$$P(U \mid R_i) = \frac{P(R_i \mid U) \times P(U)}{P(R_i)}$$

where

- $P(R_i)$ is the probability of observing risk i. This is obtained from surveys of healthcare organizations using time to occurrence of the risk factor;
- $P(U)$ is the probability of unauthorized disclosure across institutions. These data are calculated from the Incidence Database of Unauthorized Disclosures; and
- $P(R_i|U)$ shows the prevalence of risk factor i among unauthorized disclosures. These data are also available from the Incidence Database on Unauthorized Disclosures.

An example of how to apply the indirect method can be shown using the privacy incident database reported earlier (Alemi and Arya 2005). To start with, a master list of privacy violations was created from the incidence database (see Table 9.3). Four hospitals were surveyed using this master list. Table 9.3 also contains the probability of each risk factor as well as the prevalence of the security violation given the risk factor.

The overall privacy risk for the organization listed in Table 9.3 was calculated as 0.01. Table 9.4 provides the same probability at different organizations. The data in Table 9.4 can be used as benchmarks for comparing various hospitals. For example, the data show that the risk at Hospital 2 is lower than the risk at Hospital 1.

Step 5: Adjust the Probability of Security Violations Based on Incidents Elsewhere

In the previous steps, the analyst has estimated the probability of security violations within the organization based on historical incidents. To make this estimation more accurate, the analyst must adjust the probability to reflect emerging threats. These emerging threats have not occurred in the industry but have occurred elsewhere in other industries, and there are concerns that the situations are similar enough that they may occur in the organization being assessed. Here again is a kernel of truth around which the analyst might construct a speculative scenario about what might happen within the organization if the event were to occur there.

The adjustment for emerging threats can be made using the method of similarity judgment. Similarity judgment involves predicting an event

TABLE 9.3
Predicting Probability of Violations from Prevalence of Vulnerabilities

Description of Risk Factor	*Prevalence of Risk Factor in the Organization*	*Prevalence Security Violation Given the Risk Factor*
Employee views paper documents or manipulates computer passwords to view records of patients not under her care	0.0003	1
Benefit organizations or employers request employee information	0.0003	0.8805
Employees engage in whistle blowing to uncover illegal or unacceptable business or clinical practices	0.0003	0.0201
Clinician uses unsecured e-mail environment	0.0003	0.1606
Employee removes patient records from secure location or workplace without authorization	0.0003	0.88
External infection of computers/password/ network systems (e.g., computer hacker)	0.0003	0.5888
Theft of computers or hard drives	0.0003	0.5867
Sale of patient records	0.0003	1
Blackmail or extortion of organization or an employee	0.0003	1
Changes in custody or family relationships not revealed by the patient	0.0003	0.1472
Audit of business practices by outside firm without clinicians' approval	0.0003	0.4416
Business associate violates chain of trust agreement	0.0003	1
Error in patient identity during data transfer to third-party insurers	0.0014	0.0142
Caring for employees' friends and family members and discussing the care outside of the work environment	0.0014	0.2202
Clinician gathers information from patients' family and friends after the visit without the patient's consent	0.0014	1
Patient uses identity of another person to gain insurance benefits	0.0056	0.093
Patient records (paper documents) not sealed or kept in secure environment	0.0056	0.0592
Discussion of patient care with coworkers not engaged in care	0.0056	0.1218
Medical reports or records with wrong recipient information	0.1429	0.0405
Patient care discussed in a setting where others can easily hear	0.1429	0.0023

TABLE 9.4 Overall Risk of Privacy Violations Calculated from Various Vulnerabilites Within Four Organizations

	Hospital 1	*Hospital 2*	*Hospital 3*	*Hospital 4*
Rate of security violations	0.022	0.011	0.011	0.012

based on the historical precedence of a similar event. For example, before the September 11 attack on the World Trade Center in New York City, terrorists tried to attack the Eiffel Tower by flying a hijacked plane into it. The two incidents are similar in the sense that both are tall buildings with important symbolic value. Both were attacked using a passenger jet in the hopes that the jet fuel would lead to additional destruction. They are, of course, also different incidents occurring for different reasons at different times in different places. Based on the pattern of shared and unshared features between the two events, the analyst can calculate the probability that the novel event will occur. Similarity judgments can be used to extend the probability of known rare events to new situations.

Psychologists have conducted numerous experiments showing that the similarity of two situations will depend on features they share and features unique to each case (Mobus 1979). In 1977, Tversky summarized the research on similarity and provided a mathematical model for judging similarity. The similarity of two situations, i and j, can be assessed by listing the following three categories of features:

1. Features in the index case but not in the prototype, $f_{i,\text{ not } j}$;
2. Features in the prototype but not in the index case, $f_{\text{not } i,\, j}$; and
3. Features in both cases, f_{ij}.

Then similarity, S, can be measured as the count of shared and not shared features using the following formula:

$$S_{ij} = \frac{f_{ij}}{f_{ij} + a(f_{i,\text{ not } j}) + b(f_{\text{not } i,\, j})}.$$

In above formula, the constants a and b add up to 1 and are set based on whether the index case is a defining prototype. If these constants are different from 0.5, they allow the comparison case to be more like the index case than vice versa.

Once an estimate of similarity of the index case and the prototype are available, then the probability of an attack in the index case can be calculated as

$$\text{Probability of attack in index case} = \text{Probability}_{\text{prototype}} \times \text{Similarity}_{\text{case, prototype}}.$$

For example, recall the Beslan school siege in North Ossetia, Russia in September 2004. Every year on the first day of September, every school in Russia celebrates the holiday known as the Day of Knowledge. The children dress in their finest clothes and are accompanied to school by parents and other family members. On this particular holiday, 30 Chechen rebels used this tradition as an opportunity to seize the school and take more than 1,300 hostages. The siege ended two days later when Russian Special Forces stormed the building. The crisis left more than 330 civilians dead, 186 of whom were schoolchildren, and hundreds wounded.

Suppose you want to estimate the probability of a Beslan-like siege on a hospital in the United States. Using the method of similarity judgment, a risk analyst would ask, "What is the likelihood of a terrorist attack on schools in Russia?" Next would follow the question, "How similar are the conditions in Russia and the United States?" By judging the probability of an actual event and the similarity of that event to conditions existing in the United States (e.g., hospital populations), the likelihood that a hospital would be the target of a similar terrorist attack can be estimated.

The Beslan school siege is considered a prototype of how vulnerable children might be gathered and killed. Because such an attack has only occurred only once from September 2004 to May 2006, its probability of reoccurring is estimated to be 0.0009. The risk analyst needs to determine the features that a school in Russia shares with a hospital in the United States, as well as those features unique to each setting. The school and the hospital are similar in the sense that both are buildings that house a sizable number of civilians, both serve a vulnerable population, and both are publicly accessible. Here is one summary of shared and different features in the two situations:

1. Features in the index case (school) but not in the comparison case (hospital):
    a. No proximity defense
    b. No communication system available between rooms
    c. Capacity to house population into one central location
    d. School-age children
2. Features in the comparison case (hospital) but not in the index case (school):
    a. Difficulty in gathering the population into one central location
    b. Availability of security officers
    c. Presence of items that could be used for defense
3. Features shared by both cases:
    a. Large number of civilians
    b. Vulnerable population

c. Publicly accessible

This list is for the purpose of providing a brief example; obviously, additional analysis might reveal more features. Here it is assumed that the constant *a* is 0.20 and the constant *b* is 0.80, because the similarity between the two situations are quite asymmetrical. The attack on the hospital is more likely to be judged similar to the Beslan school siege than the Beslan school siege is likely to be judged similar to the attack on the hospital. The similarity of the hospital situation to the Beslan school situation is calculated as

Based on this measure of similarity of the two situations,[4] the probability of a similar attack on the hospital is calculated as

$$\text{Similarity}_{\text{hospital, Beslan school}} = \frac{3}{3 + (0.20 \times 4) + (0.80 \times 3)} = 0.48.$$

$$\text{Probability of similar attack on hospital} = \text{Probability}_{\text{Beslan attack}} \times \text{Similarity}_{\text{hospital, Beslan}},$$

$$\text{Probability of similar attack on hospital} = 0.0009 \times 0.48 = 0.0004.$$

Step 6: Report Findings to the Organization

In the final report, the probability of various types of security violations, including emerging threats, are reported. This report should identify the credible threats faced by the organization, as well as set priorities among risks to guide the organization in its preventive efforts.

A Case Example

Suppose an analyst was asked to estimate the overall risks faced by a nursing college in a university in the southern United States. In step one, the analyst articulated the decisions faced by the nursing college. These included the following:

1. Should more funds be put into protecting against computer viruses?
2. Should faculty and staff be educated about physical security and theft?
3. Should background checks be required for all prospective nursing students?
4. Should a camera surveillance of offices be implemented?

In step two, an incident database was constructed from events that had occurred at the university in the past five years. Because of the limited nature of this incident database, the analysis should be considered preliminary until confirmed against incidents in other universities. The analyst had access to dates of occurrences of various physical security incidents with the university, but the database did not contain information on computer security violations. The observed data for physical incidents was used, and the analyst supplemented it with employee's estimated rates for the time to the next information technology (IT) security incidence.

The IT risk factors for the nursing college were classified into the groupings suggested by a research study (Rezmierski et al. 2005). The employee in charge of security incidents at the nursing college was asked to estimate the number of days to various incidents, and this information was used to estimate the rates of various incidents. Table 9.5 shows the risk factors, estimated days to the event, and estimated frequency.

TABLE 9.5 Example of IT Security Violations

IT Security Violation	*Description and Possible Risk Factors*	*Estimated Days to Event*	*Probability*
Desktop security violations	This may be caused by failure to install relevant operating system or application software patches or failure to have updated virus protection. An example is the GAO Bot Outbreak.	3 months	.03
Unsolicited e-mails requesting personal information	Employees receive disguised alerts from well-known companies (e.g., a bank) requesting them to send information in order to (1) complete an application, (2) prevent a security breach, or (3) win money.	Once a week	.14
Unsolicited e-mails not requesting personal information	Employees receive e-mails advertising products. Sender's machine has guessed the employee's e-mail or has obtained the e-mail through the web. No private information is asked for. Strictly speaking, this is not a security violation but is listed here because of its potential to lead to large numbers of employees falling victim to financial scams.	Daily	1.00
Network penetration	Outside hacker obtains illegal access to the network by manipulating the system or purchasing passwords from disgruntled employees	Once in last two years	.0014

In step three, the probability of various security violations was calculated. For each security violation, the time to the event was transferred into a frequency count. For example, in the past two years, there was one occasion in which a person was able to gain access to the information on the servers. Therefore, the probability of network penetration was calculated as follows:

$$P(\text{Network penetration}) = \frac{1}{2 \times 365 + 1} = 0.0014.$$

To assess the non-IT risks for this nursing college, the analyst used the data in the five-year incidence database. Table 9.6 shows the various non-IT security violations and the dates of their occurrences.

The frequencies of events in Table 9.6 were calculated from actual observations of dates of the events in the previous five years at the university. For example, Table 9.7 shows the steps in calculating daily probability of computer theft.

First, the dates of computer theft were sorted. Then, the difference between two consecutive dates was calculated. Next, the differences were averaged to produce the average number of days until the next occurrence of the incidence. Finally, the days to the next occurrence were used to calculate a daily rate.

In step four, emerging risks were added in. The analysis was supplemented with information about shootings at the University of Arizona (UA). On Monday, October 28, 2002, Robert Flores, a nursing student

TABLE 9.6 Observed Frequencies of Security Violations

Category of Risk Factor	*Number of Incidents*	*First Reported Date*	*Last Reported Date*	*Average Days Between Occurrences*	*Daily Rate*
Theft of computer	21	7/1/1999	11/29/2004	99	0.010
Theft of other equipment	36	2/5/1999	8/10/1999	63	0.016
Theft of personal property	2	7/12/2001	7/11/2003	365	0.003
Property damage	26	10/7/1999	10/7/2004	73	0.013
Vehicle accident on premise	10	10/27/2000	8/3/2005	193	0.005
Damage from natural causes	40	12/26/1999	6/30/2005	52	0.019
incidents hazardous materials	1	10/10/2003	10/10/2003	726	0.001

TABLE 9.7 Sample Calculation of Daily Rate of Security Violations

Date of Theft of Computers	*Time Between Consecutive Thefts**
7/1/1999	14.00
7/15/1999	146.00
12/8/1999	55.00
2/1/2000	191.00
8/10/2000	34.00
9/13/2000	133.00
1/24/2001	231.00
9/12/2001	86.00
12/7/2001	26.00
1/2/2002	64.00
3/7/2002	141.00
7/26/2002	52.00
9/16/2002	16.00
10/2/2002	147.00
2/26/2003	257.00
11/10/2003	128.00
3/17/2004	97.00
6/22/2004	31.00
7/23/2004	5.00
7/28/2004	124.00
11/29/2004	—

Average time between thefits	98.900
Standard deviation	73.421
Count of events	21
Daily rate	0.010

at UA, who apparently was angry at having been barred from taking a midterm exam, entered the classroom where the exam was taking place and shot and killed two professors. It was discovered later that a third nursing professor had also been killed in her office on another floor of the building. After killing his professors, the student killed himself. According to reports of nursing staff and fellow students (Rotstein 2002), the student often tangled with professors and disrupted class by asking inappropriate questions and challenging teachers. In the weeks leading up to the shooting, the student had failed one class and was in danger of failing a second. In April of 2001, a nursing staff member reported to the university police that the student had conveyed to staff that he was depressed and suicidal, and that he may take action against the College of Nursing in retaliation for the perceived lack of respect and assistance he received from his professors. Others also reported that the student had bragged about obtaining a concealed weapons permit. In a letter sent to the *Arizona Daily Star* before his death, the student reported a troubled childhood and stated that he was experiencing a great deal of stress in his personal life because of health problems and a recent divorce. He described being pushed to the breaking point by his recent poor performance at school and the possibility that he would fail out of the nursing program.

This incident caused many universities to reexamine security strategies, fearing a similar attack on their campuses. Before a university expends large amounts of time, effort, and money toward preventing such an attack, however, it would be useful to assess the likelihood that such an attack may occur on campus. The method of similarity judgment was used to estimate the likelihood of this incidence at the nursing college in this case example. To estimate the likelihood of a shooting at the nursing college, the analyst first needed to determine the likelihood of reoccurrence of the UA shooting. Next, the analyst needed to assess the similarity of the conditions between the nursing college and UA.

The probability of reoccurrence of the UA shooting was estimated to be at least once in the past four years (0.0007). Next, the analyst identified the features that the nursing college shares with UA, as well as those features unique to each setting.

Recall the formulation of the similarity between the two schools:

1. Features in UA but not in the nursing college, $f_{\text{UA, Not college}}$:
   a. Large enrollment (61,000 students)
2. Features in the nursing college but not UA, $f_{\text{College, Not UA}}$:
   a. Mostly working students
   b. Potential students screened with a background check
3. Features shared by both colleges, $f_{\text{College, UA}}$:
   a. Easily accessible
   b. Large population of students, faculty, and staff
   c. Campus police
   d. Standards for student academic performance
   e. Focus on nursing or health science

The analyst measured similarity using the count of shared and not shared features:

$$S_{\text{College, UA}} = \frac{f_{\text{College, UA}}}{f_{\text{College, UA}} + (a \times f_{\text{College, Not UA}}) + (b \times f_{\text{UA, Not College}})}$$

The analyst used the estimate 0.20 for the constant a and the estimate 0.80 for constant b. The similarity of the nursing college situation to the UA situation was calculated as

$$\text{Similarity}_{\text{College, UA}} = \frac{5}{5 + (0.20 \times 1) + (0.80 \times 2)} = 0.74.$$

To calculate the probability of a similar event occurring at the nursing college, the analyst multiplied the probability of the UA shooting reoccurring by the similarity between UA and the nursing college:

$$\text{Probability of school shooting at nursing college} = 0.0007 \times 0.74 = 0.0005.$$

In the final step, a report should prepared for the nursing college's leadership group, providing them with the list of security violations. The leadership group was asked to think through the relative frequency of various violations and decide how to distribute their limited security funds.

Summary

Recall the three criticisms of objective focused risk assessment: rare probabilities cannot be estimated, probabilistic analysis is too time consuming, and emerging threats will be missed. These criticisms are not valid. It has been shown by way of examples that it is easy and practical to assess the probability of rare events through the use of various probability tools (e.g., time to event, importance sampling). It has also been shown that emerging new threats can be added to the analysis through similarity judgments.

Focused risk analysis has a distinct advantage over comprehensive and consensus-based approaches: it is more grounded in reality, and is not based on speculations regarding potential risks but on actual experienced incidents within the enterprise and across the industry. In this fashion, the proposed approach may be more accurate than a consensus-based approach. Credible threats can be identified from actual incidents, allowing organizations to set realistic priorities in their efforts to protect against security and privacy violations.

The focused risk assessment is based on analysis of actual incidents within the industry or outside it; in this sense, it starts with a kernel of truth. An incident database is used to focus the assessment on risk factors that have occurred in at least one other healthcare organization or elsewhere in the world. In contrast, comprehensive and consensus-based assessments are often based on imagined risks that might mislead organizations to protect against events that may never occur. In doing so, they may waste precious security funds. Even worse than a one-time waste is the prospect that when another consultant, with a more active imagination and a more vivid assessment tool, shows up, the healthcare organization is catapulted to invest more—chasing elusive and esoteric security targets. Because imagination is limitless, there is no end to how much should be spent on security and which vulnerability is more important. Like a child, the organization ends up fighting imaginary foes. Risk assessment, instead of helping the organizations focus on high-value targets, misleads them to pursue irrelevant targets. When analysis is based on real vulnerabilities and threats, an organization can focus on probable risks and rationally prioritize and limit investment in security controls.

Review What You Know

1. How can the probability of a rare event be measured? Describe at least two methods for doing so.
2. If an event occurred once five years ago, what is its minimum daily probability of occurrence?
3. Suppose last year, computer thefts occurred on March 10, September 1, and October 6 in your organization; what is the average number of days to reoccurrence of the computer theft? How will your estimate of the average length of days to computer theft be different if you assume that there will be a theft at start of next year on January 1. What is the daily probability of occurrence of computer theft (give a range based on your different assumptions)?
4. Calculate the probability that a shooting will occur within a hospital by reviewing media reports on the web regarding these incidents. List the dates of the shootings and calculate the probability of the time to the event.

Rapid-Analysis Exercises

Assess the probability of unauthorized disclosure and security violations at one hospital and clinic by following these steps:

1. Interview at least one person in the organization to collect data on prevalence of various risk factors using the instrument available at the Chapter 9 section of this book's companion web site at ache.org/DecisionAnalysis.
2. Use time between events to assess the daily prevalence of risk factors.
3. From the information on industry patterns in Table 9.3, estimate the overall probability of unauthorized disclosure for your hospital or clinic.

TABLE 9.8 Worksheet for Reporting Risks

Category of Risk Factor	*Number of Incidents*	*First Reported Date*	*Last Reported Date*	*Average Days Between Occurrences*	*Daily Rate*
Theft of computer					
Theft of other equipment					
Theft of personal property					
Property damage					
Vehicle accident on premise					
Damage from natural causes					
Hazardous materials incidents					
Desktop security violations					
Unsolicited e-mails requesting personal information					
Unsolicited e-mails not requesting personal information					
Network penetration					

4. For your organization, interview your contact person and record responses on Table 9.8.
5. Use the information in the first four rows of the table to calculate the daily probability of various types of security violations.
6. Provide a report on what should be the top three priorities of the clinic or hospital.

Audio/Visual Chapter Aids

To help you understand the concepts of security-risk analysis, visit this book's companion web site at ache.org/DecisionAnalysis, go to Chapter 9, and view the audio/visual chapter aids.

Notes

1. This research was supported in parts by the National Capital Region Critical Infrastructure Project (NCR-CIP), a multi-university consortium managed by George Mason University, under grant #03-TU-03 by the U.S. Department of Homeland Security's Urban Area Security Initiative, and grant #2003CKWX0199 by the U.S. Department of Justice's Community Oriented Policing Services Program. The views expressed are those of the authors, and do not necessarily reflect those of the Department of Homeland Security or the Department of Justice.
2. See http://www.symantec.com/index.html.
3. See http://nvd.nist.gov.
4. Please note that this is not the same as the similarity of the Beslan school incident to the hospital situation, which is

$$\text{Similarity}_{\text{Beslan school, hospital}} = \frac{3}{3 + (0.20 \times 3) + (0.80 \times 4)} = 0.44.$$

References

Alemi, F., and V. Arya. 2005. "Objective Analysis of Privacy Risks." [Online information; retrieved 11/7/2005]. http://gunston.doit.gmu.edu/healthscience/730/RiskAnalysis.asp.

Apostolakis, G. E., and D. M. Lemon. 2005. "Screening Methodology for the Identification and Ranking of Infrastructure Vulnerabilities Due to Terrorism." *Risk Analysis* 25 (2): 361–76.

Becker, E. S., W. T. Roth, and M. Andrich. 1999. "Explicit Memory in Anxiety Disorders." *Journal of Abnormal Psychology* 108 (1): 153–163.

Bell, T. E., and K. Esch. 1989. "The Space Shuttle: A Case Study of Subjective Engineering." *IEEE Spectrum* 26 (6): 42–6.

Bonnabry, P., L. Cingria, F. Sadeghipour, H. Ing, C. Fonzo-Chrite, and R. E. Pfister. 2005. "Use of a Systematic Risk Analysis Method to Improve Safety in the Production of Pediatric Parenteral Nutrition Solutions." *Quality Safety Health Care* 14 (2): 93–8.

Cahill, L., and J. L. McGaugh. 1998. "Mechanisms of Emotional Arousal and Lasting Declarative Memory." *Trends in Neuroscience* 21 (7): 194–9.

Chang, S. E., M. Shinozuka, and J. E. Moore. 2000. "Probabilistic Earthquake Scenarios: Extending Risk Analysis Methodologies to Spatially Distributed Systems." *Earthquake Spectra* 16 (3): 557–72.

Cohen, B. L. 2003. "Probabilistic Risk Analysis for a High-Level Radioactive Waste Repository." *Risk Analysis* 23 (5): 909–15.

Colglazier, E.W., and R. K. Weatherwax. 1986. "Failure Estimates for the Space Shuttle." In *Abstracts for Society Analysis Annual Meeting*, 80. McLean, VA: Society for Risk Analysis.

Cooke, R. M. 1991. *Experts in Uncertainty: Opinion and Subjective Probability in Science*. New York: Oxford University Press.

Cooke, R. M., and E. Jager. 1998. "A Probabilistic Model for the Failure Frequency of Underground Gas Pipelines." *Risk Analysis* 18 (4): 511–27.

DeRosier, J., E. Stalhandske, J. P. Bagain, and T. Nudell. 2002. "Using Health Care Failure Mode and Effect Analysis: The VA National Center for Patient Safety's Prospective Risk Analysis System." *Joint Commission Journal of Quality Improvement* 28 (5): 248–67.

Ellwart, T., M. Rinck, and E. S. Becker. 2003. "Selective Memory and Memory Deficits in Depressed Inpatients." *Depression and Anxiety* 17 (4): 197–206.

Environmental Protection Agency. 1976. *Reactor Safety Study Oversight Hearings before the Subcommittee on Energy and the Environment of the Committee on Interior and Insular Affairs, House of Representatives.* 94th Cong., 2d sess., June 11.

Ewing, R. C., C. S. Palenik, and L. F. Konikow. 2004. Comment on "Probabilistic Risk Analysis for a High-Level Radioactive Waste Repository" by B. L. Cohen. *Risk Analysis* 24 (6): 1417.

Gardner, W. L., C. L. Pickett, and M. B. Brewer. 2000. "Social Exclusion and Selective Memory: How the Need to Belong Influences Memory for Social Events." *Personality and Social Psychology Bulletin* 26 (4): 486–96.

Garrick, B. J., and S. Kaplan. 1999. "A Decision Theory Perspective on the Disposal of High-Level Radioactive Waste." *Risk Analysis* 19 (5): 903–13.

Gray, G. M., and D. P. Ropeik. 2002. "Dealing with the Dangers of Fear: The Role of Risk Communication." *Health Affairs* 21 (6): 106–16.

Haimes, Y. Y., and T. Longstaff. 2002. "The Role of Risk Analysis in the Protection of Critical Infrastructures Against Terrorism." *Risk Analysis* 22 (3): 439–44.

Heidelberger, P. 1995. "Fast Simulation of Rare Events in Queueing and Reliability Models." *ACM Transactions on Modeling and Computer Simulation (TOMACS)* 5 (1): 43–85.

Kaplan, S., and B. J. Garrick. 1981. "On the Quantitative Definition of Risk." *Risk Analysis* 1 (1):11–27.

Kaczmarek, Z. 2003. "The Impact of Climate Variability on Flood Risk in Poland." *Risk Analysis* 23 (3): 559–66.

Keefer, D. L. 2001. "Practice Abstract." *Interfaces* 31 (5): 62–4.

Kemeny, J. 1979. *Report of the President's Commission on the Accident at Three Mile Island.* Washington, DC: Government Printing Office.

Kollar, J. J., B. C. Lipton, W. T. Mech, A. D. Pelletier, D. S. Powell, E. C. Shoop, R. S. Skolnik, G. G. Venter, D. L. Wasserman, T. A. Weidman, and S. Ringsted. 2002. *Terrorism Insurance Coverage in the Aftermath of September 11th.* Washington, DC: American Academy of Actuaries. [Online report; retrieved 10/11/05] http://www.actuary.org/pdf/casualty/terrorism_may02.pdf.

Leask, A., V. Delpech, and J. McAnulty. 2003. "Anthrax and Other Suspect Powders: Initial Responses to an Outbreak of Hoaxes and Scares." *New South Wales Public Health Bulletin* 14 (11–12): 218–21.

Lewis, H. W., R. J. Budnitz, A. W. Castleman, D. E. Dorfan, F. C. Finlayson, R. L. Garwin, L. C. Hebel, S. M. Keeny, R. A. Muller, T. B. Taylor, G. F. Smoot, F. von Hippel, H. Bethe, and W. K. H. Panofsky. 1975. "Report to the American Physical Society from the Study Group on Light-Water Reactor Safety." *Review of Modern Physics* 47 (Suppl. 1): S1–S123.

Mai, S., and C. Zimmerman. 2003. *Risk Analysis: Tool for Integrated Coastal Planning.* Proclamation of the 6th International Conference on Coastal and Port Engineering in Developing Countries, Columbo, Sri Lanka.

Mobus, C. 1979. "The Analysis of Non-Symmetric Similarity Judgments: Drift Model, Comparison Hypothesis, Tversky's Contrast Model and His Focus Hypothesis." *Archiv Fur Psychologie* 131 (2): 105–136.

Moore, D. R. J., B. E. Sample, G. W. Suter, B. R. Parkhurst, and T. R. Scott. 1999. "A Probabilistic Risk Assessment of the Effects of Methylmercury and PCBs on Mink and Kingfishers Along East Fork Poplar Creek, Oak Ridge, Tennessee, USA." *Environmental Toxicology and Chemistry*, 18 (12): 2941–53.

Ortwin, R. 1998. "Three Decades of Risk Research: Accomplishments and New Challenges." *Journal of Risk Research* 1 (1): 49–71.

Pate-Cornell, M. E., and P. S. Fischbeck. 1993. "Probabilistic Risk Analysis and Risk-Based Priority Scale for the Tiles of the Space Shuttle." *Reliability Engineering and System Safety* 40 (3): 221–38.

———. 1994. "Risk Management for the Tiles of the Space Shuttle." *Interfaces* 24 (1): 64–86.

Planning Research Corporation. 1989. *Independent Assessment of Shuttle Accident Scenario Probabilities for Galileo Mission and Comparison with NSTS Program Assessment.* Los Angeles: Planning Research Corporation.

Rasmussen, N. C. 1981. "The Application of Probabilistic Risk Assessment Techniques to Energy Technologies." *Annual Review of Energy* 6:123–38.

Rezmierski, V. E., D. M. Rothschild, A. S. Kazanis, and R. D. Rivas. *Final Report of the Computer Incident Factor Analysis and Categorization (CIFAC) Project.* Ann Arbor, MI: Regents of the University of Michigan. [Online report; retrieved 10/28/05]. http://www.educause.edu/ir/library/pdf/CSD4207.pdf.

Rogovin, M., and G. T. Frampton. 1980. *Three Mile Island: A Report to the Commissioners and to the Public.* Washington, DC: Government Printing Office.

Rotstein, A. H. 2002. "Shooting Leaves Four Dead at University of Arizona." *The Daily Texan:* World & Nation, October, 29.

Sadiq, R., T. Husain, B. Veitch, and N. Bose. 2003. "Distribution of Arsenic and Copper in Sediment Pore Water: An Ecological Risk Assessment Case Study for Offshore Drilling Waste Discharges." *Risk Analysis* 23 (6): 1309–21.

Safie, F. M. 1991. "A Statistical Approach for Risk Management of Space Shuttle Main Engine Components." In *Probabilistic Safety Assessment and Management: Proceedings of the International Conference on Probabilistic Safety Assessment and Management.* New York: Elsevier Science Publishing Co., Inc., 13–8.

———. 1992. "Use of Probabilistic Design Methods for NASA Applications." *American Society of Mechanical Engineers Symposium on Reliability Technology.* New York: American Society of Mechanical Engineers, 17–24.

———. 1994. "A Risk Assessment Methodology for the Space Shuttle External Tank Welds." *Annual Proceedings on Reliability and Maintainability Symposium.* Anaheim, CA: Reliability and Maintainability Symposium, 230–4.

Schmidt, S. R. 2004 "Autobiographical Memories for the September 11th Attacks: Reconstructive Errors and Emotional Impairment of Memory." *Memory and Cognition* 32 (3): 443–54.

Schwarz, G., and A. Tversky. 1980. "On the Reciprocity of Proximity Relations." *Journal of Mathematical Psychology* 22 (3): 157–75.

Science Applications International Corporation. 1995. *Probabilistic Risk Assessment of the Space Shuttle.* Washington DC: NASA.

Siegel, M. 2005. *False Alarm: The Truth About the Epidemic of Fear.* Hoboken, NJ: John Wiley and Sons.

Siegel, P. S., D. M. McCord, and A. R. Crawford. 1982. "An Experimental Note on Tversky's Features of Similarity." *Bulletin of Psychonomic Society* 19 (3): 141–2.

Slob, W., and M. N. Pieters. 1998. "A Probabilistic Approach for Deriving Acceptable Human Intake Limits and Human Health Risks for Toxicological Studies: General Framework" *Risk Analysis* 18 (6): 787–98.

Taylor, C., A. Krings, and J. Alves-Foss. 2002. "Risk Analysis and Probabilistic Survivability Assessment (RAPSA): An Assessment Approach for Power Substation Hardening." Paper presented at the ACM Workshop on Scientific Aspects of Cyber Terrorism, Washington, DC.

Tversky, A. 1977. "Features of Similarity." *Psychological Review* 84 (4): 327–52.

Union of Concerned Scientists. 1977. *The Risk of Nuclear Power Reactors: A Review of the NRC Reactor Study.* Cambridge, MA: Union of Concerned Scientists.

U.S. Nuclear Regulatory Commission. 1975. *Reactor Safety Study, WASH-1400.* Washington, DC: U.S. NRC.

———. 1983. *PRA Procedure Guide: A Guide to the Performance of Probabilistic Risk Assessments for Nuclear Power Plants, NUREG/CR-2300.* Washington, DC: U.S. Nuclear Regulatory Commission.

Voortman, H. G., P. van Gelder, and J. K. Vrijling. 2002. *Risk-Based Design of Large Scale Flood Defense Systems.* 28th International Conference on Coastal Engineering, Cardiff, Wales.

CHAPTER

10

PROGRAM EVALUATION

David H. Gustafson and Farrokh Alemi

Large-scale evaluations of health and social service programs are commonly initiated to help policymakers decide on the future direction of programs. They often examine issues such as the following:

- Approval of the program and enrollment of the patients (e.g., elapsed time from announcement of the funding to enrollment of first patient);
- Correspondence between what was approved and what was done (e.g., the percent of program objectives planned that were actually implemented);
- The demand for the proposed program (e.g., the ratio of patients to the service capacity);
- Description of the patients (e.g., the number and demographic background of patients);
- Provider satisfaction (e.g., measures of conflict among providers and satisfaction with care);
- Satisfaction with the program (e.g., patient satisfaction surveys); and
- Affect on patient outcomes (e.g., measures of patients' mortality, morbidity, or health status);

Not surprisingly, with this kind of interest, program evaluation has become a big business and an important field of study; program evaluations are requested and funded by virtually every department of health and social services, not to mention many legislatures, governors, and city administrations.

The basic concept of evaluating social and healthcare programs, as shown in Figure 10.1, is straightforward. A program is expected to meet certain performance standards (A). The program actually performs at a level (B) that may equal or exceed the standards or may fall short because of flaws or unexpected environmental influences. Actual performance is compared to expected performance (C), and decisions are made about which, if any, of the discrepancies are worrisome (D). The findings are explained and interpreted to decision makers (E), and changes are introduced in either system performance or the expectations of it (F).

This book has a companion web site that features narrated presentations, animated examples, PowerPoint slides, online tools, web links, additional readings, and examples of students' work. To access this chapter's learning tools, go to ache.org/DecisionAnalysis and select Chapter 10.

Although the basic concepts of evaluation are simple, actual implementation can be quite complex, and numerous evaluation techniques and philosophies have been introduced over the years (Alemi 1988). The major approaches are categorized as experimental, case study, and cost-benefit analysis.

Some researchers have advocated an experimental approach, with carefully designed studies using experimental and control groups, random assignment of subjects, and pre- and post tests (Reynolds 1991).

Variations on this experimental theme often remove the random assignment criterion. These "quasi-experimental" designs interject alternative explanations for findings (Campbell and Stanley 1966). Many process improvement efforts can be thought of as quasi-experimental studies (Benedetto 2003; Alemi, Haack, and Nemes 2001). An experimental evaluation is not always necessary, but when it is, random assignment must be an essential element of it.

Another school of thought advocates examining case studies (Barker and Barker 1994; Alemi 1988; Brown 2003), arguing that case studies are superior to experiments because of the difficulty of identifying criteria for experimental evaluation. Further, experiments require random subject assignment and pre- and post tests, both of which are impractical because they interfere with program operation. Case studies use unobtrusive methods to examine a broad range of objectives and procedures that are sensitive to unintentional side effects. This approach helps administrators improve programs instead of just judging them. Some case studies report on services offered and the characteristics of their use, while others are less concerned with the physical world and emphasize the values and goals of the actors. Their reports tend to contain holistic impressions that convey the mood of the program. Any evaluation must contain case studies to help people really understand and act on the conclusions. In the context of continuous quality improvement, the importance of case studies is emphasized by insisting on expressing the problem in the "customer's voice."

Cost-benefit analysis evaluates programs by measuring costs and benefits in monetary terms and calculating the ratio of costs to benefits (Neumann 2005; Weinstein et al. 1996). This ratio is an efficiency statistic

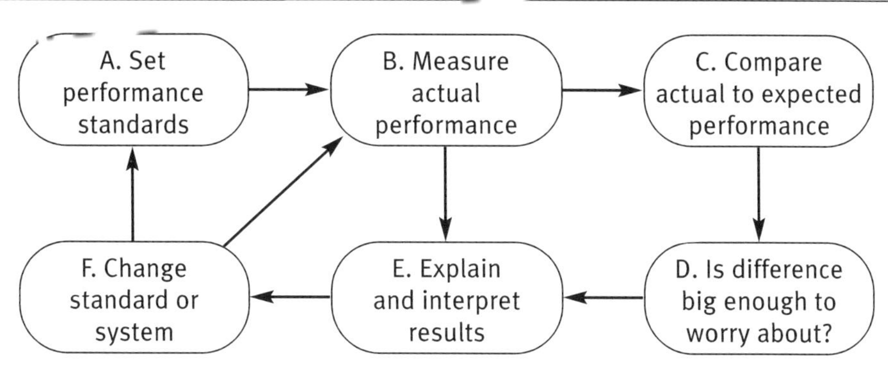

FIGURE 10.1 Schematic Representation of Program Evaluation

showing what is gained for various expenditures. There are many types of cost-benefit analysis. Some analyses assume that the market price of services fairly and accurately measures program benefits; others measure benefits on the basis of opinion surveys. Variations on the cost-benefit theme involve comparisons that do not translate everything into a dollar equivalent. The critical characteristic of those studies is an ability to compare what you get against what it costs to get it.

Many Evaluations Are Ignored

Although program evaluations take a good deal of time and money, their results are often ignored (Hoffmann and Graf von der Schulenburg 2000; Drummond 1994). Even if interesting data are collected and analyzed, evaluations have no effect if their results are not directly relevant and timely to a decision. Often, evaluation reports present a variety of unrelated findings and thus confuse rather than clarify the decision maker's choices. Despite calls for evidence-based practice, many clinicians ignore small and large evaluation studies (Zeitz and McCutcheon 2003).

Evaluation studies with little effect generally began with a poor design. An evaluation can gain influence if the evaluator understands and focuses on the options, values, and uncertainties of the decision makers. To provide the kind of evaluation that supports policy formation, relevance to the decision must be designed at the start, not tacked on at the end. Edwards, Gutentag, and Snapper (1975) wrote:

> Evaluations, we believe, exist (or perhaps only should exist) to facilitate intelligent decision making . . . an evaluation research program will often satisfy curiosity. But if it does no more, if it does not improve the basis for

> decisions about the program and its competitors, then it loses its distinctive character as evaluation research and becomes simply research (p. 140).

Decision-Oriented Evaluation Design

Certain design factors can increase the relevance of an evaluation to the actual decision making. The evaluators should do the following:

- *Identify the primary users of the evaluation.* Often, evaluators say their findings are intended for policymakers, not particular individuals. The evaluators do not contact an individual policymaker because they consider such person's views irrelevant or they perceive that such individuals hold their positions temporarily, while the policy issue and the evaluation task remain more or less permanent. It is best to name the decision makers before designing evaluation studies to meet their needs. Asking decision makers is preferred even if these individuals will not be on the job when evaluation results become available because decision makers' information needs are often dictated by their positions, not by their idiosyncratic preferences. Even though decision makers change, their needs remain stable, and identifying the needs of a single decision maker is not a waste of effort because it will help meet the needs of future decision makers.
- *Identify the decision-making needs of decision makers, and provide information to meet their needs.* Gustafson and Thesen (1981) found that once decision makers' information needs were prioritized in order of importance, the top 65 percent of the priorities had nothing to do with the type of questions addressed by typical evaluation data. Decision makers tend to seek help on issues that depend more on values and expectations than on objective statistics. Although program statistics cannot be ignored, program evaluations should provide information that will actually influence decisions.
- *As part of the evaluation, suggest options that creatively address the issues.* Too often, evaluations produce evidence about the strengths and weaknesses of the existing system, touching only briefly on what improvements could be made. An effective evaluation must devote considerable effort to identifying improvements that will remove the weaknesses.
- *Identify and attempt to reduce the most important uncertainties involved in the system being evaluated.* Frequently, a system performs well under some conditions and poorly under others. Attempts to improve system performance are limited by the inability to predict

when true differentiating conditions will arise. Evaluators should identify the differentiating conditions, develop means to predict when they will arise, or propose system improvements that are less susceptible to variations in those conditions.

- *Explain how they reached their results.* Statistical analysis can satisfy detached, rational decision makers, but many policymakers find that examples underscore the justification for conclusions in a more persuasive manner than rational and statistical arguments alone. Such examples can be constructed by careful evaluation of the program. To explain the evaluation results, examples should allow analysts to observe, experience, and describe how the system actually operates. Succinct examples can make an evaluation report "come alive" and help decision makers feel and understand the consequences of their decisions at several levels. The use of examples has three benefits: (1) it permits you to describe how the system actually functions; (2) it permits you to compare actual operation to intended operation; and (3) if done by qualified personnel, it omits the need to assess the adequacy of the system's operation.
- *Examine the sensitivity of the evaluation findings to assess their practical significance.* With a sufficiently large database, almost any difference can be statistically significant. But small differences, even if statistically significant, may not matter. Analysts should conduct a sensitivity analysis to see how erroneous the assumptions can be before they cause the decision makers to act mistakenly. Evaluation studies can include sensitivity analyses but rarely do.
- *Present results more quickly and when they can be most useful.* Too often, decisions must be made before an evaluation is complete. Analysts should present reliable preliminary findings to decision makers as they go along. This shows that they are sensitive to the timing of a decision, particularly in terms of knowing the critical moments in the policy process. Reliable information that could influence policy almost always surfaces during an evaluation and not only at its end. If evaluators know the timing of a decision, they can give input when it is most useful. The decisions will be made anyway, and policymakers will act on whatever information they have.

In summary, program evaluation should be tied to the decision-making process. The remainder of this chapter presents a nine-step strategy for such a decision-oriented evaluation design. This presentation will be clarified by referring to an evaluation of the nursing home quality assurance process conducted by Gustafson and his colleagues (Gustafson, Fiss, and Fryback 1981; Gustafson et al. 1990).

Continued rises in nursing home costs in the United States have stimulated increasing debate about how regulation can improve the industry. Some critics find the government ineffective at evaluating nursing homes (Winzelberg 2003). These critics argue that current surveys of nursing home quality are too frequent, are too intensive, and have little relation to the health status and functional ability of nursing home residents. Gustafson, Fiss, and Fryback (1981) were asked to evaluate the process of surveying nursing home quality (this work was continued in Gustafson et al. 1990), and this chapter uses their experience to illustrate how a decision-oriented evaluation is done.

Step 1: Identify the Decision Makers

The first step in planning an evaluation is to examine the potential users and to invite them to devise the plan of action. In the nursing home example, three groups were expected to use the evaluation results: (1) the state government, to decide what program to implement; (2) the federal government, to decide whether to support the state's decision and whether to transfer aspects of the project to other states; and (3) several lobbying groups (nursing home associations), to choose their positions on the topic. The evaluators identified individuals from each group, asked them to collaborate with the evaluation team, and kept them informed of progress and preliminary conclusions throughout the study.

Step 2: Examine Concerns and Assumptions

Next, the evaluators talked to the chosen decision makers (the program administrator and experts on the program, for example) to determine their concerns and assumptions and to identify the potential strengths, weakness, and intended operations of the program.

In the nursing home example, a decision maker who was concerned about the paperwork burden for quality assurance deemed the effort excessive and wasteful. A second decision maker was concerned with the cost of the quality assurance process and worried that it would divert money from resident care. A third was more concerned that quality assurance funds be distributed in a way that helped not only to identify problems but also to facilitate solutions. This person preferred to find solutions that would bring nursing homes into compliance with regulations. A fourth decision maker felt that the quality assurance process should attend not only to clients' medical needs but also to their psychological and social needs. All of these divergent objectives were important because they suggested where to look while designing a quality assurance process to address the decision makers' real needs.

The evaluators also helped identify and clarify each decision maker's assumptions. These assumptions are important because, regardless of accuracy, they can influence decisions if not challenged. One decision maker believed the state must play a policing role in quality assurance by identifying problems and penalizing offending homes. Another person believed the state should adopt the role of change agent and take any necessary steps to raise the quality of care, even if it had to pay a home to solve its problems. Arguments for and against these philosophies about the role of government were examined, and although new data on these issues were not collected, the final report reviewed others' research on the matter.

Step 3: Add Your Observations

Another important method of examining a program is to use one's own observations. The perceptions of decision makers, while very useful for examining problems in detail, do not prove that problems exist, only that they are perceived to exist. Thus, it is important to examine reports of problems to see that they are, indeed, real problems. Members of the evaluation team should watch the system from beginning to end to create a picture of its functioning. A system analyst should literally follow the quality assurance team through a nursing home and draw a flowchart of the process.

Although observational studies are not statistically valid, they can add substantial explanatory power and credibility to an evaluation and allow you to explain failure and suggest improvements. A valuable side effect of such observations is that you will gather stories describing specific successes and failures. These stories have powerful explanatory value, often more than the statistical conclusions of the evaluation. The observations not only suggest how and where to modify the program, but they also indicate areas that should be targeted for empirical data collection.

Step 4: Conduct a Mock Evaluation

The next step is performing a mock evaluation, which is a field test to refine the evaluation protocol and increase efficiency. The mock evaluation keeps the decision maker informed and involved. Too often, decision makers first see the results of the evaluation when reading the final report. While this sequence probably allows enough time to produce a fine product, time alone guarantees neither quality nor relevance. It is preferable to inform the decision maker about the findings as the project proceeds, because information being gathered could influence the decision. Decision makers will want access to this information. The mock evaluation lets the decision maker determine which areas require more emphasis, allowing you to alter your approach while you have time.

A mock evaluation is similar to a real one except that experts' opinions replace much of the data. This "make-believe" evaluation helps estimate how much money and time are needed to complete the evaluation. It also changes the data collection procedures, sample-size requirements (because a more realistic estimate of variance in the data is gained), and analysis procedures. Finally, the mock evaluation gives a preview of likely conclusions, which allows decision makers to tell whether the projected report will address the vital issues as well as identify weaknesses in the methodology that can still be corrected.

Critics of such previews wonder about the ethics of presenting findings that may be proven wrong by careful subsequent observation. But supporters counter by questioning the ethics of withholding information that could inform policy. These questions represent two extreme positions on a difficult issue. It is true that preliminary results may receive more credibility than they deserve. Moreover, decision makers may press to alter the evaluation design to prevent reaching embarrassing conclusions. Those dangers may be outweighed by the alternatives of producing irrelevant data, missing critical questions, or failing to contribute valuable information when it could help the policy debate.

In the nursing home example, after the decision makers had read the mock report, they were asked to speculate about how its findings might affect their actions. As the evaluation team described its preliminary findings, the decision makers explained their possible courses of action and listed other information that would increase the evaluation's utility.

It is important to make sure that evaluation findings lead to action. Decision makers can react in many ways to various findings. Some consider negative findings a sufficient basis for changing their opinions and modifying the system, while others continue to adhere to existing opinions. If your findings do not motivate the decision makers to change the system, this is a signal that you could be collecting the wrong data. At this point, you can decide to collect different data or analyze it more appropriately. The goal remains to provide information that really influences the decision maker's choices.

In the nursing home study, the evaluation team observed several nursing home surveys, talked with interested parties, developed a flowchart of the process, and then asked the group to consider what they would do differently if the evaluation suggested that current efforts were indeed effective. The question was then repeated for negative findings on various dimensions. The discussion revealed that the experts, like others in the field, believed existing quality assurance efforts were inefficient and ineffective, and these people expected the evaluation to confirm their intuition. They thought evaluation findings would make a difference in the course of action they would follow. In other words, they were certain about the effectiveness of the current system but uncertain about how to improve it. This is an important distinction, because an evaluation study that only gauged the effectiveness of the current system would confirm their suspicions but not help them act. What they needed was a study that would pave the way for change, not just to criticize a system that was clearly failing.

At this point, the evaluation team and its advisory group developed an alternative method of nursing home quality assurance that helped reallocate resources by focusing on influencing the few problematic homes, not the majority of adequate ones. A brief nursing home survey was designed to identify a problem home and target it for more intensive examination. Then, an evaluation was designed to contrast this alternative approach to the existing method of evaluation. Thus, the mock evaluation led to the creation of an alternative system for improving nursing home quality; instead of just evaluating quality of the current system, the team compared and contrasted two evaluation systems.

The mock evaluation is a preview that helps the decision makers see what information the evaluation will provide and suggest improvements that could be made in the design. "Showing off" the evaluation also makes the decision makers more likely to delay their decision making until the final report is complete.

Step 5: Pick a Focus

Focus is vital. In the planning stage, discussions with decision makers usually expand the scope of the upcoming evaluation, but fixed resources force you to choose which decision makers' uncertainties to address and how to do so. For example, further examination of the potential effect of the evaluation of nursing home quality assurance revealed a sequence of decisions that affected whether evaluation findings would lead to action. The state policymakers were responsible for deciding whether to adopt the proposed changes in quality assurance. This decision needed the approval of federal decision makers, who relied on the opinions of several experts as well as on the evaluation. Both state and federal decisions to modify the quality assurance method depended on a number of factors, including public pressure to balance the budget, demand for more nursing home services, the mood of Congress toward deregulation, and the positions of the nursing home industry and various interest groups. Each of these factors could have been included in the effort, but only a few were selected because of budget constraints.

Some factors in the decision-making process may be beyond the expertise of the evaluation team. For example, the evaluators might not be qualified to assess the mood of Congress. Although the evaluation need not provide data on all important aspects of the decision process, the choice not to provide data must be made consciously. Thus, the analyst must identify early in the process which components to include and which to exclude as a conscious and informed part of evaluation planning.

Sloppy analyses are not being advocated here. Rather, evaluations often operate on limited budgets and thus must allocate resources to produce the best product without "breaking the budget." This means that specificity in some areas must be sacrificed to gain greater detail elsewhere.

Step 6: Identify Criteria

Now the evaluation team and decision makers set the evaluation criteria, based on program objectives and proposed strengths and weakness of the program. (See Chapter 2 for a discussion of how to identify evaluation criteria, or attributes; see Chapter 6 to see how the analysis can be done using a group of decision makers.)

The nursing home evaluation focused on a number of questions, one of which was the difference between the existing method of quality assurance and the alternative method. The following criteria were used to evaluate this issue:

- *Relation to regulatory action.* The quality assurance effort should lead to consistent regulatory actions.
- *Ease of use.* Administering quality assurance should interfere with delivering nursing home care no more than necessary.
- *Reliability.* The quality assurance effort should produce consistent findings, no matter who does the reviews.

- *Validity.* The findings should correlate with adverse outcomes of nursing home care (such as an increasing rate of deterioration in residents' ability to attend to their daily activities).
- *Influence.* Quality assurance should change the way long-term care is delivered.
- *Cost.* The cost of conducting quality assurance must be measured to allow the selection of the most cost-effective method.

In the nursing home example, an evaluation design was created to divide the state into three regions. In the lower half of the state (and the most populous), nursing homes were randomly assigned to control and experimental conditions, after ensuring that an equal number of proprietary nursing homes and nonprofit nursing homes, of similar sizes and treating similar patients, would be placed in each group. The northern half of the state was divided into two regions, one receiving the new regulatory method and one not. This was done to observe how the management of the regulatory process would change the results. Such random assignment greatly increased the credibility of the evaluation.

A second aspect of design was the measures used. Previously, a nursing home's quality was judged on the basis of the number of conditions, standards, and elements found out of compliance. However, it was apparent that radical differences in the severity of violations could take place within a level (e.g., element). It was decided to convene a panel of experts to numerically rate the severity of different violations.

Step 7: Set Expectations

Once the evaluation design was completed, decision makers were asked to predict the evaluation findings and express what they expect to find. This request accomplished two things. First, it identified the decision makers' biases so the team could design an evaluation that responded to them. Second, it gave a basis for comparing evaluation findings to the decision maker's expectations, without attributing them to specific people. The effect of evaluation results is often diluted by hindsight. Reviewers might respond to the results by saying, "That is what I would have expected, but. . . ." Documenting expectations in advance prevents such dilution.

In the nursing home example, decision makers expected that the alternative method would be slightly better than the current method, but they were surprised at how much better it performed. There were substantial cost savings as well as improvements in effectiveness. Because their expectations had been documented, their reactions were more akin to "Aha!" than to "That's what we expected." This helped create a momentum for change.

Step 8: Compare Actual and Expected Performance

In this phase, data are collected to compare actual and expected performance. The observed findings are compared to the decision maker's expected findings. (For more information on data collection and statistical comparison, consult the many books on evaluation that cover these topics in detail.) There are a variety of ways this can be done. One common way is to replace actual and expected performance comparisons with a comparison of the control (or currently operating) and experimental (new) methods.

Another way is to use statistical process control tools. First, a control chart is created, showing progression of time in the *x*-axis. Three lines are plotted: One line shows the actual observed performances of the program, and the other two lines show the upper and lower control limits based on the expected performance of the program. When the observed rate is outside the control limits, a statically significant change in the program is signified.

Step 9: Examine Sensitivity of Actions to Findings

Sensitivity analysis allows you to examine the practical effect of your findings. In this step, decision makers were asked to describe the various courses of action they would have taken if they had received specific evaluation findings. Then they were asked to consider what they would have done upon receiving different findings. Once the threshold above which the actions would change was identified, the probability that the findings could contain errors large enough to cause a mistake was calculated. Using the nursing home example, the evaluation might have revealed that one method of quality assurance was 5 percent more expensive than another. Decision makers might determine that savings of 20 percent would induce them to change their decision. In this case, the decision makers would be asked to identify a threshold, say 15 percent, above which they would change their decision. The evaluation team would then calculate the probability that the findings contained an error large enough to exceed the threshold. In other words, the team would then state the chance that a reported 5 percent difference in cost is indeed a 15 percent difference in cost.

Sensitivity analysis allows decision makers to modify their confidence in the evaluation findings. If the findings suggest that the reported practical differences are real and not the result of chance, then confidence increases. Otherwise, it decreases.

Summary

This chapter has provided a step-by-step approach to using decision analysis in program evaluation. The primary uses for the evaluation are identified. The decision makers' assumptions are identified, and information is provided to meet the need. A particular focus is selected, data are gathered, and the program's performance is compared to expected outcomes. The sensitivity of the conclusions are examined, and new options are proposed. A decision analytic design engages decision makers throughout the effort and actively focuses on data that are likely to lead to action. One advantage of the proposed approach is the extensive involvement of decision makers in various components of the evaluation.

Review What You Know

1. Is it necessary to identify one or more decision makers before conducting a program evaluation as described in this chapter? Why or why not?
2. Why should a program evaluation focus on decisions? Why not focus on cost or improvements in access to care or some other feature?
3. What is the point of doing mock evaluations? What are the advantages?
4. How does a decision analytic evaluation select criteria used for evaluation?
5. What are the steps in a decision analytic evaluation?
6. What is the point of doing a sensitivity analysis in a decision analytic evaluation?
7. Should an evaluator speed up the preparation of a report? Why or why not?
8. Why should an evaluator collect information about a policymaker's expectations before presenting evaluation reports?

Rapid-Analysis Exercises

This exercise is designed to help you decide whether you should evaluate a service and how you should do so. For many of the questions, there is no right or wrong answer. Just provide an answer that fits your preferences. To proceed, you must have a specific service in mind, either a service where you work or a service where you are a customer. Assume that you are the manager of this service. The purpose of the activity is to help you become more aware of your own thoughts and reservations about conducting an evaluation of services.

This exercise is in three parts. In the first part, you will think about the need for program evaluation. In part two, you will design a way of evaluating your customers' satisfaction with your service. In the last part, you will contrast your design with what was covered in the chapter and, in this manner, gain insights about some of the ideas expressed in the chapter. Before proceeding, identify the particular service you will evaluate.

Part 1

Evaluation takes time and money. To maintain independence, an evaluation of the effect of your service is best done by independent groups of investigators. Other evaluations (e.g., market studies, studies of patient satisfaction with your service) can be done in-house. No matter who does the evaluation, it still requires much planning, data collection, analysis, and reporting. These activities could compete with your ability to focus your funds and time on organizing and improving the service. Sometimes evaluations are not done because the effects of the services are known or can be deduced from the experiences of others. The following questions will help you understand why you may be ambivalent about conducting an evaluation of your services:

1. What reservations do you have about conducting an evaluation of your service?
2. Is there sufficient evidence in the literature or in the industry to suggest that what you are doing will work well for patients of different backgrounds?

If you think about it, evaluation could have many benefits. It could tell you and your clients that the service is effective in changing lives. It can tell you how to improve, and everyone—even the best among us—needs to improve. It can help you convince third-party payers to pay for your service. In this section, you are asked a number of questions about the implications of not evaluating the service.

3. Would it help your efforts to market your service if you knew more about the people who are currently using your service and how they feel about it?

4. Describe how a survey of your clients could help you improve the service or improve the way it is marketed.
5. Would patients who use your service ask for the evaluation of the service (particularly when there is news coverage of unique events), or have your patients already evaluated your reputation by the time they come to the service?
6. Would your efforts to market the service to third-party payers be hurt if you do not have data that the service works (e.g., that it saves money, improves access, or improves quality of health services)?
7. Inside your organization, would your career be affected if you do not have data to show that what you did was reasonable? In other words, do you have a lot of support from different managers so long as the service makes money, or is the utility of the service already being questioned?
8. What might go wrong if you fail to evaluate the service? Think through the next six months to the next two years. Describe a situation where you would say "Oops, I wished I had evaluated the effect of our service."
9. Think harder. Is there some opportunity missed or negative consequences that may happen to you or to your organization as a consequence of failing to evaluate your service?

The following questions are designed to help you determine whether you should evaluate your service, what type of evaluation would be most useful, and who should conduct it:

10. Now that you have gotten this far, how do you feel about the evaluation and the type of questions that it should address?
    - There is no need for an evaluation.
    - Evaluate market, including characteristics and sizes of patient groups attracted.
    - Evaluate patients' satisfaction with service.
    - Evaluate effect of service on patients' health status and lifestyles.
    - Do other types of evaluations.
11. Do you feel that you have the sufficient training or experience to conduct the evaluation yourself, or would you like help on how to evaluate your service?

Part 2

This part is intended to help you evaluate the satisfaction with your program services. As before, you must have a specific service in mind before proceeding.

Think through the goal of the evaluation survey. Sometimes, purchasers are interested in repeated evaluation efforts that not only document problems but also show a systematic effort to resolve them. You may also engage in an evaluation to help you find and fix problems. In this case, you are not so much interested in reporting the problems you find but in fixing them and going on. There are many other reasons too.

1. What is your real reason for wanting to know if consumers are satisfied with your service?

One of the first issues you need to think through is who should do the work. Sometimes it is useful to engage a third party, which will help convince purchasers and other reviewers of the data that independent evaluations were done. If you evaluate your own efforts, there is always a suspicion that you may not report the whole story. In addition, some third-party surveyors can benchmark your service against your competitors. For example, they can report that your service is among the top 5 percent of all services. Purchasers and consumers like benchmarked data. At the same time, asking others to help you evaluate is time consuming and expensive, and it may interfere with keeping your activities secret until it is publicly released.

2. Given these issues, who do you think should evaluate your service? Why?

Next, you need to determine the type of evaluation and how often it should be conducted. This depends in part on what questions you want answered. If, for example, you want to know which target group (e.g., people of certain age or gender) is most satisfied with your service, then an occasional cross-section analysis is sufficient. In a cross-section analysis, you would survey the patients after they have been exposed to your service. Cross-section analysis can also be used to benchmark your service against other services. If you plan to regularly survey your clients over time, then you need a longitudinal study. These types of studies are best if you want to know whether exposure to your service changed the level of satisfaction patients have over time.

3. Do you think you may need to conduct a longitudinal or a cross-sectional study?
4. How often do you want to evaluate the satisfaction with your service?

Satisfaction surveys can be misleading in many ways. One possibility is that improvement in satisfaction may be related to other events and not to your service. For example, patients' lifestyle adjustments may change their satisfaction with your service. To control for this type of error, it is important to contrast the improvement against a control group that has been exposed to another service. Another source of error could be that, over time, respondents are learning the system more and thus are more satisfied with the services they are using. Dissatisfied individuals are unlikely to use your service. Surveying only users of your services may mislead you by painting a rosy picture of clients' satisfaction. To control for these types of errors, it is important to contrast your services with others and to explicitly look for customers who are not repeat users.

5. What steps will you take to ensure that changes in patient care mix are not misleading you?

Other sources of errors are also possible. Campbell and Stanley (1966) highlight a list of common errors in survey research. Given the various sources of error, you need to choose for yourself how important it is to have an accurate picture of clients' satisfaction with your service. At the extreme, you can randomly assign people to two services: yours and an alternative placebo service. Random assignments control for most types of errors. But random assignment is expensive and, in some occasions, blind assignment may be unethical. Subjects have to volunteer to be assigned to the experimental or a placebo service, and subjects may refuse to participate. Another approach is repeated evaluation of satisfaction over time. It provides a time series of data that control for some errors. Because subjects have self-selected to be part of these studies, the result may be rosier than if all subjects were included. The least accurate analysis is to do studies without any comparison group.

6. Should your analysis consist of randomly assigned control groups, repeated evaluations over time, or no control group?

Obviously, you will survey the people who received your service, but you can also survey others to serve as a comparison group for you. If you do so, you would need to determine which type of comparison group you will include. If you need a preponderance of evidence, track a control group over time and use it as your comparison group. If you need data that are beyond reasonable doubt, then choose a control group that is randomly assigned.

7. Will you survey others who have not used your service as a comparison group?
8. If so, will you track a control group over time or use a group that is randomly assigned?

Next, you need to determine what you want to ask. Some of the items in satisfaction surveys include the following:

- Overall satisfaction with quality of the services
- Ease of use of the services
- Satisfaction with the integration of the services with other health services
- Accuracy, comprehensiveness, usefulness, and timeliness of the information and services received
- Comfort received
- Skills gained from cognitive services and support groups

You do not need to include all of the above items, nor do you need to limit your surveys to above items. There are many data banks of surveys. Keep in mind that standardized surveys allow you to benchmark your data against others. In contrast, doing your own survey helps you focus on patients' reactions to innovations in your effort. You can tailor your own surveys to fix your needs and therefore get more for the effort you are putting in.

9. What questions are you planning to ask?

It is neither necessary nor reasonable to survey all patients who use your service; instead, you can sample. *Sampling* helps reduce the data collection burden on both the patients and the analyst. The size of the sample depends on what you are trying to conclude. If there is a lot of variability in patients' satisfaction with your service, you need larger samples. If you plan to compare your service with others and the two efforts are very similar, you need larger data. More important than the size of the survey is whether it represents the population. Getting many patients to respond does not correct for the lack of a representative sample. This is one case in which more is not always better. The point of sampling is to get a representative sample of people who receive your service. Small and large samples can both be representative. The key is to examine whether there are systematic differences among people who respond and those who do not. Some examples of nonrepresentative designs include the following:

- *Surveying only those who complete your service.* Most dissatisfied patients will abandon the service before reaching the end.
- *Surveying patients in a particular month.* Patients' preferences and types of illness may be seasonally different.

You should randomly select a percentage of patients (not to be mistaken with randomly assigning patients to the service, which is a much harder task). This gives an equal chance that any particular patient may be included. In some circumstances, you may wish to over sample segments of the population. When segments of your population are small, you need to over sample these segments so that you can obtain an accurate estimate of their satisfaction. Otherwise, too few of them will be in your sample to provide an accurate picture. Suppose few teenagers visit your service. If you want to know about their satisfaction with your service, you will need to over sample teenagers. Thus, you may sample every ten adults but every five teenagers. Over sampling helps get a more accurate picture of small subgroups of patients using your service.

10. Which sampling strategy do you wish to implement?
11. Why do you expect that satisfied or dissatisfied clients will be reached in this fashion?
12. How you plan to verify whether your sample represents the population to which you want to generalize?

Many choices are available for data collection. You can have the survey done online and automatically. In these types of surveys, a computer calls or sends an e-mail to your clients. You can also survey participants by mail, by telephone, or in person. The mode of conducting the survey may affect the results. Online, computerized telephone, and mailed surveys are self-administered. Patients are more likely to report deviant social behavior in self-administered surveys. Online surveys (if connected to an automatic reminder) have a larger response rate than offline surveys. Online surveys are less expensive than offline surveys. Among offline surveys, face-to-face interviews are most expensive but allow for longer interviews.

13. Given the trade-offs of different modes of surveys (e.g., online, face-to-face, mailed, or telephone) which is your preferred approach, and why?

How you conduct your survey will have a lot to do with its success. You should alert the respondents that you plan to survey them before you actually send them a survey. This is preemptive reminder for people who forget to respond. In this fashion, the respondents will hear about you at least four times, when you (1) invite them to participate in the survey, (2) alert them that the survey is upcoming, (3) send them the survey, and (4) remind nonrespondents to complete the survey.

The invitation to participate in a survey should highlight who is conducting the survey, what the goal of the survey is, how long it should take to complete the survey, and how nonresponse will affect the overall conclusions.

14. What will you say in your invitation to participate?

The alert of the upcoming survey should include an appreciation of respondent's willingness to participate, the day the survey will be sent, and the importance of timely responses.

15. What will you say in the alert of the upcoming survey?

A reminder to nonrespondents often includes another copy of the survey. With online surveys, it is often necessary to make sure that respondents can answer questions quickly and without much download time. In fact, if you are tracing the person through e-mail, then it is best to embed the survey in the e-mail. With mailed surveys, you should include a self-addressed, stamped envelope.

16. What will you say in your reminder to participate?
17. What method will you use to send the second copy of the survey?

No matter how you do the survey, you should provide a real benefit for the respondent in completing the survey. Altruism and voluntary requests get you far, but not far enough. Think through what questions you can add that will make the respondent feel happier and more cared for at the end of the survey. Many providers combine satisfaction surveys with surveys of patients' health status or lifestyle appraisals. Patients get the benefit of a free health appraisal and evaluation while they complete the satisfaction surveys.

18. Why should your potential respondents take time away from their busy schedules to answer your questionnaire? In other words, what will they gain from completing your survey?

The language you use for the survey is important. Keep in mind that your services are open to many people from different backgrounds, and people are more likely to respond to a questionnaire prepared in their native language.

19. What language will you use for the survey?

Before you can analyze the data, you need to code the data (i.e., assign numbers to responses). When coding the data, you should include different codes for

- no responses to any questions in the survey;
- skipped questions;
- unclear or unusable responses; and
- responses of N/A (not applicable).

Analyze the missing data codes first. If a large percent of responses is missing, then it is doubtful that you can use the survey to arrive at any conclusions. If certain patient groups tend to skip specific questions, then the survey might have a systematic bias.

20. What response rate do you think is adequate to consider the survey useful?
21. What types of patterns might indicate a systematic bias?

If you are conducting online data collection, then there is no need to spend time entering the data into the computer. If you have done mailed, telephone, or in-person surveys, you must enter the data into the computer. This is often a tedious process. To make sure that the data are correct, enter the data twice and verify the difference between the two data sets.

Another step taken in cleaning the data is to check for inconsistent or out-of-range responses. If responses 1 through 5 are expected, but response 7 is given, then the response 7 is considered out of range and erroneous. Similarly, if earlier in the survey the client indicated that he is male and later that he is pregnant, then an inconsistent response is detected. Spend time cleaning the data. It will help you when it comes to interpreting the results.

22. How would you prepare the data for analysis?

To analyze the data, begin with descriptive statistics. Check each variable for skewness, range, mode, and mean to determine if the responses seem reasonable. Next, plot the data. Satisfaction surveys usually have a number of scales. Each scale is the average of responses to a number of questions. The idea is that if there are different ways of asking the same question, then one may have a more reliable scale. If so, then data may have a normal distribution. Scale responses should look like an upside down "U" shape. Statistical theory suggests that averages of more than four numbers will tend to have a normal distribution.

23. What do you expect to be the distribution of your data?

After you have completed your descriptive data analysis and everything makes sense to you, then you should conduct other analyses. If you have a cross-sectional design, then you may use cross-tabulation to display the data and use statistical methods (e.g., a chi-square test) to examine the significance of the differences you observe in a table.

24. How do you plan to analyze the data?
25. What will the final figures and tables look like (prepare mock-ups with hypothetical data)?

Part 3

Planning for program evaluation requires you to think through your needs and activities, which you did in parts 1 and 2. Now, explain how your plans are different from the steps described in this chapter.

1. What is missing from your plans that, according to this chapter, is important in decision analytic approaches to program evaluation? List all of the steps described in this chapter and, for each step, describe if it has been addressed in part 1 and 2 of the assignment.
2. Does the decision analysis approach give you a perspective that might otherwise be missing from a program evaluation (e.g., sensitivity to the timing of decisions, the need to focus on a decision maker, the need to focus on a specific decision with various options, or the need for a sensitivity analysis)?
3. How could you do a mock evaluation as part of your efforts to survey client satisfaction?
4. How could you make sure that decision makers' expectations are assessed before your data are reported?
5. If the decision maker is under time pressure, what steps will you take to make sure that your findings are available in time or that the decision maker is aware of what you are working on so she may wait for the results.

Audio/Visual Chapter Aids

To help you understand the concepts of program evaluation, visit this book's companion web site at ache.org/DecisionAnalysis, go to Chapter 10, and view the audio/visual chapter aids.

References

Alemi, F. 1988. "Subjective and Objective Methods of Program Evaluation." *Evaluation Review* 11 (6): 765–74.

Alemi, F., M. R. Haack, and S. Nemes. 2001. "Continuous Improvement Evaluation: A Framework for Multisite Evaluation Studies." *Journal for Healthcare Quality* 23 (3): 26–33.

Barker, S. B., and R. T. Barker. 1994. "Managing Change in an Interdisciplinary Inpatient Unit: An Action Research Approach." *Journal of Mental Health Administration* 21 (1): 80–91.

Benedetto, A. R. 2003. "Six Sigma: Not for the Faint of Heart." *Radiology Management* 25 (2): 40–53.

Brown, P. 2003. "Qualitative Methods in Environmental Health Research." *Environmental Health Perspectives* 111 (14):1789–98.

Campbell, D. T., and J. C. Stanley. 1966. *Experimental and Quasi Experimental Design for Research.* Chicago: Rand McNally.

Drummond, M. 1994. "Evaluation of Health Technology: Economic Issues for Health Policy and Policy Issues for Economic Appraisal." *Social Science and Medicine* 38 (12): 1593–600.

Edwards, W., M. Gutentag, and K. Snapper. 1975. "A Decision-Theoretic Approach to Evaluation Research." In *Handbook of Evaluation Research*, edited by E. L. Streuning and W. Gutentag. London: Sage Publications.

Gustafson, D. H., C. J. Fiss, Jr., and J. C. Fryback. 1981. "Quality of Care in Nursing Homes: New Wisconsin Evaluation System." *Journal of Long Term Care Administration* 9 (2): 40–55.

Gustafson, D. H., F. C. Sainfort, R. Van Konigsveld, and D. R. Zimmerman. 1990. "The Quality Assessment Index (QAI) for Measuring Nursing Home Quality." *Health Services Research* 25 (1 Part 1): 97–127.

Gustafson, D. H., and A. Thesen. 1981. "Are Traditional Information Systems Adequate for Policy Makers?" *Health Care Management Review* 6 (1): 51–63.

Hoffmann, C., and J. M. Graf von der Schulenburg. 2000. "The Influence of Economic Evaluation Studies on Decision Making: A European Survey. The EUROMET Group." *Health Policy* 52 (3): 179–92.

Neumann, P. J. 2005. *Using Cost-Effectiveness Analysis to Improve Health Care: Opportunities and Barriers.* New York: Oxford University Press.

Reynolds, J. 1991. "A Reconsideration of Operations Research Experimental Designs." *Progress in Clinical and Biological Research* 371:377–94.

Winzelberg, G. S. 2003. "The Quest for Nursing Home Quality: Learning History's Lessons." *Archives of Internal Medicine* 163 (21): 2552–6.

Weinstein, M. C., J. E. Siegel, M. R. Gold, M. S. Kamlet, and L. B. Russell. 1996. "Recommendations of the Panel on Cost-Effectiveness in Health and Medicine." *JAMA* 276 (15): 1253–8.

Zeitz, K., and H. McCutcheon. 2003. "Evidence-Based Practice: To Be or Not to Be, This Is the Question!" *International Journal of Nursing Practice* 9 (5): 272–9.

CHAPTER

11

CONFLICT ANALYSIS

Farrokh Alemi, David H. Gustafson, and William Cats-Baril

Attitudes toward conflict have shifted. Conflict, once considered a problem, is now seen as a potentially positive and creative force. Conflict should be managed, rather than eliminated. Effective management of conflict depends on an analysis that points the way to constructive outcomes—to win-win solutions.

The idea of a decision-analysis framework for examining and resolving conflicts is not new. Theoretical models with specific prescriptions have long been discussed in the literature (Raiffa 1982). Conflict analysis is a methodology to increase all parties' understanding of the conflict. It includes not only a mathematical formula but also behavioral advice on what to do and when. It is a methodology to support the process of conflict resolution by addressing the basic sources of conflict: lack of understanding, lack of information, and distorted communication. After these roadblocks are disposed of, conflict is broken down into its component issues, which can be traded off. If a negotiation over the components of the conflict succeeds, each party achieves a victory on the issues it deems important.

Application of Conflict Analysis

Conflict analysis may be applied in different situations:

- To assemble conflicting parties to find general areas of agreement and a solution that meets the concerns of all parties
- To help a neutral observer or mediator understand the issues and priorities of the parties to a conflict
- To help one party clarify its position and perhaps role-play the opposing positions; this helps clarify the opposition's values and perceptions, enabling one side to understand the opposition's viewpoint and to develop a negotiating strategy

This book has a companion web site that features narrated presentations, animated examples, PowerPoint slides, online tools, web links, additional readings, and examples of students' work. To access this chapter's learning tools, go to ache.org/DecisionAnalysis and select Chapter 11.

Analysis of conflict can be useful in several situations. First, conflict analysis is useful if several constituencies recognize that a conflict must be resolved and are willing to take the necessary steps. An example is when department heads meet to resolve their conflict about the budget. Second, analysis can also be used if one party wants a deeper understanding of the conflict. For example, a clinician negotiating an agreement with a health maintenance organization (HMO) might want to explore various contract provisions. If a constituency cannot or will not participate in the analysis, a group of "objective outsiders" should be asked to role-play it. While such refusal or inability to participate may reduce the chances that a chosen treaty will be implemented, having proxies is better than omitting pertinent viewpoints from the analysis. Note that it is helpful if the objective outsiders are highly regarded by the missing constituency.

Who should be invited to participate in the analysis depends on the purpose of the analysis. If a manager wants to explore how the other side might react to various proposals without committing to an action, the analysis must be performed with a group of objective outsiders. But if the purpose is to raise awareness about the problem or to reach an agreement on it, the analysis should involve as many actual parties to the conflict as possible.

A related point of discussion is the preference to meet alone with each constituency. Conflict analysis is a process to increase the understanding of each constituency's position, increase available choices in subsequent negotiations, and identify different ways of solving the conflict by finding areas of possible agreement with the opponents. Many of these goals can be better realized in private meetings of constituencies. Group meetings can follow but should not precede individual model-building sessions. When people in conflict meet before conflict is understood, they may stress their disputes instead of their agreements and escalate the conflict to personal issues. They may force each other into a corner, reducing the possibility of later compromise. It is better to wait and meet after various points of views are better understood and the possibility of miscommunications is reduced.

Assumptions Behind Conflict Analysis

The premises underlying conflict analysis are as follows:

1. *People have cognitive biases that become more acute under conflict or crisis.* When negotiations are complex (meaning that they are based on many issues), these cognitive limitations prevent full consideration of possible solutions.
2. *Preconceptions and false assumptions impair the ability to make the trade-offs that can lead to a solution.* Each party may erroneously assume that they know the priorities of the other. Asking for the priorities can reduce these misconceptions. When two parties negotiate, some conflict is caused by their differences but other conflicts are caused by miscommunications. Analysis reduces conflict caused by poor communication.
3. *A conflict is easier to grasp if the situation is broken into components (some of which may include little or no conflict).* Many parties that see each other in conflict are surprised to find out that they have large areas of agreement.
4. *Individuals can specify their values and prioritize them by using a structured process.* Using the procedures described in Chapter 2, preferences can be modeled even when people are in conflict.
5. *The decision maker can learn about every viewpoint by modeling each party separately.* When one party is not available, the analyst can interview observers who can role-play the values, preferences, and priorities of the absent parties.
6. *The analyst can reduce conflict caused by miscommunication, provide insight into the thinking of each party, and identify solutions overlooked by both parties.* A conflict analyzed is a conflict understood. The analyst can emphasize that there are wide areas of agreement so the conflict does not escalate. The analysis injects rationality into highly charged situations and helps each party gain new insights. The analyst can use models of parties to identify better solutions that are often overlooked by both parties.

When thinking about managing conflict, the analyst must always consider that conflict might lead to a higher level of tension where the potential for losses is increased. This is the escalation of conflict, a debilitating syndrome with many deleterious effects. The sources of escalation are a lack of understanding among the parties, a lack of information about the opponent's position, and an emphasis on bargaining so that one party wins and the other loses. Conflict analysis counteracts these problems by increasing communication, emphasizing a problem-solving attitude, offering a joint definition of the problem, reducing the influence of ideology, and pointing the parties toward win-win solutions.

Conflicts can become so heated and the constituencies so stubborn that rational approaches cannot manage them. Often, however, all sides realize that a decision must be made and that a better understanding of one another's position is essential. In that case, it becomes helpful for the parties to know the goals, attitudes, values, motivations, and levels of aspiration of the parties; the nature of the vital issues in the conflict and the options available to resolve them; and the consequences of taking each possible action. Unfortunately, research suggests that people are sometimes inconsistent in their judgment, often unaware of their own values, and certainly unable to explain their opponents' positions accurately (Kenny and DePaulo 1993; de Dreu and van Knippenberg 2005; Hammond, Keeney, and Raiffa 1998).

The Methodology

Analysis of conflict consists of the three major phases (as shown in Table 11.1), which can be broken down into ten steps. The first phase helps the analyst understand the underlying issues and gain a perspective on the background of the conflict. In the second phase, the analyst explores the problem by refining and decomposing the preliminary goals into specific components, which are called "issues." In the third phase, the analyst explores solutions to the entire conflict by analyzing treaties. The third phase of analysis begins by asking the constituencies to weight the relative importance of the various issues and to state preferences for possible levels of resolution. The analyst then packages one level of resolution for each issue into a treaty and scores it to see how well it meets each constituency's needs. In the next step, the analyst searches for the optimum treaty for all parties (or for a specific party if that is the purpose). Then, the analyst convenes all parties to search for a consensus resolution.

An Example

The application of conflict analysis will be illustrated by way of an example. Healthcare managers face conflict in many situations. Making budget allocations involves resolving conflicts among the manager's team (Bruckmeier

TABLE 11.1
Summary of the Conflict Analysis Methodology

Phase	Step	Action	Purpose
Understand the problem	1	Identify constituencies and their spokespeople	To define the coalitions and identify individuals who will later develop the conflict model and choose treaties
	2	Analyze assumptions	To obtain a general understanding of the problem and to identify ideological and technical sources of conflict
Structure the problem	3	Perform an in-depth interview with one or more objective outsiders	To refine the goals identified in step 1, check understanding of the issues and different set of values involved, and begin exploring grounds for resolution
	4	In separate sessions with each constituency, identify issues and levels of resolution	To develop the conflict model and identify key levels of resolution that lead to an overall compromise
	5	Assess the importance of issues and the value of resolution levels	To quantify the importance and preference of the component issues and the levels of resolution
Explore the solution	6	Form and score treaties	To generate a set of feasible solutions and explore Pareto-optimal solutions
	7	Analyze the treaties	To generate treaties that are likely to resolve the conflict
	8	Develop a strategy of negotiation	To increase the likelihood of a positive outcome
	9	Present results to all constituents	To generate an acceptable treaty and develop guidelines to implement the treaty or agree on further actions in the resolution process

2005). Often, interdisciplinary providers have role conflicts, and managers are called upon to resolve these tensions (Shannon 1997). Managers face conflicts in merger negotiations (Dooley and Zimmerman 2003), settlement of lawsuits disputes (Dauer 2002), labor-management negotiations (Alemi, Fos, and Lacorte 1990), and many other similar situations. The example used in this chapter is a discussion of how managers can improve community relationship by understanding the conflict in the community about their services. In particular, the focus is on a community's conflict about the requirement of parental consent before family-planning services are provided to adolescents. A hospital administrator who is developing a family-planning service must structure the service to reflect the views of many constituents as well as a growing market demand.

Phase 1: Understand the Problem

Step 1: Identify Constituencies and Spokespeople

Constituencies—people or groups that stand to gain or lose as a result of a conflict—can be identified in several ways, such as by examining lists provided by lobbying organizations, by reviewing testimony on past legislation, by inviting local chapters of national organizations to a discussion, and by interviewing key individuals by telephone. Commonly, many groups with various persuasions must be taken into account. However, the value systems of these differing groups as they relate to family planning may be similar enough to be characterized by just two or three models. Such a simplification is a significant help in devising a useful solution. In the example, parents, clergy, physicians, health educators, social workers, and women's rights advocates might be grouped in ways they are comfortable. The analyst can decide whether groups can be lumped into one constituency by asking several prominent organizations to assign priorities to a set of goals about the conflict. This empirical approach works well if all relevant groups are surveyed.

A common mistake is to canvass only those groups that have lined up against each other. Although the first glance might suggest that only two groups are in opposition, further analysis may identify other important players. Using the example, at first it appears that just two constituencies are involved in the conflict: the "antiabortion forces" and the "family-planning advocates." However, further examination might unearth a third group, which may be called the "concerned parents"—people who believe their teenage children are mature enough to make correct decisions if given balanced, unbiased information. These concerned parents care mostly about their children's well-being, and if they have an ideology on abortion, they do not want it to influence their children's actions.

Once the preliminary analysis is finished, the analyst must identify a spokesperson to represent each constituency participating in the conflict analysis. The analyst needs at least three types of spokespeople: the proponents and opponents of the conflict and objective outsiders. The third group is valued for having a perspective that differs from that of the constituencies. In contrast, if policymakers do not want to negotiate with a constituency but merely wish to increase their understanding of the conflict, the analysis can be performed using only objective outsiders instead of a spokesperson.

Spokespeople should be good at identifying issues and solutions and should be comfortable with the task of quantifying preferences. While later in the process the analyst may want to include individuals with the institutional power to implement a compromise, during the analysis phase the analyst needs people who are willing to break the problem into its components and who are sensitive, insightful, and articulate.

A nomination process to identify spokespeople begins by identifying five or six nominators—people who know the leaders and insightful people in the field and can identify individuals who might adequately represent a constituency. It is good practice to select only nominees who are suggested by several nominators because this indicates the person is widely respected. While in general having many people consider somebody to be an expert will signify that person's credibility, even the most widely respected will have opponents and the most knowledgeable will have cynics.

When talking with the nominees, the analyst can motivate them to participate by mentioning the following:

- Who nominated them (make sure to get permission to use the nominator's name)
- What the project is about
- Why their participation is important
- What will and will not be done with the results
- How their names will be used
- What tasks will expected of them
- How long each task will take, and when it will occur
- What payment (if any) they will receive

In general, three spokespeople (one from each constituency) are sufficient, although there may be good reasons, such as attrition, to identify more nominees. During a long process, some spokespeople may drop out because of other commitments or loss of interest. The analyst must beware of running out of spokespeople before concluding the analysis. A second reason for having more than one representative is that in a complex analysis, especially one involving a series of technical and ethical issues, a single spokesperson may be unable to convey the full spectrum of a constituency's position.

Step 2: Analyze Assumptions

After the preliminary analysis is finished and the spokespeople have agreed to participate, the analyst must do some homework. This is because conflict about the definition or solution of a problem often arises from sharp disagreement over a fundamental factor that is not obvious to even the stakeholders themselves. Some conflict is caused by unconscious assumptions. The analyst must bring these assumptions to the surface for examination.

To elicit the assumptions, the analyst must gain as much information as possible about each constituency's views. Leaflets, brochures, advertisements, position papers, legislative hearings, and data used by a constituency to buttress its position are all valuable clues. Interviews may also be useful, but more often than not assumptions are so ingrained that people accept them unconsciously and have difficulty articulating them. People are commonly surprised by their assumptions once they are made explicit.

Throughout this process, analysts should look for recurring catchwords or slogans in a constituency's statements. Slogans are chosen for their emotional content; they contain a wealth of information about the constituency's values. In the example of parental notification about family planning services for adolescents, constituency 1 said, "I want my children to have the courage to say no." Constituency 2 said, "Let's stop children from having children." Although such statements simplify the conflict, they certainly give the flavor of the competing positions. This tone allows the analyst to devise whether the debate is emotional or technical, and whether it concerns ethics or money. Again, remember that at this stage the analyst is trying to understand where the different constituencies are coming from and summarize their positions.

Table 11.2 shows some assumptions behind the world views of constituencies 1 and 2. A close reading shows that assumptions can be classified as contradictory and noncontradictory. Constituency 1's assumption that access to contraceptives lures teenagers into sex directly contradicts constituency 2's assumption that access to contraceptives does not increase sexual activities. Clearly, the two assumptions cannot both be true at the same time. A noncontradictory pair of assumptions is also shown. While constituency 1 assumes that administration and red tape will soak up as much as 90 percent of the funds, constituency 2 assumes that the cost-benefit ratio of family-planning programs is excellent. These assumptions seem to be in opposition to each other, but both can be true at once.

TABLE 11.2
Catchphrases and Assumptions of Two Constituencies

	Constituency 1	*Constituency 2*
Catchphrases	Government has too much control.	Let's stop children form having children.
	I want my children to have the courage to say no.	Contraception is better than unwanted pregnancies.
Assumptions	Administration and red tape will eat up as much as 90 percent of the funds.	The cost-benefit ratio in family-planning programs is excellent.
	Contraception is dangerous, and people are misinformed about its effects.	Lack of pregnancy allows minors to take advantage of other possibilities (education, employment, etc.).
	Parents do a better job of providing sexual education.	Parents do not provide adequate sexual education.
	Morality is the best contraceptive.	Counselors in family-planning agencies provide the most persuasive influence against premarital sex.
	Access to contraceptives lures teenagers into sexual activities.	Access to contraceptives does not increase sexual activities.
	The decision to have sex is a good opportunity for establishing communication between parents and children.	Confidentiality is crucial in obtaining family-planning services.

It is crucial that the constituencies perceive the analyst to be a fair individual who is sensitive to their values. To accomplish this, the analyst should use the same terminology as the constituency and restrain from evaluating the validity of ascertains. The analyst can ask clarifying questions but not make any judgment regarding the response.

Phase 2: Structure the Problem

After the analyst has identified the constituencies and their general goals and assumptions, and the spokespeople have agreed to participate, it is time to model the conflict. In this phase, the analyst breaks down the conflict into its components and then quantifies each one. These components are the goals of each constituency, the issues that form the heart of the conflict and that must be addressed to resolve it, and the possible levels of resolution for each issue.

Step 3: Conduct In-Depth Interviews

During this phase, the analyst will have two sets of meetings, one with objective outsiders and one with the spokespeople for each constituency. Performing in-depth interviews with a few objective outsiders is an excellent way of preparing and rehearsing before the actual sessions with the spokespeople. Objective outsiders need not be experts in the subject matter—they can be trusted associates who are acquainted with the problem and not intimately involved with its solution. These people are chosen for their analytical skills, candor, and knowledge of the issues. The sessions with the objective outsiders give the analyst a preliminary conflict model that serves as a starting point for the constituency sessions.

During both the proxy interviews and the spokespeople group sessions, the analyst should do the following:

1. *Discuss the problem in general terms and note examples of goals, issues, and levels of resolution.* The analyst asks questions to help define the problem and ensure that its key elements are understood.
2. *Ask for descriptions of the parties.* Who are the proponents? Who are the opponents? How do they view the conflict? What would each side like to see in terms of a resolution? Why?
3. *Ask for an exhaustive list of the issues that are dividing the sides to make sure they are as independent of each other as possible (i.e., there is no overlap).* What is the underlying conflict? On which issues do the opponents agree or disagree? Which issues must be resolved for the sides to reach agreement?

4. *Ask for a list of all levels of resolution for each issue.* What is this side's position on the issue? What solutions might it accept? What solutions are totally unacceptable? Why are the levels considered in this way? Some levels will be preferred by one side, and other levels by the other side. Some levels will be compromises that are not preferred by any side but may be acceptable to all. The analyst tries to identify as many levels of resolution as possible on each issue, even though only a few may be considered in the final analysis. The reason for seeking so many levels is to promote the development of creative levels of resolution.

A private meeting of each constituency is held to obviate the risky and possibly dysfunctional step of assembling the opponents before the analyst knows the depth and nature of the conflict. Later, after the conflict-analysis model has been formed and some trade-off resolutions have been mapped out, the constituencies may be assembled to search for solutions, or treaties.

Step 4: Identify Issues and Levels of Resolution

Issues are the basic building blocks of conflict; they are fundamental factors that must be understood and addressed to reach resolution. Once the issues are identified, the analyst can classify them on a continuum from agreement to disagreement. This allows the concentration to be on finding acceptable compromises or trade-offs on intensely disputed issues. The classification may reveal, for example, that the constituencies agree on several issues, that they are mildly opposed on others, and that the conflict really concerns just a couple of issues. This makes the conflict appear more manageable and focused and thus simplifies its resolution.

If disputed issues are not ripe for resolution because their political time has not arrived, or if they are too thorny to be resolved, the analyst can try to develop a partial solution by concentrating on more tractable issues. Either way, separating the conflict into component issues allows the analyst to localize the problem to specific areas and to use resources to solve problems more effectively.

Finally, the levels of resolution—the specific actions, laws, and services that can resolve an issue—must be identified. Typically, constituencies identify levels of resolution that range from optimal to unacceptable. This step tells the analyst what each constituency is considering or fearing in terms of suitable and unsuitable solutions, and it serves as a foundation for generating new solutions.

Let's return to the example of the issue of parental notification. Suppose that after performing these interviews with two objective outsiders and meeting with the spokespeople, the list of goals include reducing unwanted pregnancies, teaching children to be responsible, preserving the family, and reducing the number of abortions.

Furthermore, suppose the interviews reveal that the conflict can be distilled into two issues: (1) which components of family planning should be available to minors and (2) under what conditions. Suppose also that both constituencies agree that any family-planning program must have at least three components:

1. Education should include such topics as values, morals, biological processes, birth control, decision making, goal setting, sex roles, pregnancy, and parenting skills.
2. Counseling should focus on some of the same issues as education but should also involve more interaction between the provider and client. The focuses of counseling might include crises, pregnancy, abortion, elective non-parenthood, and preparation for childbirth.
3. Services might include birth control, adoption, abortions, prenatal care, sexually transmitted disease testing and treatment, and financial assistance.

With this information, the analyst is now in a position to explore the issues at the heart of the conflict. In this example, the crucial issues are as follows:

- Should values and morals be taught when delivering family-planning services?
- Should counseling of adolescents start from the position that premarital sex among adolescents is bad?
- Which is more important, allowing easy access to services or having services controlled by organizations that have what are considered high morals?
- What are the optimum technical qualifications of the family-planning personnel?
- Who, if anybody, should regulate the provision of family-planning services to adolescents?

Once the issues have been identified, the objective outsiders and spokespeople are asked, separately, to define a set of feasible resolutions to each issue. A set of issues and their possible levels of resolution are listed in Table 11.3.

Once the issues and levels of resolution have been formulated by the full group of spokespeople, they must be checked, detailed, and rephrased in separate sessions with spokespeople from each constituency. It is critical

TABLE 11.3 Issues and Levels of Resolution

	Issues		*Levels of Resolution*
A	To what extent should family-planning programs try to convince clients that adolescent sex is bad?	A1	Should not do so
		A2	Should be available to clients
		A3	Should be required of all clients
		A4	Should be a fundamental part of every service of a family-planning program
B	To what extent should family-planning programming be oriented toward strengthening the family?	B1	Not at all
		B2	Depends on the client
		B3	Always, with all clients
C	What limitations to access to family-planning programs should exist for adolescents?	C1	No parental notification
		C2	Parental notification before counseling or services
		C3	Parental permission before counseling or services
D	What type of supervision should be required for people who provide family-planning services to adolescents?	D1	Social work supervision
		D2	Physician supervision
		D3	Theologian supervision
		D4	Experience as parent of adolescent
E	What organization (with what moral qualifications) should be allowed to deliver family-planning services?	E1	Nonprofit
		E2	Educational
		E3	Governmental
		E4	Healthcare (doctor's office or hospital)
		E5	Religious
F	Who should regulate the provision of family-planning services for adolescents?	F1	Peer review
		F2	Local government
		F3	State government
		F4	Federal government
		F5	Community

to obtain a consensus on the phrasing and substance of all issues and levels of resolution from all parties before proceeding. Note that at this time the goal is to have all of the constituencies agree on the components of the conflict, not on a solution to it. In many conflicts, merely listing the issues and the possible levels of resolution reduces the conflict.

Step 5: Elicit Weights and Preferences

In this step, the analyst helps each constituency estimate the importance of various issues and the values assigned to different resolutions of those issues. Methods to elicit weights and preferences are found in the Chapter 2 (see also Ryan et al. 2001). Two sets of parameters need to be estimated. First, the analyst must identify the values of the different resolutions to each constituency. This is done by listing the various levels from least to most preferred and then assigning the most preferred option the value of 100 and the least preferred option the value of 0. All resolutions in between the best and worst levels are assigned proportional values. Alternatively, if more precision is needed, the double-anchored estimation method can be used, in which the most preferred level is assigned 100, the least preferred level is assigned 0, and the spokesperson is asked to rate the remaining levels.

The relative priorities between the issues are assigned using the method of ratio estimates. The spokesperson is asked to list the issues in order of importance; the least important issue is assigned a value of 10. The spokesperson is then asked to rate how much more important the next issue is (e.g., ten times as important). The process is continued until all issues are judged relative to one issue of lesser importance. The ratio judgments are then used to assign a score to each issue. The scores are divided by the total of all the scores to produce the weight for each issue. This manner of developing issue weights ensure that the weights for issues are constrained to add to one; thus, if the spokesperson weights one issue heavily, he is forced to weight other issues as less important.

When multiple spokespeople are involved for one constituency, and if they differ in their estimates or weights for issues or values of different resolution levels, then they are asked to discuss their differences and come to a consensus. If their differences are small, responses from different spokespeople for the same constituency are averaged. Note that during the discussion among the spokespeople, the analyst might find certain factions of a constituency to be more amenable to compromise; this is signaled by the faction that has priorities similar to the opposing parties. In the extreme cases, the analyst might find that the spokespeople on one side actually represent several positions, not just one. If so, the analyst may need to develop a distinct model for each position.

Table 11.4 shows the resulting weights and value scores for the different constituencies in the example.

Once levels of resolution for all issues have been identified and the weights and preferences assessed, it is useful to do an initial review. For instance, preserving the family is important to constituency 1 and of

TABLE 11.4
Weight and Value Scores of Two Constituencies in the Family-Planning Example

Issues		Levels of Resolutions		Issue Weight		Resolution Value	
				Constituency 1	*Constituency 2*	*Constituency 1*	*Constituency 2*
A	To what extent should family-planning programs try to convince clients that adolescent sex is bad?	A1	Should not do so	0.14	0.07	0	100
		A2	Should be available to clients			30	90
		A3	Should be required of all clients			80	20
		A4	Should be a fundamental part of every service			100	0
B	To what extent should family-planning programming be oriented toward strengthening the family?	B1	Not at all	0.20	0.04	0	100
		B2	Programs available			30	90
		B3	Programs required			90	20
		B4	Built into all components			100	0
C	What limitations to access to family-planning programs should exist for adolescents?	C1	No parental notification	0.25	0.48	0	100
		C2	Parental notification before counseling or services			80	10
		C3	Parental permission before counseling or services			100	0

TABLE 11.4
(continued)

Issues		Levels of Resolutions		Issue Weight		Resolution Value	
				Constituency 1	*Constituency 2*	*Constituency 1*	*Constituency 2*
D	What type of supervision should be required for people who provide family-planning services to adolescents?	D1	Social work supervision	0.11	0.14	0	100
		D2	Physician supervision			60	50
		D3	Theologist supervision			100	30
		D4	Experience as parent of adolescent			50	0
E	What organization (with what moral qualifications) should be allowed to deliver family-planning services?	E1	Nonprofit	0.23	0.16	0	100
		E2	Educational			60	30
		E3	Governmental			30	15
		E4	Healthcare (doctor's office or hospital)			80	10
		E5	Religious			100	0
F	Who should regulate the provision of family-planning services for adolescents?	F1	Peer review	0.07	0.11	0	100
		F2	Local government			90	20
		F3	State government			40	30
		F4	Federal government			10	40
		F5	Community			100	0

relatively little importance to constituency 2. This suggests that resolutions that enhance the family might be included in the model as long as they do not impair other goals. For example, family-planning organizations could teach parenting skills to parents of adolescents or could develop educational and counseling programs to teach adolescents to get along with their families.

Phase 3: Explore Solutions

Step 6: Form and Score Treaties

A *treaty* is a set of resolutions for each issue in the conflict: one level of resolution per issue. Each resolution has a particular value to the constituency, and each issue has been given a priority by each constituency. The goal is to find a treaty—a combination of resolutions—that has a high value score for all constituencies.

Calculate the value of a treaty by multiplying the value of one level of resolution by its issue importance weight, continuing in this way for all issues, and then summing the results. In the example, suppose family-planning legislation passed with the following levels of resolution (as shown in Table 11.4):

- A2: Programs stress the negative aspects of adolescent sex.
- B2: Programs to strengthen the family would be required in any adolescent family-planning service.
- C2: Parents must be notified when an adolescent uses a family-planning program.
- D2: All providers of family-planning services must have medical qualifications.
- E2: Educational institutions will carry out family-planning programs.
- F3: State governments must regulate family-planning programs.

The value of this treaty is calculated by multiplying the relative importance weight of an issue by the value assigned to the level of resolution, then adding across all issues. That is, the score of treaty k for constituency c is equal to

$$k_c = \sum_{i=1,\ldots,n} W_{ci} \times V_{cij},$$

where

- k_c is the score for treaty k (a set of levels of resolution for all n issues) evaluated for constituency c;
- W_{ci} is the importance weight of issue i for constituency c;

- V_{cij} is the value of level of resolution j to issue i for constituency c;
- n is the number of issues underlying the conflict;
- i is the issue number; and
- j is the resolution level within the issue.

For constituency 1, the value of the treaty described above is

$$(.14 \times 30) + (.20 \times 30) + (.25 \times 80) + (.11 \times 60) + (.23 \times 60) + (.07 \times 40) = 53.4.$$

For constituency 2, the value of the treaty is

$$(.07 \times 90) + (.04 \times 90) + (.48 \times 10) + (.14 \times 50) + (.16 \times 30) + (.11 \times 30) = 29.8.$$

How good is this treaty? Can both constituencies improve their positions? These questions are addressed in the next section.

The point of analyzing treaties is to identify those treaties that are acceptable to all parties. A large number of treaties are typically available—in this example on parental notification, 4,800 treaties could be formed. In general, the number of possible treaties n is equal to:

$$n = \Pi_{i=1,\ldots,n}\, x_i,$$

where x_i is the number of levels of resolution attached to issue i, and n is the number of issues.

One way to reduce the number of possible treaties is to look at only two values: the best and worst resolutions for each issue. In these circumstances, the number of possible treaties becomes two to the power of the number of issues involved. With the model on family-planning services, the possible number of treaties with the best and worst levels is 2^6, or 64 possible treaties. This reduces the number of possible treaties, but how could one choose among these remaining treaties?

Step 7: Analyze Treaties

A treaty is Pareto optimal if it allows one party to get as much as possible without damaging the opponent's position, and vice versa. This concept of mutual improvement is called the Pareto-optimality criterion (Raiffa 1982). Pareto optimality is reached when one side cannot improve its position without degrading the position of its opponents. In Figure 11.1, the circled treaties are Pareto optimal, and all other treaties are not. All of the treaties outside the circle can be improved for at least one party (without depreciating the position of the other party) by moving to a treaty in the circle.

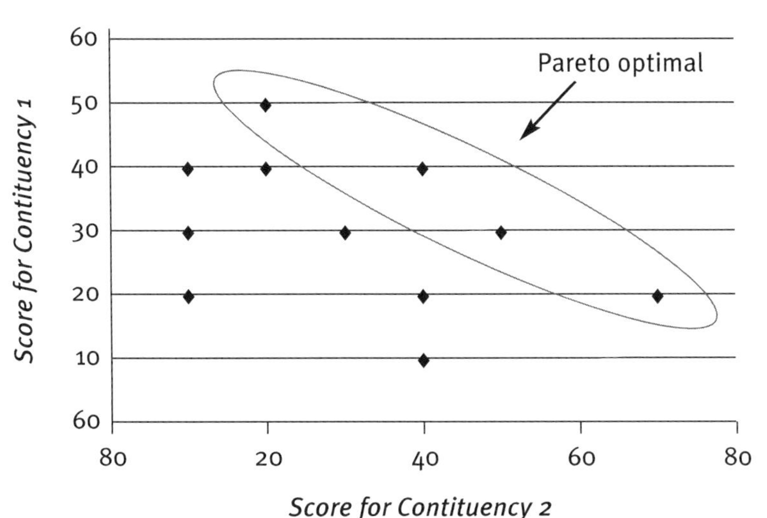

FIGURE 11.1 Value Scores for Two Constituents and Pareto-Optimal Treaties

In a graph of the value of treaties to two constituencies, an analyst can find the Pareto-optimal treaties by connecting a line from the treaty having the maximum possible value to one constituency to the treaty having the maximum possible value to the other constituency. Typically, these are treaties having the value of 100 to one constituency and zero to the other. If there is conflict between the two constituencies, all treaties should fall below this line. The treaties closest to the line are Pareto optimal.

The purpose of analyzing treaties is to devise a few that are acceptable to all constituencies and that can recast the conflict as a win-win situation. The analyst and constituencies should explore all trade-offs and compromises in a cooperative manner.

The examination of alternative treaties is an iterative process that can be simplified by using computer programs. The important point is that understanding the relative importance of issues and levels of resolution often allows one to find treaties that trade off and improve the outcome for everybody.

It is common to approach conflict resolution by seeking a compromise on each issue in turn. Yet compromising on issues one by one can lead to inferior solutions. Suppose that both sides in the example negotiate and settle on something in between the two extremes for all issues (i.e., something close to value of 50, halfway between 0 and 100). Table 11.5 shows the resulting treaty and the total value of the treaty to each constituency. The value of this treaty for constituency 1 is 53.4 and for constituency 2 is 29.8.

TABLE 11.5
Value of Satisfying Both Constituencies on All Issues Related to Family-Planning Services

	Issues		*Levels of Resolutions*	*Issue Weight*		*Resolution Value*	
				Constituency 1	*Constituency 2*	*Constituency 1*	*Constituency 2*
A	To what extent should family-planning programs try to convince clients that adolescent sex is bad?	A2	Should be available to clients	0.14	0.07	30	90
B	To what extent should family-planning programming be oriented toward strengthening the family?	B2	Programs available	0.20	0.04	30	90
C	What limitations to access to family-planning programs should exist for adolescents?	C2	Parental notification before counseling or services	0.25	0.48	80	10

TABLE 11.5
(continued)

Issues		Levels of Resolutions		Issue Weight		Resolution Value	
				Constituency 1	*Constituency 2*	*Constituency 1*	*Constituency 2*
D	What type of supervision should be required for people who provide family-planning services to adolescents?	D2	Physician supervision	0.11	0.14	60	50
E	What organization (with what moral qualifications) should be allowed to deliver family-planning services?	E2	Educational	0.23	0.16	60	30
F	Who should regulate the provision of family-planning services for adolescents?	F3	State government	0.07	0.11	40	30
	Overall treaty score					53.4	29.8

An alternative approach, called *logrolling*, may be useful in selecting treaties. In logrolling, gains in some issues are traded off against losses in other issues, so each party can win those it considers most important. Researchers have found that conflict-resolution processes that allow logrolling lead to more Pareto-optimal settlements and higher value to each participant than processes based on issue-by-issue compromises (Harinck, De Dreu, and Van Vianen 2000; Bazerman et al. 2000). Logrolling's advantages over compromising within each issue are that it

- defuses ideological disputes,
- increases Pareto optimality,
- satisfies both parties better,
- encourages looking at the big picture, and
- does not divide the original conflict into several separate conflicts.

If one side wins issue *x*, the losers may try all the harder to win issue *y*. The very nature of the procedure encourages the parties not to search for the best overall solution.

Let's examine logrolling with data from the family-planning program design. Table 11.6 provides a treaty in which the constituency that cares most about an issue receives the best possible resolution on that issue. The values for this treaty would be 57 and 73, improving the satisfaction of both constituencies over the treaty in Table 11.5. Thus, this type of logrolling should be encouraged at the expense of compromising on issues one by one. Logrolling produces Pareto-optimal treaties, in which no one can improve her situation further without hurting other participants. In fact, an easy way to identify all possible Pareto-optimal treaties is to connect the following three points in Figure 11.1 to each other: (1) the treaty where one constituency gets all it wants, (2) the treaty where the opponent gets all it wants, and (3) the treaty arrived at by logrolling. A line then connects these three points; the treaties close to the line are all Pareto optimal.

Step 8: Develop a Strategy of Negotiation

Coming up with an agreed-upon conflict model is a big achievement in itself. The opposing constituencies have been delineated, the conflict has been specified, the structure of the model (goals, issues, and levels of resolution) has been defined, and the value structures of the constituencies have been articulated. Now, the constituencies are assembled for the first time. The delay emphasizes the need for each constituency to understand its own position before discussing it with its opponents. To minimize conflict caused by a lack of understanding of one's own position, analysts spend a great deal of time clarifying what those positions are and what feasible treaties might look like.

TABLE 11.6
Result When Each Constituency Is Allowed to Win on Issues They Care Most About

		Issue Weight		Resolution Value	
Issues	*Levels of Resolutions*	*Constituency 1*	*Constituency 2*	*Constituency 1*	*Constituency 2*
A To what extent should family-planning programs try to convince clients that adolescent sex is bad?	A4 Should be a fundamental part of every service	0.14	0.07	100	0
B To what extent should family-planning programming be oriented toward strengthening the family?	B3 Always, with all clients	0.20	0.04	100	0
C What limitations to access to family-planning programs should exist for adolescents?	C1 No parental notification	0.25	0.48	0	100

TABLE 11.6
(continued)

Issues		Levels of Resolutions		Issue Weight		Resolution Value	
				Constituency 1	*Constituency 2*	*Constituency 1*	*Constituency 2*
D	What type of supervision should be required for people who provide family-planning services to adolescents?	D1	Social work supervision	0.11	0.14	0	100
E	What organization (with what moral qualifications) should be allowed to deliver family-planning services?	E5	Religious	0.23	0.16	100	0
F	Who should regulate the provision of family-planning services for adolescents?	F1	Peer review	0.07	0.11	0	100
	Overall treaty score				57		73

Now it is time to choose a course of action. Note that at this point the parties have agreed on the issues and feasible levels of resolution, but not on preferred resolutions. It is unlikely that agreement will be reached on all these matters, because some issues are purely ideological, but it is realistic to aim for agreement on certain issues and levels of resolution and to hope to compromise on the rest. The following discussion offers suggestions and guidelines for increasing the probabilities of success at this stage.

Because the issues and levels of resolution have been agreed upon, the emphasis of the meeting is to reduce differences of perception and judgment on the relative importance of disputed issues and levels. But which issue should be addressed first? The answer arises from an examination of the source of the disagreements, which the analyst performs before the plenary meeting. The source of disagreements can be classified along a continuum ranging from purely ideological to purely technical.

The analyst must determine the order in which to present the issues to the constituencies. It might help to classify the issues as follows:

1. *Issues about which parties agree regarding the level of resolution.* Because there are no disagreements, each party's utility can be maximized by allowing the best solution for either party.
2. *Issues where parties agree on the importance of the issue.* In these circumstances, a compromise must be reached by finding some resolution between the preferred choices of the two parties within the issue.
3. *Issues where parties disagree on the importance of the issue.* In these circumstances, the party that considers the issue to be less important may be willing to give up on the issue entirely in return for gains on other issues that are more important to the party.

The presentation order matters. The process should start with those issues on which the constituencies agree regarding the level of resolution. Starting here establishes a mood of goodwill and cooperation; all parties get what they want. Then, issues where both parties disagree on the level of resolution should be presented. Two strategies are followed here. If the two parties agree on the importance of the issues, they are encouraged to consider a compromise within each issue. If the two parties disagree on the relative importance of the issues, the parties are encouraged to swap gains in one issue against losses in another. This is the most difficult set of discussions and should be presented at the end. The presentation order should start with easy issues on which there is agreement and move to difficult issues in which there are significant value differences.

One way to decide on the order of the issues to discuss is to examine the difference in weights assigned by the constituents. Issues with large ranges contain more conflict. For example, in Table 11.4, the biggest conflict is in "To what extent should family-planning programming be oriented toward strengthening the family?" The difference in weights in this issue is 0.16 points, larger than for any other issue. It is likely that a discussion of this issue will contain most of the conflict. The more disagreement and polarization there is about an issue, the larger the range (or variance) of the weights on it, and thus the later in the discussion it should be presented. As before, this ordering typically implies dealing with purely technical issues first and then moving gradually to the more ideological issues.

Why spend so much time determining the order in which to present and discuss issues? Primarily because when the parties assemble, they can create such an explosive atmosphere that it is good to get some agreement on some issues as quickly as possible. If a feeling of accomplishment and understanding can be instilled, the constituencies may suspend or water down their negative preconceptions of the other side and adopt a constructive, problem-solving attitude. Also, if a controversial issue cannot be resolved, the fact that some issues were settled diminishes the frustration of deadlocked negotiations and assures the constituencies that their efforts were at least partially successful.

Throughout the negotiations of differences, the analyst must keep in mind the Pareto-optimal treaties that were developed earlier with the objective outsiders. If negotiations are deadlocked, the analyst uses the fair treaties to generate a breakthrough. These Pareto-optimal treaties can prove that one constituency can improve its satisfaction without damaging the satisfaction of its opponents.

Finally, it is important to end the meeting with a concrete plan for action. If the analyst succeeded in bringing about an overall resolution and drafting a final treaty, then actions to implement this treaty should be agreed upon. On the other hand, if no treaty or only a partial treaty was obtained, the analyst should list actions that will continue the conflict analysis and resolution. Remember that conflict analysis is being done with spokespeople who must sell the resulting agreement to their constituencies.

Step 9: Present Results to all Constituents

The conflict analysis methodology is a strategy to increase the understanding of the underlying sources of conflict. This section shows how an analysis can de-escalate a conflict and increase the probability of a negotiated settlement to conflicts that seem intractable. Analysis checks this escalation by

- preventing the parties from negotiating on the overall treaty until some agreements have been reached;
- discussing issues in a sequence that minimizes frustration; and
- dividing the conflict into component issues and increasing the probability of finding a few areas of agreement.

Parties to escalating conflicts frequently forget their initial concerns and turn to trying to beat each other. The parties may think about saving face, getting even, teaching the others a lesson, or showing others that they can't get away with this. At this point, they more closely resemble a battered prizefighter than a reasonable participant in a public policy debate. When this stage has been reached, the conflict is likely to expand to other areas where it should not logically exist.

Escalation is likely to increase the number and size of the issues under dispute, as well as the hostile and competitive relations among the parties. The opponents may pursue increasingly extreme demands or objectives, using more and more coercive tactics. At the same time, whatever trust existed between the parties is likely to corrode. The ultimate stage in escalation is reached when the parties think differences exist across many issues, even some that were created solely for the sake of bargaining. A feeling of frustration settles in, along with the impression that the parties are incompatible, that compromise is impossible, and that a fight for total victory is the wisest course.

Where substantial differences exist, parties must ventilate their feelings toward each other and talk about the issues dividing them before they can seek a solution that integrates the positions of all important parties. That is, a ventilation phase generally needs to precede an integration phase. Analysis encourages, and actually demands, that parties state their positions, their perception of the sources of conflict, and their assumptions. The model-building phase usually has a cathartic effect, alleviating hostility and creating an atmosphere conducive to such an integration phase.

Conflict escalates when decision makers fail to evaluate their positions, when they are caught in self-fulfilling prophecies of biased misperceptions, and when the communication itself is distorted by distrust and hostility. Analytical approaches can prevent conflict from escalating (Raiffa, Richardson, and Metcalfe 2003) by improving communication and enhancing understanding of the underlying issues.

Summary

This chapter describes a methodology to reduce conflict and build consensus. It consists of identifying the constituencies, their assumptions, and the appropriate spokespeople to represent their position; identifying the issues underlying the conflict and possible levels of resolution; developing and analyzing treaties; and following a structured process of negotiation and consensus building to agree on a final treaty. A summary of the methodology is shown in Table 11.1.

The main sources of conflict escalation are a lack of understanding among the parties, a lack of information about the opponent's position, and an emphasis on bargaining behavior. An analysis of conflict addresses these problems by using a joint definition of the problem, emphasizing win-win solutions, and helping to minimize the impact of ideological differences by identifying areas of agreement. The logrolling procedure described in this chapter allows each party in the conflict to win in issues they care most about and lose in issues they care the least about.

The conflict analysis methodology promotes consensus building by underscoring the importance of a clear and structured resolution process, by eliciting an understanding of the positions held by the constituencies, and by finding potential trade-offs among them.

Rapid-Analysis Exercises

1. Using the data in Table 11.4, generate 20 possible treaties and calculate the value score for each constituency. Plot your data and show the treaties that are Pareto optimal in bold.
2. Produce a list of at least six issues and the possible resolutions for each issue for either resolving an end-of-life conflict among family members or negotiating a compensation employment package. Assign what you think are the appropriate weights and values that the parties would have assigned to these issues. Use the format of Table 11.7 to report the issues, the issue resolutions, the values of each resolution, and the importance of each issue to both constituents.
3. Using logrolling and your assigned weights, identify a Pareto-optimal solution to the conflict.
4. The data in Table 11.8 were obtained from three people opposed to family planning. Estimate what values are associated with the attribute levels. Make sure your estimates for values on each attribute are normalized to range from 0 to 100. (Please review the convention on constructing single-attribute value functions described in step 5 in Chapter 2.)

TABLE 11.7
Worksheet for Rapid-Analysis Exercise

Issues		*Levels of Resolutions*		*Issue Weight*		*Resolution Value*	
				Constituency 1	*Constituency 2*	*Constituency 1*	*Constituency 2*
A	Description of issue A	A1	Description of worst resolution of A			0	
		A2	Intermediate resolution of A				
		A3	Intermediate resolution of A				
		A4	Best resolution of B			100	
B	Description of issue B	B1	Description of worst resolution of B			0	
		B2	Intermediate resolution of A				
		B3	Intermediate resolution of A				
		B4	Best resolution of B			100	

TABLE 11.8
Data on One Issue from Three Respondent Opposed to Family Planning

Issues		Levels of Resolutions		Constituency 2		
				Respondent 1	*Respondent 2*	*Respondent 3*
A	To what extent should family-planning programs try to convince clients that adolescent sex is bad?	A1	Should not do so	0	0	20
		A2	Should be available to clients	20	30	0
		A3	Should be required of all clients	50	80	100
		A4	Should be a fundamental part of every service	100	100	60

Audio/Visual Chapter Aids

To help you understand the concepts of conflict analysis, visit this book's companion web site at ache.org/DecisionAnalysis, go to Chapter 11, and view the audio/visual chapter aids.

References

Alemi, F., P. Fos, and W. Lacorte. 1990. "A Demonstration of Methods for Studying Negotiations between Physicians and Health Care Managers." *Decision Sciences* 21 (3): 633–41.

Bazerman, M. H., J. R. Curhan, D. A. Moore, and K. L. Valley. 2000. "Negotiation." *Annual Review of Psychology* 51:279–314.

Bruckmeier, K. 2005. "Interdisciplinary Conflict Analysis and Conflict Mitigation in Local Resource Management." *Ambio* 34 (2): 65–73.

Dauer, E. A. 2002. "Alternatives to Litigation for Health Care Conflicts and Claims: Alternative Dispute Resolution in Medicine." *Hematology/Oncology Clinics of North America* 16 (6): 1415–31.

De Dreu, C. K., and D. van Knippenberg. 2005. "The Possessive Self as a Barrier to Conflict Resolution: Effects of Mere Ownership, Process Accountability, and Self-Concept Clarity on Competitive Cognitions and Behavior." *Journal of Personality and Social Psychology* 89 (3): 345–57.

Dooley, K. J., and B. J. Zimmerman. 2003. "Merger as Marriage: Communication Issues in Post Merger Integration." *Health Care Management Review* 28 (1): 55–67.

Hammond, J. S., R. L. Keeney, and H. Raiffa. 1998. "The Hidden Traps in Decision Making." *Harvard Business Review* 76 (5): 47–8, 50, 52 passim.

Harinck, F., C. K. De Dreu, and A. E. van Vianen. 2000. "The Impact of Conflict Issues on Fixed-Pie Perceptions, Problem Solving, and Integrative Outcomes in Negotiation." *Organizational Behavior and Human Decision Processes* 81 (2): 329–58.

Kenny, D. A., and B. M. DePaulo. 1993. "Do People Know How Others View Them? An Empirical and Theoretical Account." *Psychological Bulletin* 114 (1): 145–61.

Raiffa, H. 1982. *The Art and Science of Negotiation*. Cambridge, MA: Harvard University Press.

Raiffa, H., J. Richardson, and D. Metcalfe. 2003. *Negotiation Analysis: The Science and Art of Collaborative Decision Making*. Cambridge, MA: Belknap Press.

Ryan, M., D. A. Scott, C. Reeves, A. Bate, E. R. van Teijlingen, E. M. Russell, M. Napper, and C. M. Robb. 2001. "Eliciting Public Preferences for Healthcare: A Systematic Review of Techniques." *Health Technology Assessment* 5 (5): 1–186.

Shannon, S. E. 1997. "The Roots of Interdisciplinary Conflict Around Ethical Issues." *Critical Care Nursing Clinics of North America* 9 (1): 13–28.

CHAPTER

12

BENCHMARKING CLINICIANS

Farrokh Alemi

In hiring, promoting, and managing clinicians, managers often need to understand the efficiency and effectiveness of clinical practices. To accomplish this, they need to benchmark clinicians, usually on the basis of risk-adjusted expected cost. This chapter describes how to organize benchmarking efforts.

Why Should Clinicians Be Benchmarked?

Managers are focused on the survival of their organization, which often translates to two overarching objectives: improve productivity and increase market share. Clinicians' decision making affects both the organization's productivity and its market share. Poor clinicians are bad for the patient and for the organization. Inefficient clinicians increase the cost of care for everyone. Clinicians with poor quality of care affect the reputation of the organization and, de facto, its market share. Managers who ignore poor quality of care among their clinicians and focus on nonclinical issues are failing to see the real causes of their organization's malaise. If a manager is serious about improving the long-term financial performance of her organization, she has no choice but to address clinicians' practice patterns.

For a long time, managers have avoided addressing the quality of clinical decisions on the grounds that they do not have sufficient training to understand these decisions and because such managerial interventions would be an unwelcome intrusion in the patient-provider relationship. But are these criticisms valid? Do managers need to know medicine to understand practice patterns?

Managers can profile physicians by looking at the outcomes of their patients. They may not understand how a patient should be managed but they certainly can understand patient outcomes such as mortality, morbidity, satisfaction, health status, and numerous other measures. Managers can then compare clinicians to each other and see who is performing better. Across encounters and over time, the manager detects patterns and uses

This book has a companion web site that features narrated presentations, animated examples, PowerPoint slides, online tools, web links, additional readings, and examples of students' work. To access this chapter's learning tools, go to ache.org/DecisionAnalysis and select Chapter 12.

this information to bring about lasting changes in practice patterns. Typically, the information is provided back to a group of clinicians who identify and propagate the best practices.

The concern that benchmarking intervenes in physician and patient relationships might be a red herring. After all, practice profiles are constructed after the fact, when the patient is gone. Practice profiles do not indicate how an individual patient should be managed; rather, they identify patterns across individual visits. In short, these profiles leave the management of individual patients in the hands of the physician. There is no interference in these clinical decisions. No one tells the clinician to prescribe certain drugs or to avoid certain surgeries for a specific patient. Practice profiles document the net effect of the physician on groups of patients; these profiles provide information about a clinician's performance overall.

Practice profiles can help patients select the best clinicians. Managers need to act responsibly about who they hire and promote and practice profiles can inform them. Providers can use practice profiles to learn from each other. Patients, managers, and providers can use practice profiles, if accurate profiles can be constructed and easily communicated to them.

How Should Benchmarking Be Done?

In benchmarking, a clinician's performance is compared to the expected outcomes of her peers. This expectation is set in many different ways. This section reviews some typical methods.

Benchmarking Without Risk Adjustment: Comparing Clinicians to the Average Performance of Peers

The most common benchmarking method is to compare a clinician to the average performance of his peers. A statistical procedure for the analysis of the means of two samples (mean of outcomes for the clinician and mean of outcomes for the peer providers) is well established. Excel software contains a tool for such analysis. Analysts can use these procedures to see if the difference in means is statistically significant.

An example may demonstrate this type of benchmarking. Callahan, Fein, and Battleman (2002) set out to benchmark the performance of 123 internal medicine residents at the New York-Presbyterian Hospital in New York City. The outcomes examined included the following:

- Patients' satisfaction as measured by telephone interviews of at least ten patients of the resident;
- Disease-management profiles for an average of 7 patients with diabetes and 11 patients with hypertension. Data reported included measures of patient's condition and frequency of use of various medications; and
- Faculty evaluations on seven dimensions, including
  - History taking
  - Physical examination
  - Differential diagnosis
  - Diagnostic and treatment plan
  - Healthcare maintenance
  - Compassion
  - Being a team player

Each resident received data about her individual performance compared with the mean data for his peer group (the remaining residents). Feedback was provided once every six months. Figure 12.1 shows an example of a report received by the residents. This report shows the mean for clinician X and the overall average of all remaining clinicians.

Callahan, Fein, and Battleman's (2002) benchmarking of residents was successful. The analysis identified a variety of performance patterns among residents. Some were above average and others below. Residents reacted positively to the feedback, and some considered it as the "most comprehensive evaluation" they had received to date.

But on the negative side, this benchmarking as well as all other efforts of comparing the unadjusted mean outcomes of clinicians, is flawed. It does not account for the severity of the illness of the patients of the clinicians. On the surface, all patients may have the same illness and can be categorized together; but in reality, some patients, even those with the same disease, are sicker than others. Logically, worse outcomes are expected for sicker patients. Clinicians treating sicker patients will have below average outcomes, not because of their performance but because they started with patients who had poorer prognoses. Naturally, many clinicians question benchmarking efforts on the grounds that these efforts do not adequately account for the differences in their patient populations. To avoid these errors and to address the concerns of clinicians regarding apple-to-apple comparisons, it is important to adjust for differences of case mix among the clinicians.

FIGURE 12.1 Comparing One Resident's Performance on Satisfaction with the Average of Other Residents

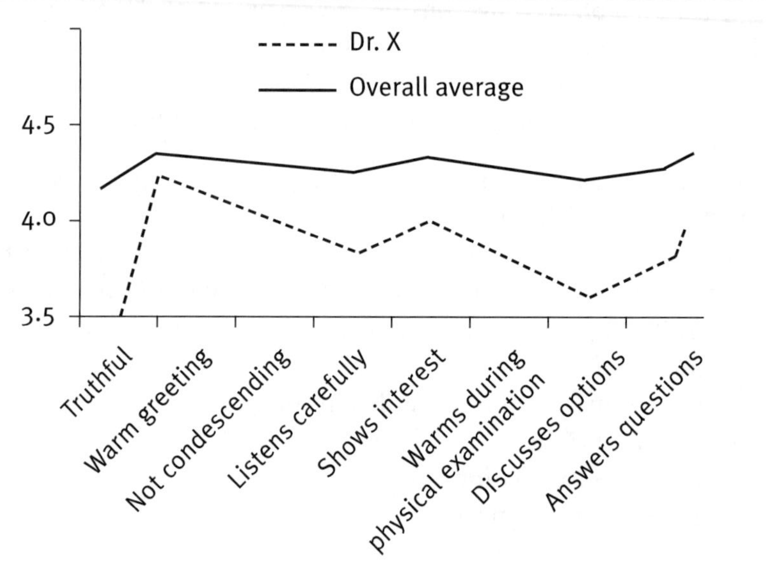

SOURCE: Callahan, M., O. Fein, and D. Battleman. 2002. "A Practice-Profiling System for Residents." *Academic Medicine* 77 (1): 34–9. Used with permission.

Risk-Adjusted Benchmarking: Comparing Clinicians to Peers on Patients of Similar Severity of Illness

Three methods of comparing clinicians on similar patients are presented here; the choice of which to use will depend on what data are available. In the first approach, the performance of the peer providers is simulated on the patients of the clinician being evaluated. First, the severity of each patient is noted and the probability of having patients in a particular severity group is calculated. If P_i is the probability of observing the patient in the severity group i, and $O_{i,\ \text{clinician}}$ is the average outcome for the clinician for severity group i, then the following formula is used to calculate expected outcomes for the clinician, $O_{\text{clinician}}$:

$$O_{\text{clinician}} = \sum P_i \times O_{i,\ \text{clinician}},$$

where i = low, medium, and high severity.

Next, the analyst projects the performance of peer providers on the type of patients seen by the clinician being evaluated. This is done by weighting the outcomes of peer providers according to the frequency of patients seen by the clinician being evaluated:

$$O_{\text{peer providers}} = \sum P_i \times O_{i,\ \text{peer providers}},$$

where i = low, medium, and high severity.

Note that in the above formula, the probability of observing a patient in a severity category comes from the clinician's practice and not from the peer provider's practice.

For example, consider that a clinician and her peers have had the outcomes displayed in Table 12.1. Is this clinician better or worse than the peer providers? To answer this question, the analyst must compare the expected outcomes for the clinician to the expected outcomes for the peer providers simulated on the same patients as the clinician.

The first step is to calculate the probability of finding a patient in a different severity grouping. This is done by dividing the number of patients in a severity group by the total number of patients seen by the clinician being evaluated. The probability of having a low severity patient is 20/120, a medium severity patient is 30/120, and a high severity patient is 70/120. This clinician mostly sees severely ill patients. Once the probabilities are calculated, the second step is to calculate the expected length of stay of the patients of the clinician being evaluated:

$$O_{\text{clinician}} = (20 \div 120) \times 3.1 + (30 \div 120) \times 3.4 + (70 \div 120) \times 5.2 = 4.4 \text{ days.}$$

To understand if 4.4 days is too high or too low, the analyst needs to compare this clinician's performance to her peer providers. But the peer providers do not see patients who are as severely ill as those of the clinician being evaluated. To simulate the performance of the peer providers on the patients seen by the clinician, the analyst uses the frequency of severity among that clinician's patients to weight the outcomes of the peer providers:

$$O_{\text{peer providers}} = (20 \div 130) \times 4.1 + (30 \div 120) \times 3.0 + (70 \div 120) \times 4.5 = 4.1 \text{ days.}$$

The clinician whose data are being analyzed seems to be less efficient than the average of her peer group. Note that in both analyses the same frequency of having low, medium, and high severity patients is used. Therefore, the differences cannot be caused by the severity of patients. Of

TABLE 12.1 Severity-Adjusted Comparison of the Performance of Several Clinicians

	Clinician		*Peer Providers*	
Severity of Patients	*Number of Patients*	*Average Length of Stay of Patients*	*Number of Patients*	*Average Length of Stay of Patients*
Low	20	3.1	80	4.1
Medium	30	3.4	10	3.0
High	70	5.2	10	4.5

course, the analysis can be misleading if the classification of patients into various severity groups is faulty or if observed differences are caused by random variations and not by real practice differences. But if the classification of patients into severity groups is correct, the fact that the projected length of stay for peer providers was lower than the clinician suggests that peer providers may be more efficient.

Risk-Adjusted Benchmarking: Comparing Clinicians to Expected Prognosis

Another way to construct meaningful risk-adjusted benchmarks for a practice is to compare observed outcomes against what would be expected from patients' prognoses. A patient's prognosis can be estimated from the patient's severity on admission (as shown in Chapter 2 by the construction of a severity index), from the patient's self-reported expectation, or from the judgment of other clinicians. Once the patient's prognosis is known, the observed outcomes can be compared and variations from the expected prognosis can be noted. For example, assume that using the Acute Physiological Chronic Health Evaluation severity index you have predicted the expected length of stay of 30 patients to be as indicated in Table 12.2.

The first step in comparing the observed and expected values is to calculate the difference between the two. Then, the standard deviation of the difference is used to calculate the *Student's t-test*. The Student t-test is used to decide if the differences between observed and expected values are statistically significant. Excel provides a program for calculating the Student's t-test in paired observations. Assume that you have obtained the results shown in Table 12.3 by using this program.

The analysis showed that the length of stay of patients of this clinician were lower than the expected values on admission. Therefore, this clinician's practice is more efficient than the expectation.

Risk-Adjusted Benchmarking: Comparing Clinicians When Patient's Severity of Illness Is Not Known

As the previous two sections have shown, in any benchmarking effort it is important to make sure that you compare clinicians on the same type of patients; otherwise, it would be like comparing apples to oranges. Every provider sees a different patient. The typical approach is to measure the severity of the illness of the patient and build that into the analysis. For example, in the first approach, patients were divided into broad categories of severity (low, medium, and high) and care provided within each category was compared. In the second approach, patients' severity of illness was used to forecast their prognoses and compare this forecast to observed outcomes. Both methods are built on access to a reliable and valid measure of

TABLE 12.2 Expected and Observed Length of Stay

Case Number	Length of Stay Expected	Length of Stay Observed	Difference	Case Number	Length of Stay Expected	Length of Stay Observed	Difference
1	5	4	1	16	4	4	0
2	7	3	4	17	6	3	3
3	6	4	2	18	3	5	−2
4	4	3	1	19	7	5	2
5	6	4	2	20	3	5	−2
6	8	6	2	21	6	5	1
7	6	3	3	22	3	4	−1
8	4	4	0	23	5	4	1
9	4	3	1	24	3	4	−1
10	3	3	0	25	5	4	1
11	7	3	4	26	3	4	−1
12	4	4	0	27	5	4	1
13	5	3	2	28	3	3	0
14	6	3	3	29	4	4	0
15	4	4	0	30	5	5	0

TABLE 12.3 Comparison of Expect and Observed Values Using Student-Statistics in Excel

	Expected	*Observed*
Mean	4.80	3.90
Variance	2.10	0.64
Observations	30.00	30.00
Pearson Correlation	0.10	
Hypothesized Mean Difference	0.00	
Degrees of freedom	29.00	
Student's t-test	3.11	
$P(T \le t)$ one-tail	0.00	
Critical one-tail	1.70	
$P(T \le t)$ two-tail	0.00	
Critical two-tail	2.05	

the severity of illness. However, sometimes such measures are not available or available measures do not adequately measure the full spectrum of the severity of the patient's illness. This section provides an alternative method of benchmarking that does not require the availability of a valid and accurate severity index.

When no severity index is available, an analyst must still make sure that apples are compared to apples by matching the patients seen by different providers feature by feature. The expected outcome for the clinician being evaluated is calculated as

$$O_{\text{clinician}} = \sum P_{j,\ldots,m}\, O_{j,\ldots,m,\ \text{clinician}} \quad \text{for all values of } j_{,\ldots,m},$$

where

- $j_{,\ldots,m}$ indicates a combination of features j through m;
- $P_{j,\ldots,m}$ indicates the probability of these features occurring; and
- $O_{j,\ldots,m,\ \text{clinician}}$ indicates the clinician's outcomes when these features are present.

The expected outcome for the peer providers is calculated in a similar fashion, with one difference:

$$O_{\text{peer providers}} = \sum P_{j,\ldots,m}\ O_{j,\ldots,m,\ \text{peer providers}} \text{ for all values of } j_{,\ldots,m}.$$

In this calculation, the probabilities are based on the frequency of features among the patients seen by the clinician being evaluated, but the outcomes are based on the experience of peer providers. By using this formula, the analyst is simulating what the expected outcomes would have been for peer providers if they had the same patients as the clinician being evaluated.

An example can demonstrate the use of this procedure. Table 12.4 shows 20 patients of one clinician and 24 patients of her peer providers. These patients were admitted to a hospital for myocardial infarction (MI). In each case, two features were recorded: existence of a previous MI and presence of congestive heart failure (CHF). Obviously, a patient with a previous MI and with CHF has a worse prognosis than a patient without these features. The analyst needs to separate outcomes for patients with and without specific characteristics.

An *event tree* can be used to organize the data. An event tree is a decision tree without a decision node. Each feature can be used to create a new branch in the event tree. For example, the event tree for the patients seen by the clinician is provided in Figure 12.2.

Using the data in Table 12.4, the analyst can group patients and calculate the probabilities and average cost for clinician's patients. Figure 12.3 shows the result.

The expected length of stay for the patients of the clinician being evaluated is 5.4 days. This is obtained by folding back the tree to the root node. Starting from the right (the highlighted area in the formula), each node is replaced with the expected length of stay:

$$\text{Expected length of stay} = \underbrace{[6 \times 0.65 + 5 \times (1 - 0.65)]}_{\text{Expected value for top node to the right}} \times (0.85) + \underbrace{(4 \times 1.0 + 0)}_{\text{Expected value for bottom node to the right}} \times (1 - 0.85) = 5.4.$$

TABLE 12.4 Patients of the Clinician and Peer Providers May Differ in Severity of Illness

Clinician's patients				*Peer Provider's Patients*			
Case No.	*Previous MI*	*CHF*	*Length of Stay*	*Case No.*	*Previous MI*	*CHF*	*Length of Stay*
1	Yes	Yes	6	1	Yes	Yes	6
2	Yes	No	5	2	Yes	Yes	6
3	Yes	Yes	6	3	No	Yes	4
4	Yes	Yes	6	4	No	No	3
5	Yes	Yes	6	5	No	Yes	4
6	Yes	No	5	6	No	Yes	4
7	Yes	Yes	6	7	Yes	Yes	6
8	Yes	No	5	8	Yes	Yes	6
9	Yes	Yes	6	9	Yes	Yes	6
10	Yes	No	5	10	Yes	Yes	6
11	Yes	Yes	6	11	Yes	Yes	6
12	No	Yes	4	12	No	No	3
13	No	Yes	4	13	No	Yes	4
14	No	Yes	4	14	No	Yes	4
15	Yes	Yes	6	15	No	Yes	4
16	Yes	Yes	6	16	No	Yes	4
17	Yes	Yes	6	17	No	Yes	4
18	Yes	No	5	18	No	No	3
19	Yes	No	5	19	Yes	No	5
20	Yes	Yes	6	20	Yes	Yes	6
				21	Yes	Yes	6
				22	Yes	Yes	6
				23	Yes	No	5
				24	No	Yes	4

Procedures for folding back a tree were described the Chapter 5. To simulate how the same patients would have been cared for under the care of peer providers, the event tree is kept as before, but now the average length of stay of each patient grouping is replaced with the average length of stay of patients of the peer providers. Table 12.5 provides the average length of stay of patients seen by peer providers.

If one combines the event tree from the clinician's patients and the outcomes of peer providers, the result is the graph in Figure 12.4.

The expected stay (obtained by folding back the tree in Figure 12.4) of the patients of the peer providers is 5.4 days. Thus, the clinician being evaluated and the peer provider have similar practice patterns. Note that if the event tree had not been changed to reflect the probabilities of patients seen by the clinician, the expected length of stay for patients seen by the provider would have been 5.75 days; this would have led to the erroneous conclusion that the clinician is more efficient than his peer. This example

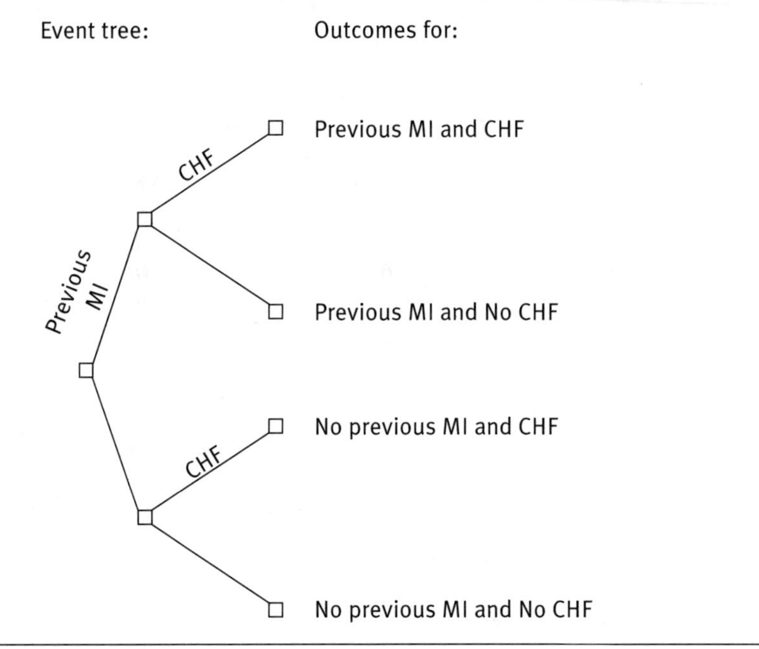

FIGURE 12.2 An Event Tree for the Clinician's Patients

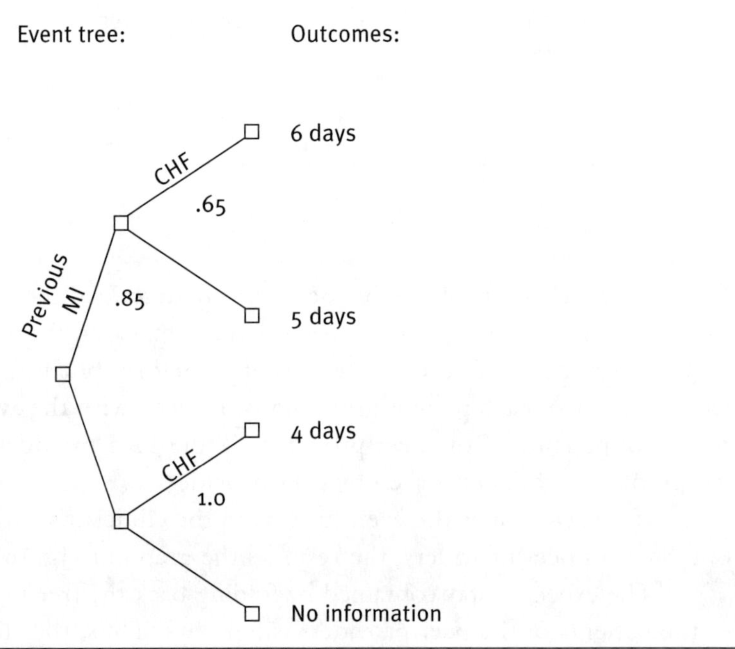

FIGURE 12.3 The Probability and Length of Stay for Different Patient Groups Seen by Clinician

highlights the importance of simulating the performance of peer providers on the patients seen by the clinician.

As the number of features increase, the number of data points that fall within each path on the decision tree becomes smaller. Soon, most

TABLE 12.5 Length of Stay and Probability of Observing Various Types of Patients Among Peer Providers' Patients

		Previous MI	
		No	*Yes*
CHF	*No*	3 days .13	5 days .08
	Yes	4 days .38	6 days .42

FIGURE 12.4 Projected Performance of Peer Providers on the Clinician's Patient

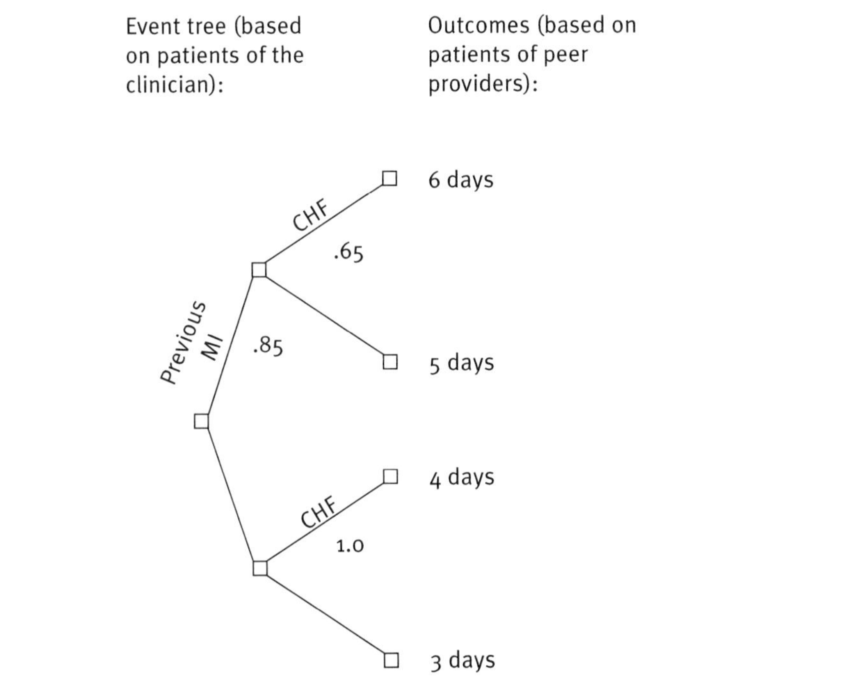

paths will have no patients. Many peer providers' patients cannot be matched on all features to the clinician's patients. When the features available do not match, the analyst can use expected outcomes to replace missing information. For example, consider if the only feature available among the clinician's patients was the presence of previous MI. No information was available on CHF for these patients. Now the event node available on the clinician's patient is as shown on the left of Figure 12.5. In addition, the outcomes for the peer providers need to be calculated as the expected outcomes. Note that from Table 12.5 and for patients of the peer providers,

FIGURE 12.5 Projecting Peer Providers' Performance on the Clinician's Patient When Only "Previous MI" Feature Is Available

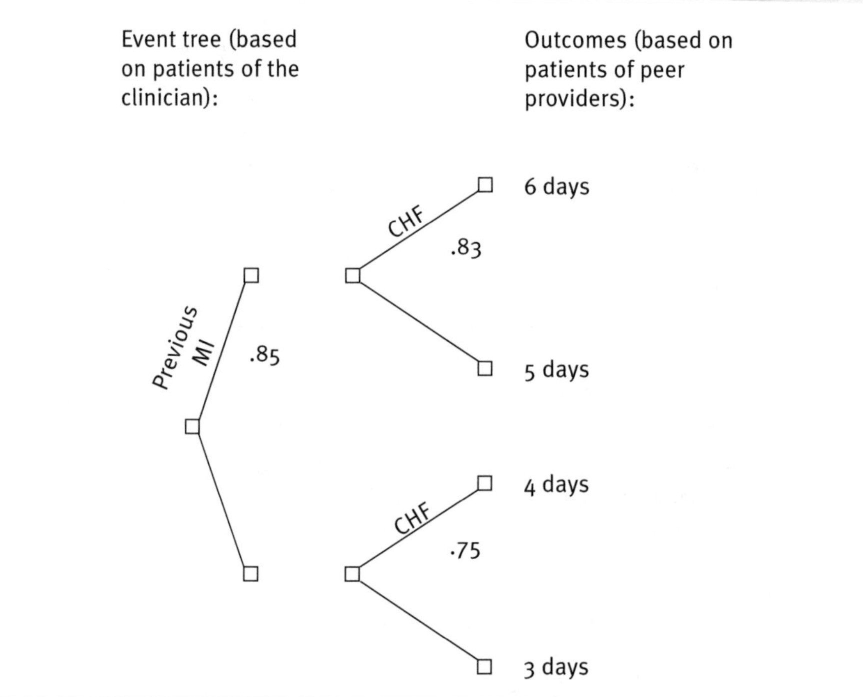

the probability of CHF for patients who have had a previous MI is calculated as

$$\text{Probability of CHF given a previous MI} = \frac{.42}{.08 + .42} = .83.$$

Similarly, the probability of CHF for patients who have not had a previous MI can calculated as

$$\text{Probability of CHF given no previous MI} = \frac{.38}{.13 + .38} = .75.$$

Figure 13.5 shows these probabilities and the outcomes used to calculate the expected outcome of the peer providers on patients seen by the clinician being evaluated.

The expected outcome for the peer providers is given as

$$O_{\text{peer providers}} = .85 \times .83 \times 6 + .85 \times (1 - .83) \times 5 + (1 - .85) \times .75 \times 4 + (1 - .85) \times (1 - .75) \times 3 = 5.5 \text{ days.}$$

One way to think about this procedure is that you have simulated the performance of peer providers on the patients of the clinician being evaluated by replacing the probabilities with the corresponding values from the clinician's experience whenever such probabilities are available. When such values are not available, you should continue to use the probabilities from the experience of peer providers.

It is also possible that some features are found in the patients seen by the clinician being evaluated but not among the patients seen by the peer providers. In these circumstances, the expected outcome for peer providers is calculated on the basis of the event tree of the clinician being evaluated, and truncated to features shared among the clinician and the peer providers. Thus, if it is not clear among the peer providers' patients if they had CHF, then the event tree used to simulate the performance of peer providers is based on the experience of the clinician but without the CHF feature. In this fashion, the clinician and the peer providers can be compared even when features of some of the patients do not match the others' features.

When no features are shared between the patients seen by the clinician being evaluated and the patients seen by peer providers, the procedure provides an unadjusted comparison of the mean of the two groups. As the number of features shared between the two groups increases, there are more adjustments for the severity of illness of the patients.

What Are the Limitations of Benchmarking?

When the number of features on which patients of the clinician and peer providers must be matched increases, a visual display of the data through a decision tree is no longer feasible. Furthermore, because no two cases are likely to match on all features, strict feature-by-feature comparisons are not possible. In these situations, a modified approach is needed. One such modification is to weight patients in the clinician's care according to the similarity of these patients to the peer provider cases. Tversky (1977) proposed a method of assessing the similarity of two patients by examining features they share and features they do not share. Alemi, Haack, and Nemes (2001) used Tversky's approach to compare patients with similar, but not exactly the same, features.

When, because of a large number of features, decision trees are not used for benchmarking clinicians, they remain useful as a method of explaining how the analysis was done. The tree structure helps clinicians get a sense that like patients are being compared to each other. It reassures them that the analysis has followed their intuitions about comparing similar patients to each other.

Is it Reasonable to Benchmark Clinicians?

Risk assessment is not as benign as it first looks. When a clinician's performance is measured and the clinician is provided with feedback, several unintended consequences may occur:

1. *Measurement may distort goals.* Clinicians may improve their performance on one dimension but inadvertently deteriorate on another. For example, if the manager emphasizes length of stay, clinicians may improve on this measure but inadvertently increase the probability of rehospitalization because they have sent patients home too early. People tend to focus on what is measured and may ignore other issues. To avoid this shortcoming, it is important to select the benchmarking goals broadly and to select multiple benchmarks.
2. *Measurement may lead to defensive behavior.* Clinicians may put their effort or time in defending their existing practices as opposed to improving them. To avoid this pitfall, it is important to engage the clinicians in selecting the performance indicators and the severity index. Managers can ask clinicians what they want to be evaluated on and how they wish to measure the severity of their patients. Furthermore, it is important to make sure that feedback to each clinician is provided privately and without revealing the performance of any single peer provider. It is okay to share the average of the peer providers, as long as the identity of each provider remains anonymous. The focus of feedback should be on everyone, not just on the clinicians with poor performance. An environment needs to be created where no one is blamed and all clinicians are encouraged to seek improvements as opposed to argue about the results.
3. *Inadequate measure of severity may mislead the analysis.* A poor severity index, one that is not predictive of the patients's prognosis, might give the impression of severity adjustment but in reality be no better than a random guess of outcomes. In these circumstances, an unadjusted benchmark is better because at least it does not give the appearance of what it is not. To avoid this pitfall, it is important to select a severity index that has high predictive power.
4. *Too much measurement may lead to too little improvement.* Sometimes analysts who conduct benchmark studies take considerable time to collect information and analyze it. In these circumstances, too little time may be spent on discussing the results, selecting a new course of action, and following up to make sure that the change is an improvement. It is important to keep in mind that the goal of benchmarking is improvement. Conducting an accurate analysis is only helpful if it leads to change and improvement; otherwise, it is a waste of time.

For more details about the risk of benchmarking, see Iezzoni 1997; Hofer et al. 1999; and Krumholz et al. 2002.

Presentation of Benchmarked Data

Presenting benchmarked data should be done in a fashion that helps clinicians improve their practices as opposed to act defensively. Poorly presented information leads to unnecessary and never-ending debates about the accuracy of the information presented. The Agency for Healthcare Research and Quality, the Centers for Medicare and Medicaid Services, and the Office of Personnel Management sponsored a working group on how to talk about healthcare quality.[1] The group made a number of suggestions on the presentation of benchmarked information. The following is a modification of the group's suggestion to fit within the context of benchmarking clinicians.

Before the Meeting

Check the Data

A simple mistake in benchmarked data will undermine the perception of the validity of the entire data set. To avoid this, check the accuracy of the data thoroughly before the meeting, making sure that all variables are within range and that missing values are appropriately handled. Prepare histograms of each individual variable in the analysis and review them to make sure they seem reasonable.

Prepare Graphs and Pictures

To help clinicians have an intuitive understanding of statistics, it is important to provide them with visual displays of data. Show data and summary statistics using bar charts and *x-y* plots.

Plan to Do it in Person

It is important to present benchmarked information in person to clinicians, allowing open question-and-answer periods. The presentation session should be scheduled ahead of time and well in advance.
Prepare handouts for discussion during the session. Distribute handouts to participants ahead of the meeting. Make sure that handouts are stamped "draft" and that the date of final report is clearly reported.

Prepare Stories

Supplement numeric data with anecdotal information that conveys the same message. Make sure that the anecdotes do not reflect judgments about quality of care but focus on the data being reported (i.e., patient's condition or patient outcomes). Provide an example of a typical patient complaint (usually in the form of a short video- or audiotape). It is important to weave the story or the anecdotal data with the voice of the customer.

At the Meeting

Confidential Evaluation

Make it clear that the evaluation is confidential. If you are talking to a group of clinicians, do not identify who is the best or worst. The analyst may let each clinician privately know how they performed against the group, but should not provide this information publicly.

Brief Introduction

Make a brief introduction of the purpose of the session. Introduce your project team, and ask clinicians to introduce themselves. Even if they know each other, still ask them to introduce themselves so they feel more comfortable in the meeting setting.

Limitations of Benchmarking

Acknowledge the limitation of the practice profiling method. Explicitly say that numbers could be misleading if the measures of severity are not adequate or the sample size is small. Point out that the focus should be on improvement and not measurement issues.

Start with a Customer's Story and Voice

Start the meeting by playing a brief tape of a customer talking in her own words about what happened to him. Use both positive and negative vignettes.

Present the Data and Not the Conclusions

Present the findings without elaboration about causes or explanations. Do not give advice about how clinicians can do things differently. Say, for example, "Data show that patients stay longer in our hospital than in comparable hospital" rather than "You should shorten the time it takes to discharge hip fracture patients." It is up to the clinicians to change and decide how to change; benchmarking just points out the variation in outcomes and facilitates the clinicians to focus on specific issues. What clinicians do depends on them. During the presentation, the analyst guides the clinicians through the data. The data and not the analyst help clinicians to arrive at a conclusion and to act.

Ask for Input

Explicitly ask for the audience's evaluation of the data after each section of the report is presented. Allow the clinicians to talk about the data by pausing and staying quiet. Say, for example, "Data show large variations on how long it takes us to discharge a patient with hip fracture. What do you think about that?" Pause and let participants talk about the variation in hip fracture data. The point is not to troubleshoot and come up with solutions on the spot but to discuss the issues and think more about causes.

Accept Criticism

The analyst should not defend the practice profiling method, the benchmarking effort, or any aspect of the analysis. Let the work speak for itself and accep suggestions for future improvements. Shift the discussion from blaming the study to what can be done to improve in the future.

Thank the clinicians for their time and describe next steps (e.g., "I will correct the report and get it back to you within a week.").

Plan for the Next Step

After the Meeting

After the meeting is complete, the analyst should summarize the comments made during the meeting and append it to the report. Also, the analyst should describe the resources that were available to the clinicians (e.g., travel funds that were provided to attend meetings for a presentation of best practices).

Revise the Report

Send a written report to each clinician. Please note that reports have a way of lasting well beyond the time for which they were generated. Make sure that all providers' identities are removed.

Distribute the Report

Ask the clinicians to comment on the following:

Ask for Feedback

1. What worked well regarding the practice profiles, and what needed improvement?
2. Do clinicians plan to change their practice? If so, in what way?
3. Was it worthwhile to gather data and do benchmarking? Why or why not?

Once the reports have been completed and distributed and after the analyst has asked for feedback, it is time to schedule the next round of benchmarking.

Announce the Next Report

Summary

This chapter outlines the use of decision analysis for benchmarking clinicians. Clinicians associated with poor quality of care negatively impact the organization by decreasing productivity and market share. Clinicians can be evaluated by examining patient outcomes, such as morbidity or client satisfaction, so that managers can compare the performance of clinicians without infringing upon the doctor-patient relationship. Several methods for benchmarking clinicians are described in this chapter, including benchmarking with and without risk adjustment. Benchmarking without risk adjustment compares clinicians to the average performance of peers. Benchmarking with risk adjustment compares clinicians to peers based on patients of similar severity of illness; when severity of illness is not known, patients of two clinicians can be matched feature by feature, creating an event tree. The use of an event tree allows an analyst to evaluate what will happen if one physician would have taken care of another clinician's patients.

Review What You Know

In the following questions, assume that you have collected data for two clinicians, Smith and Jones, and constructed the decision trees in Figure 12.6:

1. What is the expected length of stay for patients of each of the clinicians?
2. What is the expected cost for Dr. Smith if he were to take care of patients of Dr. Jones?
3. What is the expected cost for Dr. Jones if she were to take of patients of Dr. Smith?

Rapid-Analysis Exercises

Through Medline, select a disease area where a decision analysis of preferred course of action is available. Suppose you would like to benchmark three clinicians who are practicing in this area. Using the analysis found, carry out the following activities:

1. Design the forms you would use to collect information about patient's severity of illness (base the severity index on a measure published in the literature) and patient outcomes (use a standardized instrument).
2. Complete the forms for ten hypothetical patients using arbitrary answers.
3. Create a report analyzing the data.
4. Prepare for the presentation of your data (anecdotes telling customer's story, graphs, text of the presentation) using the procedures outlined in the chapter.

Audio/Visual Chapter Aids

To help you understand the concepts of benchmarking clinicians, visit this book's companion web site at ache.org/DecisionAnalysis, go to Chapter 12, and view the audio/visual chapter aids.

Note

1. See http://www.talkingquality.gov/docs/section1/default.htm.

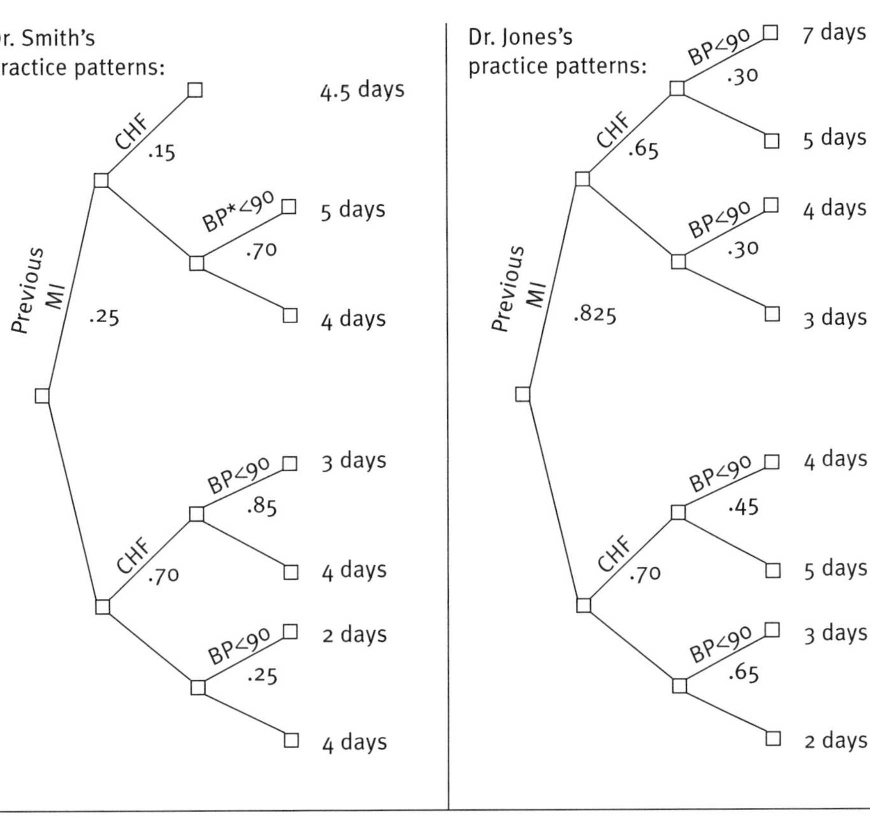

FIGURE 12.6 Practice Patterns of Two Doctors

* BP = blood pressure.

References

Alemi, F., M. R. Haack, and S. Nemes. 2001. "Continuous Improvement Evaluation: A Framework for Multisite Evaluation Studies." *Journal of Healthcare Quality* 23 (3): 26–33.

Callahan, M., O. Fein, and D. Battleman. 2002. "A Practice-Profiling System for Residents." *Academic Medicine* 77 (1): 34–9.

Hofer, T. P., R. A. Hayward, S. Greenfield, E. H. Wagner, S. H. Kaplan, and W. G. Manning. 1999. "The Unreliability of Individual Physician 'Report Cards' for Assessing the Costs and Quality of Care of a Chronic Disease." *JAMA* 281 (22): 2098–105.

Iezzoni, L. I. 1997. "The Risks of Risk Adjustment." *JAMA* 278 (19): 1600–7.

Krumholz, H. M., S. S. Rathore, J. Chen, Y. Wang, and M. J. Radford. 2002. "Evaluation of a Consumer-Oriented Internet Health Care Report Card: The Risk of Quality Ratings Based on Mortality Data." *JAMA* 287 (10): 1277–87.

Tversky, A. 1977. "Features of Similarity." *Psychological Review* 84 (4): 327–52.

References

CHAPTER

13

RAPID ANALYSIS

Farrokh Alemi

Analysis takes time and reflection. People must be lined up and their views sought. Ideas need to be sorted through. Data need to be collected, stored, retrieved, examined, and displayed. Calculating the formulas, writing the report, and presenting the findings takes time—and it should. All of this delays a decision maker's access to the final report. Often at the end of this grueling effort, analysis identifies the need for further inquiry, and therefore it creates more delays for decision makers. Something should be done to speed up analysis. Rushing through an analysis is not advocated here, but keep in mind that a late report is a wasted analysis. Timing matters. When reports are late, policymakers and managers may have to decide without the full benefit of the analysis, and many do.

This chapter focuses on how an analysis could be done more quickly without sacrificing its quality. Clearly, doing a thoughtful analysis takes time. There is no point to hurry and produce a suboptimal analysis. But there are ways to complete the analysis faster and yet maintain the quality of the work. An examination of what takes time in the analysis process suggests places where one can speed up the work without affecting the quality of the report. One could imagine analysis consisting of four distinct phases:

1. Preparation
   a. Arrange for contracts and mandate to start
   b. Coordinate kickoff meeting to clarify the purpose and scope of the analysis
   c. Find relevant experts and decision makers
   d. Design study instruments and survey forms
2. Data collection
   a. Collect observations
   b. Collect experts' opinions
   c. Store data
3. Analyze data
   a. Retrieve data
   b. Clean the data (classify data, check distribution and range of data, edit data)

This book has a companion web site that features narrated presentations, animated examples, PowerPoint slides, online tools, web links, additional readings, and examples of students' work. To access this chapter's learning tools, go to ache.org/DecisionAnalysis and select Chapter 13.

   c. Examine the accuracy of the data (check for errors in logic or in transfer of data)
   d. Examine whether experts are in consensus
   e. Calculate expected values or model scores
   f. Calculate the correspondence between the model and experts' judgments
4. Presentation
   a. Distribute draft report
   b. Prepare presentation
   c. Get input from audience before meeting
   d. Present results at meeting

If each of these phases can be speeded up even a little, then the whole analysis can be completed more quickly. This chapter addresses how this can be done.

Phase 1: Speed Up Analysis Through More Preparation

Thorough preparation can lead to significant time savings in conducting an analysis. This section lists specific recommendations regarding what should be done to be better prepared.

Step 1: Draft the Final Report at the Start

One of the simplest steps an analyst can take to reduce the time from the start of the project (signing the contract) to the end of the project is to do more thorough planning. In particular, it is helpful to draft the final report (the introduction, methods section, results section), with all related tables and appendices at the start of the project (Alemi et al. 1998). Obviously, the data will not be available to fill the report, but one could put in best guesses for the data. This exercise speeds up an analysis in several ways. First, it communicates precisely to decision makers what the final results will look like. Second, it reduces confusion and saves the time spent on clarifying the procedures of the analysis. Third, it clarifies to the analyst what data are needed and identifies the sources of these data. Finally, it clarifies what procedures should be followed to produce the tables and figures in the report. Obviously, the data and the final report will be different, but the exercise of putting the report together at the beginning of the project goes a long way in making sure that only relevant data are collected and that time is not wasted on diversions.

A good example of drafting the report before the data are available is the process of generating automatic content on the web. The text of the report is prepared ahead of the data collection, and portions of the report that depend on specific data are left as a variable to be read from a database. When the data are available, the final report is generated automatically.

Step 2: Avoid Group Kickoff Meetings

Another step that can speed up preparations is to meet individually with decision makers, even before the full kickoff meeting. Individual meetings are easier to arrange and require less coordination. Furthermore, as discussed in the Chapter 6, individual meetings facilitate larger face-to-face meetings later in the process.

Step 3: Get Access to the Right Experts Who Have Access to the Right Data

A third step is to search for external experts who understand the situation clearly and do not require additional time to orient themselves. On any topic, numerous experts are available. Finding the right expert is difficult but important in saving time and gaining access to resources that only the expert has access to. Automated methods of finding experts in a particular topic are widely available. One such tool is the Medline database (see http://www.nlm.nih.gov/medlineplus). One could search a topic in Medline and find authors who have published on the topic. Most articles include contact information for the author. In this fashion, one could quickly put together a list of experts in a topic—no matter how narrowly it is defined. For example, suppose the analyst needs to examine merger between two hospitals. First, the analyst accesses the PubMed search page (www.pubmed.gov). Here, a search for "hospital mergers" can be conducted. Next, PubMed will display the articles relevant to the search query. The analyst examines the results and notes the authors. Finally, PubMed will display the authors' affiliations and contact information after a search result is selected. These steps are shown in Figure 13.1.

In addition to searching the Medline databases, it may be useful to search CRISP, a database of National Institutes of Health funded projects (see http://crisp.cit.nih.gov). CRISP is useful in identifying researchers

FIGURE 13.1 Three Steps to Identifying Relevant Subject Matter Experts

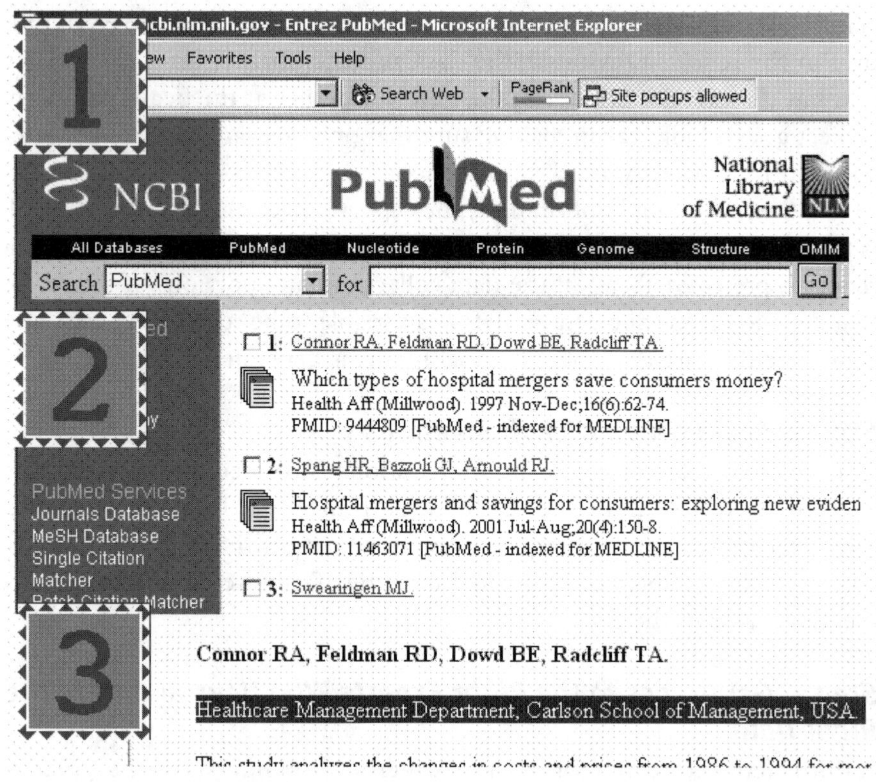

who are currently collecting data. Many have likely thought through the issue being analyzed and may have preliminary data that could be useful. Finally, search Google's scholar database (see http://scholar.google.com) for names of people who might have special expertise or knowledge of the issue being modeled.

Once a preliminary list has been identified, the analyst contacts members of the list and asks them if they are aware of others who are doing research in this area, who might have access to specific databases, or who might be able to provide valid opinions on estimates needed in the analysis. The important advice is to use automated databases to widely search for one or two people who best fit the planned analysis. Choosing the right person can significantly improve your access to various pieces of information and, in the process, reduce the time it takes to complete the analysis.

Phase 2: Speed Up Data Collection

Often, the data needed for the analysis are not available and must be collected or deduced from data that are available. There are numerous steps in which the analyst can reduce the data collection time (Alemi et al. 1998). Following is a description of these steps.

Step 4: Collect Only the Needed Data

No one sets out to collect data they do not need, but many do so anyway. When one compares the data used in reports and data collected, there is a great deal of difference between the two. Much data are collected but not reported. Some of this discrepancy is because one cannot anticipate the results of data collection. Occasionally, one collects data only to learn that the findings do not merit reporting. But sometimes one can anticipate what data will be relevant and reduce data collection by dropping irrelevant items. Some collect more demographics about their patients than they need to or will likely report. Others use standardized tools that collect data about various topics, most of which are not needed. Collecting more data than needed may waste time and resources. Unfortunately, the time and resources wasted are not directly experienced by the survey designer; he is often not the person who responds to the survey, collects the data, or even analyzes the data. Not surprisingly, survey designers are usually not sensitive to time pressures involved in collecting and analyzing data. But if one takes a larger perspective—the organization's perspective—the value of short surveys and quick data collections become more apparent. Short surveys will collect less data, have better response rates, and waste less of the organization's resources. In most surveys, the analyst needs to think through the various data needs carefully, making sure that the data collected will be reported and that the data missed are not needed. This chapter has already covered how preparing the final report ahead of time reduces the amount of data collected, as many pieces of data that do not make their way into the report are dropped from the data collection plans. In addition, the analyst may wish to go through each question to verify not that the response may be interesting but that the responses will be pivotal to the decision. If the findings are not directly related to a specific decision, then the analyst may want to drop the item from the data collection effort.

Step 5: Reduce the Data Collected by Sampling

One way to reduce the data collection burden is to reduce the number of patients surveyed through sampling. A representative sample allows the analyst to infer the population characteristics from the average of the sample. Typically, the larger the number of people surveyed, the longer the time for the completion of the analysis. Sometimes, months can be cut out of data collection by reducing the sample of people surveyed. Some decision makers are not familiar with sampling procedures and therefore miss the advantage of these techniques in reducing the data collection burden. They may insist on surveying all patients about their satisfaction when only a sample will do. An analyst should work with decision makers to highlight the importance of sampling and how it will reflect the population characteristics. Decision makers who are uncomfortable with sampling should be reminded that if a sensitivity analysis shows that the additional data could reverse the conclusions of the analysis, more data will be collected.

Sampling can be made more effective in at least two ways. One way is to start with a small group of people and, if unexpected results are obtained, expand the sample to a larger group of people. First, a small sample is drawn. If it leads to clear unequivocal conclusions, then no more data are collected. If the results are ambiguous, then a larger sample is drawn. Thus, for example, one may agree to sample 20 representative patients about their satisfaction with the new process. If less than 5 percent are dissatisfied, then no more samples are drawn. If more than 5 percent of the respondents are dissatisfied, then a larger sample of 50 patients is drawn. This method of two-stage sampling[1] reduces the number of patients that need to be contacted and thus reduces the time it takes to collect the information (see Posch, Bauer, and Brannath 2003; Schafer and Muller 2004).

Another method of reducing the data collection burden is to shift from sampling the event to measuring the time to the event. If an analyst needs to collect information about a phenomena that is rare, she needs to collect large samples of data to measure the frequency of the event. For example, if the analyst needs to estimate the probability of wrong-site surgery, many patients need to be reviewed before a sufficient number of wrong-site surgeries are identified to accurately measure this probability. An alternative is to calculate the probability of the event from the time between reoccurrences of the event. For example, one can radically reduce the number of patients examined by looking at the time between two wrong-site surgeries. Details of how the time between events can be used to estimate probability of the event are provided in Chapter 9. Here, it is sufficient to point out that this approach radically reduces the data collection burden (Benneyan 2001a; 2001b).

Step 6: Replace Data Collection with Observations of Others

When an analyst collects data, he is observing the frequency of a target event. In the absence of conflicts of interest, there are no reasons to expect that the analyst is a better observer of the event than others who are familiar with the process. In fact, one would expect that an expert familiar with the process or an employee engaged in the process may know more about what to observe, when to pay attention, and how to define the target event than an analyst, who is typically new to the process. For this reason, whenever possible, it is preferable for the analyst to rely on the observations of others as opposed to setting up her own data collection. Numerical data obtained from experts' or employees' observations of a process are often referred to as *subjective data*. When the analyst observes the same process and calculates the same data, it is referred to as *objective data*. These two labels are unfortunate because they imply that one is more accurate than the other. Note that subjective data do not refer to the likes and dislikes of a person, which are idiosyncratic and unreliable. Subjective data rely on the observations of others. Thus, a nurse's claim that patients' satisfaction has improved is based on the nurse's observation of the frequency of the patients' complaints, not on his likes and dislikes. Both subjective and objective data are suspect. Subjective opinions are distrusted when the estimator has a vested interest, the event estimated is not observed frequently by the estimator, the question asked is different from typical questions faced by the estimator, the estimator has limited expertise in the area, only one person's judgment (not a group's judgment) is sought, tools typically available (calculator and various reports) are not made available to the estimator, and estimators are not trained in the estimation process. Objective estimates are distrusted when the target event is poorly defined, the target event changes in nature over a long data-collection period, data-collection procedures are not kept consistent over time, frequent data-entry errors occur, and important nuances and exceptions are not accounted for. But if subjective opinions can be measured accurately, then subjective data can be as accurate as objective data (McManus et al. 2002; Marcin et al. 1999) and can radically reduce the data collection burden. Of course, the analyst does not need to choose between the two and can use both methods simultaneously. An example of how subjective and objective data can be combined to save time is presented later in this chapter.

Step 7: Validate Subjective Indexes on Objective Data

If experts specify the parameters of a model (e.g., the utility or probabilities in a multi-attribute value model), then there is no need to put aside data for parameter estimation; thus, the need for data is drastically reduced. For example, severity indexes can be constructed from subjective opinions and tested against objective data. When doing so, less data are needed. An objectively constructed index needs data equal to ten times the number of variables in the index. For an index with 20 variables, 200 data points are needed. In contrast, if the index is developed based on experts' opinion, then the aggregate severity score is one variable. Testing the accuracy of this single variable against objective data requires very little data: 10 to 30 cases.

Step 8: Plan Ahead for Rapid Data Collection

Data collection can be completed more quickly if various preliminary steps for data collection are taken before it is clear what data should be collected. The analyst approaches employees close to the process and alerts them that the team plans to ask them a few questions. They are told that the exact nature of the questions is not clear; but the procedures used to send the questions to them and collect the questions are explained and perhaps even practiced. Employees' consent to respond is collected, and the importance of timely response is emphasized. When the need for data becomes clear, the analyst broadcasts the questions to all who have given consent, usually through a telephone message or an e-mail, and collects the response within a few hours. For example, suppose you want to know about changes in substance abuse rates within the United States. Emergency department staff of a sample of hospitals are approached and asked to participate in the study when a specific question is e-mailed to them. Consent is obtained, and a practice run is made once every six months. Then, when the policymakers have a specific question, the network is used to obtain the response. For example, if policymakers want to know if heroin is replacing cocaine as the drug of choice, the analyst would e-mail participating emergency department staff to count the number of people who have used heroin or cocaine. Within days, the responses are collected and the analysis is provided. Of course, much time and effort goes into maintaining networks of informants and consents, but the result is spectacular: data made available when the policymaker needs it.

Step 9: Let Technology Collect the Data

Computers can now automatically call patients, find them in the community, ask them questions, analyze the responses, and fax the results to the analyst. In one study, Alemi, Stephens, and Butts (1992) asked a secretary and a computer to contact "hard to reach" persons and ask them a few questions. On average, the secretary was able to do the task in 41 hours, while the computer accomplished the same task in nine hours. Technology can help overcome the difficulty of finding people.

When technology is used to collect information from people, there is one added benefit: People are more likely to tell the truth to a machine than to a person. In surveys of drug use, homosexuality, and suicide risks, patients were more likely to report their activities to a machine than to a clinician, even though they were aware that the clinician would subsequently review the computer summary (Newman et al. 2002; Williams et al. 2000; Kissinger et al. 1999; Griest et al. 1973). Another advantage of collecting data through computer interviews is that data are immediately available, and no time needs to be spent on putting the data into the computer after collection. A number of reviews of the effectiveness of various technologies for data collection are available (see Shapiro et al. 2004; Newman et al. 2002).

Phase 3: Speed Up Data Analysis

When data are available, several steps can be taken to make the analysis go faster.

Step 10: Clean the Data and Generate Reports Automatically

To speed up analysis, the analyst puts together procedures for cleaning the data even before the data are available. At the simplest level, the analyst prepares reports of the distribution and the range of each variable. Such reports can then be examined to see if there are unusual entries. A computer program can then be prepared to run various tests on the data to make sure the responses are within range (e.g., no one with negative age) and responses do not conflict with each other (e.g., no pregnant men). The computer can examine the patterns of missing information and their reasons (i.e., not applicable, data not available, data applicable but not provided). This is typically done by calculating the mean of data items entered in previous cases and testing if the current data item is more than three standard deviations away from the mean. To ensure integrity and accuracy of data, the computer can select a random number of cases for reentry. The point is that procedures for cleaning the data can be automated early in the process so that the analyst can rapidly proceed as soon as data are available.

Another alternative that has been made possible because of the growth of web services is to allow reports to be generated from data automatically. First, the analyst drafts the report with all of the variables in the report linked to a database. Then, the analyst prepares a data collection procedure which populates the database. Third, the computer cleans the data and generates the report. This process is used in a web site, maintained by Alemi and Newhauser (2006), that tracks personal improvement. Clients who complete their personal improvement report their success and failure on the web. The data are collated by the computer, which cleans and stores the data in a web database. A report is automatically generated from the data on the web so that current and future clients can see the success rate of clients engaged in the personal improvement effort. The report is available instantaneously after the data are collected.

Step 11: Analyze Emerging Patterns Before all Data Are Available

Many readers are familiar with exit polling to predict results of elections. The same procedures can be used to anticipate data findings before a complete data set is available. One very useful tool is to predict the probability of an event from the time it takes for the event to reoccur. In this fashion, early estimates of the data can be made from just two reoccurrences of the event. If the event is rare, it takes a long time for it to reoccur. If not, it will reoccur in a short interval. By examining the interval between the event, the probability of the event can be estimated.

Step 12: Use Software to Analyze Data

One way to conduct a sensitivity analysis quickly is to use software designed to conduct decision analyses. Many of the existing software programs automatically conduct single- and two-variable sensitivity analyses. Reviews[2] of software for decision analysis are available online (Hazen 2002).

Phase 4: Speed Up Presentation

An analysis is not done until the sponsor examines the results. To speed up the presentation, several steps can be taken.

Step 13: Set Up Presentation Meeting Months in Advance

Many decision makers are busy. To arrange for their time, make an appointment many months in advance. If a presentation date is set, it will create pressure to produce the findings on time. In addition, if the project falls behind schedule, then additional resources can be brought to the task to accomplish the project on time and present it as planned. A useful tool is to calculate backwards from the presentation date and see which tasks are critical for the presentation and which tasks have slack and are not critical. Software, such as Microsoft's project management software, can help identify the critical paths so that the project can finish on time.

When a date is set for presentation, the decision maker is more aware of the report and may delay deciding on the decision until the report becomes available. Waiting is always made easier if it is clear when the wait will be over. Consider if you were asked to wait to board a flight but were not told how long the wait will be—five minutes or several days. Many find it easier to wait when they know what to expect.

Step 14: Present to Each Decision Maker Privately Before the Meeting

Even though a joint meeting is coming up, it is important to present to each decision maker separately and get their input so that the analysis can be revised in time for the meeting. As discussed in Chapter 6, research shows that obtaining a decision maker's input individually before the group meeting is important in having a successful meeting.

An Example of Rapid Analysis

One of the most complicated concepts regarding speeding up decision analysis is the process of relying on subjective opinions to speed up data collection. To illustrate this point, consider an example of how Gustafson, Cats-Baril, and Alemi (1992) combined experts' opinions with objective data to analyze a fast-moving policy decision. Gustafson was asked to predict the effect of national health insurance (NHI) programs on five low-income populations. The implementation of NHI would have profound effects on people who currently rely on federal programs administered by the Bureau of Community Health Services (BCHS) in the Department of Health and Human Services. These groups include migrant farm workers, Native Americans, mothers and children needing preventive or special care, residents of medically underserved areas, people desiring family-planning services, and those lacking adequate health insurance coverage. The unique circumstances of migrant workers and Native Americans necessitated the creation of special services responsive to their needs. If NHI results in termination of such assistance, the result could be a financial burden on current beneficiaries and a reduction in their access to care.

To accurately appraise changes that would occur under NHI, Gustafson had to find the utilization patterns of families served by the BCHS and the unit costs of services consumed. He also had to ascertain the eligibility requirements and cost-sharing provisions of the NHI proposal. Finally, he had to determine which currently used services would be included in the various NHI benefit packages. Primarily because of time constraints, he could not collect data and was confined to using the best available information.

Utilization patterns were created for individual family members (for each BCHS program) and stratified into appropriate age groups. Utilization patterns for individuals were then aggregated to achieve a family utilization description. The computer also determined the extent of coverage under different NHI schemes and compared this figure to present costs. Before directing the computer to simulate a sample of user families, Gustafson needed information on family characteristics, particularly about the population's socioeconomic and demographic status. These characteristics included such factors as the number and size of families, age and gender of family members, employment status, whether employment was longer than 400 hours per year per employer, size of employing firm, income levels, and Medicaid status. This information was primarily collected from U.S. census data on populations served by the BCHS.

The simulation also required frequency distributions of utilization rates for each of a set of health services (such as hospitalizations or prenatal visits) for each existing BCHS project. Separate distributions were created for different levels of age and income. In many cases these preliminary estimates were national averages for use of the particular service. In some cases, Gustafson decided that the best estimates of utilization came from regional sources, such as the Community Health Survey or the Mental Health Registry. The quality and reliability of these estimates were highly variable. Equally important, the available data reflected populations significantly different from BCHS users. Therefore, Gustafson brought together 80 experts to estimate the missing parameters. Some of these experts were project directors with experience caring for BCHS clients at organizations with reliable data systems; others were researchers who had studied utilization of BCHS programs.

Gustafson showed the panel of experts the utilization estimates from existing sources. Panelists were told the source of the data and were asked to revise the estimates in light of their experience. Each panel was then divided into groups of four and asked to discuss their estimates. Each group within each panel concentrated on a single user population. For example, at the community health center meeting, one table represented rural health centers, another represented small urban centers, and two others represented large urban health centers. Following their discussions, each panelist made final, independent estimates.

The revised utilization rates were aggregated into one set of estimates for each service. The aggregation across the experts was done by weighting the estimates according to the proportion of the total BCHS user population each estimate represented. For instance, the estimates of rural health center panelists received less weight than large urban health centers because fewer people participate in rural programs.

To simulate current costs to BCHS user families under NHI, Gustafson used expert-estimated distributions, the observed demographics, and the various provisions of the NHI proposal to simulate what might

TABLE 13.1 Estimated Annual Costs for Community Health Centers

	Current BCHS Cost ($)	*Costs Under NHI ($)*
Total cost of care	1,222	1,222
Payments by BCHS	64	n/a
Payments by third parties (Medicaid, Medicare, private insurance)	470	8
Payments by NHI	n/a	685
Premiums paid by users	7	92
Deductibles, copayments	109	529
Total cost to users	116	621

happen. The simulation was run for a total of 500 families. A different set of families was, of course, generated for each BCHS program. Table 13.1 depicts one sample result.

The simulation was repeated under different NHI bills and proposals and for different BCHS populations. The key surprise finding was that NHI would raise barriers to access rather than remove them, at least for several segments of the poor. A sensitivity analysis was done to see how much the estimated variables had to change before the conclusions of the analysis would change.

The point of this example was to show how a rapid analysis could be done through a combination of objective data and subjective probability. Subjective estimates from respected experts can be effective surrogates for solid empirical data.

Concluding Remarks

Technology is changing the world. Computers are faster and more available than before. Technology has changed expectations of time for analysis. If it takes only a second to search the entire web, why should an analysis take months? As media-savvy decision makers take control of healthcare organizations, they bring with them an expectation of rapid but comprehensive analysis. They see that software can reduce the data analysis time. They see that computers can reduce the data collection time. Today, most word processing and slide presentation software programs come with templates for generating reports. So, naturally, they see that templates can reduce report preparation time. When managers see that an analysis can be done in a short time, they come to expect it.

Consider the manufacturing industry in the past century. When Ford implemented industrial engineering time-and-motion studies to reduce the time it took to create cars, the entire industry changed. The cost of car production dropped and new consumers came to market. The automobile, which was previously handcrafted, was suddenly mass produced. A time-and-motion study can do the same for decision analysis. Sure, it is a unique product, but the steps in completing a decision analysis are well known and can be speeded up. You have seen some of the ideas for speeding up an analysis in this chapter. If rapid analysis is possible, if the time drops from months to days, then decision analysis will be more readily available. Naturally, the market for analysis and evidence-based decision making may grow.

Many of the ideas presented here require an analyst to spend more time thinking through the analysis. In a way, the analyst's planning time is being traded against the organization's time for collecting data, or the decision maker's waiting time. Well-planned efforts take less time to execute, but they do take more time to plan. It may be naive to think that the analyst has the extra time to spend on planning. Because the person who plans the analysis, the person who executes it, and the person who receives it may be different, rapid analysis is a burden for one person and a nirvana for another. If organizations want to produce rapid analysis, they need to set the right incentives for all parties involved. They need to recognize that not all individuals involved have the same goal.

Summary

This chapter has shown 14 ways of speeding up analysis without affecting the quality of the work:

1. Draft the final report at the start
2. Avoid group kickoff meetings
3. Get access to the right experts who have access to the right data
4. Collect only the needed data
5. Reduce the data collected by sampling
6. Replace data collection with observations of others
7. Validate subjective indexes on objective data
8. Plan ahead for rapid data collection
9. Let technology collect the data
10. Clean the data and generate reports automatically
11. Analyze emerging patterns before all data are available
12. Use software to analyze data
13. Set up the presentation meeting months in advance
14. Present to each decision maker privately before the meeting

Some of these techniques may seem pedantic; could you, for example, save much time if you reduce the data collected by one case? Other techniques may be inappropriate in some settings; for example, why rely on subjective judgments when experts disagree on the issues? Whether these techniques work and when they are effective in speeding up analyses have not been demonstrated empirically. It is not clear, for example, how much time will be saved if all 14 rules were followed. The methods of speeding up analyses are in their infancy, and much work and investigation is needed to make sure that they are effective.

Review What You Know

1. Thorough planning speeds up report creation. What are the primary reasons why drafting the final report at the start speeds up the analysis?
2. Experts are naturally familiar with the subjects of their expertise. But how could you, as a person not familiar with the field, find the right expert? What is an automated method of finding experts in a particular topic?
3. Researchers often overestimate the need for data. When is a small sample adequate?
4. Subjective and objective data can be used for research. When can subjective opinions be a reliable source of data?
5. Explain how a 200-variable model could be validated with only 50 cases as opposed to ten times the number of variables in the model?
6. Why would automated data collection not only be faster but also more accurate than data gathered by individuals?
7. All statistical sources can have problems with missing data, noise, and outliers. What is the value of setting procedures for cleaning the data even before it is collected?
8. There are ways to anticipate data findings before a complete set of data is available. How can the early estimate of the probability of an event be assessed from two observations of the event?
9. In the example analysis for the BCHS, which data were subjective and not from primary sources?

Rapid-Analysis Exercises

In groups of three, conduct a time-and-motion study of how students complete the rapid-analysis exercises in your class. Analyze at least three

TABLE 13.2
Worksheet for Reporting Time Spent in Analysis

Task	*Start Date*	*End Date*	*Total Work Hours*
1. Preparation			
• Receive assignment and understand the work to be done			
• Coordinate kickoff meeting to clarify purpose and scope of the work			
• Find relevant experts and decision makers			
• Design study instruments and survey forms			
2. Data collection			
• Collect observations			
• Collect experts' opinions			
• Store data			
3. Analyze data			
• Retrieve data			
• Clean the data (classify data, check distribution and range of data, edit data)			
• Examine accuracy of data (check for errors in logic or in transfer of data)			
• Examine if experts were in consensus			
• Calculate expected values or model scores			
• Calculate the correspondence between the model and experts' judgments			
4. Presentation			
• Prepare report and distribute draft report			
• Prepare presentation			
• Get input from audience before meeting			
• Present results at meeting			

student projects to see the time various activities take and suggest how the work can be speeded up. Table 13.2 suggests a set of tasks, although you may want to focus on other tasks as well.

In your report, analyze the total time lapsed between the start and end of each task and the total time spent working on the task. Explain why there is a difference between lapsed time and time worked on the task. For each task, describe what can be done to reduce the difference between lapsed and worked time.

Describe the prerequisites of each task by showing what needs to be accomplished before the task is started. Use a table such as Table 13.3 in your report

TABLE 13.4 Worksheet for Describing Task Prerequisites

Task	*Cannot Start Until the Following Task Is Completed*
1. Receive assignment and understand the work to be done	
2. Coordinate kickoff meeting to clarify purpose and scope of the work	
3. Find relevant experts and decision makers	
4. Design study instruments and survey forms	
5. Collect observations	
6. Collect experts' opinions	
7. Store data	
8. Retrieve data	
9. Clean the data (classify data, check distribution and range of data, edit data)	
10. Examine accuracy of data (check for errors in logic or in transfer of data)	
11. Examine if experts were in consensus	
12. Calculate expected values or model scores	
13. Calculate the correspondence between model and experts' judgments	
14. Prepare report and distribute draft report	
15. Prepare presentation	
16. Get input from audience before meeting	
17. Present results at meeting	

Review the task prerequisites to identify the critical path (these are tasks that, if delayed, would delay the completion of the project). Provide advice on how to start on critical tasks sooner and what to do to remove the dependency between the critical task and its prerequisites.

Then, review the 14 recommendations in this chapter and describe how they are the same or different from your recommendations.

Audio/Visual Chapter Aids

To help you understand the concepts of rapid analysis, visit this book's companion web site at ache.org/DecisionAnalysis, go to Chapter 13, and view the audio/visual chapter aids.

Notes

1. See Bauer, P., and W. Brannath. 2004. "The Advantages and Disadvantages of Adaptive Designs for Clinical Trials." *Drug Discovery Today* 9 (8): 351–7.
2. See the review of decision analysis software prepared by Dennis Buede for the Decision Analysis Society at http://faculty.fuqua.duke.edu/daweb/dasw.htm.

References

Alemi, F., S. Moore, L. Headrick, D. Neuhauser, F. Hekelman, and N. Kizys. 1998. "Rapid Improvement Teams." *Joint Commission Journal on Quality Improvement* 24 (3): 119–29.

Alemi, F., and D. Neuhauser. 2006. *A Thinking Person's Guide to Weight Loss and Exercise*. Victoria, BC, Canada: Trafford Publishers.

Alemi, F., R. C. Stephens, and J. Butts. 1992. "Case Management: A Telecommunications Practice Model." In *Progress and Issues in Case Management*, edited by R. S. Ashery, 261–73. Rockville, MD: National Institute on Drug Abuse.

Benneyan, J. C. 2001a. "Performance of Number-Between G-Type Statistical Control Charts for Monitoring Adverse Events." *Healthcare Management Science* 4 (4): 319–36.

———. 2001b. "Number-Between G-Type Statistical Control Charts for Monitoring Adverse Events." *Healthcare Management Science* 4 (4): 305–18.

Griest, J. H., D. H. Gustafson, F. F. Strauss, G. L. Rowse, T. P. Langren, and J. A. Chiles. 1973. "A Computer Interview for Suicide-Risk Prediction." *American Journal of Psychiatry* 130: 1327–32.

Gustafson, D. H., W. L. Cats-Baril, and F. Alemi. 1992. *Systems to Support Health Policy Analysis: Theory, Models, and Uses*. Chicago: Health Administration Press.

Hazen, G. B. 2002. "Stochastic Trees and the StoTree Modeling Environment: Models and Software for Medical Decision Analysis." *Journal of Medical Systems* 26 (5): 399–413.

Kissinger, P., J. Rice, T. Farley, S. Trim, K. Jewitt, V. Margavio, and D. H. Martin. 1999. "Application of Computer-Assisted Interviews to Sexual Behavior Research." *American Journal of Epidemiology* 149 (10): 950–4.

Marcin, J. P., M. M. Pollack, K. M. Patel, B. M. Sprague, and U. E. Ruttimann. 1999. "Prognostication and Certainty in the Pediatric Intensive Care Unit." *Pediatrics* 104 (4 Pt 1): 868–73.

McManus, R. J., J. Mant, C. F. Meulendijks, R. A. Salter, H. M. Pattison, A. K. Roalfe, and F. D. Hobbs. 2002. "Comparison of Estimates and Calculations of Risk of Coronary Heart Disease by Doctors and Nurses Using Different Calculation Tools in General Practice: Cross Sectional Study." *BMJ* 324 (7335): 459–64.

Newman, J. C., D. C. Des Jarlais, C. F. Turner, J. Gribble, P. Cooley, and D. Paone. 2002. "The Differential Effects of Face-to-Face and Computer Interview Modes." *American Journal of Public Health* 92 (2): 294–7.

Posch, M., P. Bauer, and W. Brannath. 2003. "Issues in Designing Flexible Trials. *Statistics in Medicine* 22 (6): 953–69.

Schafer, H., and H. H. Muller. 2004. "Construction of Group Sequential Designs in Clinical Trials on the Basis of Detectable Treatment Differences." *Statistics in Medicine* 23 (9): 1413–24.

Shapiro, J. S., M. J. Bessette, K. M. Baumlin, D. F. Ragin, and L. D. Richardson. 2004. "Automating Research Data Collection." *Academic Emergency Medicine* 11 (11): 1223–8.

Williams, M. L., R. C. Freeman, A. M. Bowen, Z. Zhao, W. N. Elwood, C. Gordon, P. Young, R. Rusek, and C. A. Signes. 2000. "A Comparison of the Reliability of Self-Reported Drug Use and Sexual Behaviors Using Computer-Assisted versus Face-to-Face Interviewing." *AIDS Education and Prevention* 12 (3): 199–213.

INDEX

ABOUT THE AUTHORS

Farrokh Alemi, Ph.D., is a professor of health administration and policy in the College of Health and Human Services at George Mason University in Fairfax, Virginia. His research focuses on the use of decision analysis in both individual and organizational change. His research on individual change focuses on structural life changes and on monitored self-experimentation to tailor prescriptions and healthcare interventions. His research on organizational change includes online management of patients; cost-effectiveness analysis, root-cause analysis of sentinel events such as terrorism; and physician practice profiling, for which he holds a pending patent on measuring episodes of illness. He has founded and served on the boards of TelePractice, Inc. and Interpractice, Inc., both of which focus on the online management of patients. He is a member and past president of the Health Application Section of the Institute for Operations Research and Management Science (INFORMS) and was a member of the Federal Science Panel on Interactive Communications in Health. He is currently serving as an advisor to the Substance Abuse and Mental Health Service Agency. Dr Alemi earned his doctoral degree in decision analysis, his master's degree in system analysis, and his bachelor's degree in industrial engineering from the University of Wisconsin-Madison.

David H. Gustafson, Ph.D., is a research professor at the University of Wisconsin–Madison, director of the Center of Excellence in Cancer Communications funded by the National Cancer Institute, and director of the Network for the Improvement of Addiction Treatment funded by The Robert Wood Johnson Foundation and the federal government's Center for Substance Abuse Treatment. He is also coleading a new Robert Wood Johnson Foundation program to implement evidence-based practices in addiction treatment agencies and state governments. His research focuses on the use of systems engineering methods and models in individual and organizational change. He is a Fellow of the Association for Health Services Research and of the American Medical Informatics Association, and he is also a Fellow and past vice-chair of the board of the Institute for Healthcare Improvement. He chaired the Federal Science Panel on Interactive Communications in Health, is chair of the eHealth Institute, and is a member of the Institute of Medicine Committee on Redesigning Health Insurance. Dr. Gustafson earned his doctoral, master's, and bachelor's degrees in industrial engineering from the University of Michigan-Ann Arbor.

ABOUT THE CONTRIBUTORS

William Cats-Baril, Ph.D., is a professor of information and decision sciences in the School of Business at the University of Vermont in Burlington. He has been a senior research fellow at the London School of Economics and Political Science and has been a visiting professor at several international institutions, including INSEAD in Fontainebleau, France; Reykjavik University in Iceland; the International Management Center in Budapest, Hungary; the International Executive Development Centre in Bled, Slovenia; and the China–Europe Management Institute in Beijing. Professor Cats-Baril teaches courses on business strategy, customer orientation and total quality management (TQM), and decision analysis in executive development programs in Asia, Europe, and North and Latin America. Dr. Cats-Baril is a consultant, with an international practice in TQM and program evaluation. He has trained executives in a variety of settings, including healthcare organizations, Fortune 500 companies, and government agencies. Dr. Cats-Baril has published more than 30 articles and book chapters in the management literature on business strategy, conflict resolution and negotiation, and implementation of change.

Kathryn B. Laskey, Ph.D., is an associate professor in the department of systems engineering and operations research at George Mason University in Fairfax, Virginia, where she teaches and performs research on computational decision theory. She has served on a National Academy of Sciences committee to assess the statistical validity of the polygraph and is a member of the Committee on Applied and Theoretical Statistics of the National Academy of Sciences. Dr. Laskey received her doctoral degree in statistics and public affairs from Carnegie Mellon University in Pittsburgh, Pennsylvania, her master's degree in mathematics from the University of Michigan-Ann Arbor, and her bachelor's degree in mathematics from the University of Pittsburgh.

Jennifer A. Sinkule is a doctoral candidate in clinical psychology at George Mason University in Fairfax, Virginia. Her clinical work is focused on multicultural adolescents and adults, many of whom are new or recent immigrants and refugees to the United States. She has participated in a statewide needs assessment for traumatic brain injury, contracted by the Pennsylvania

State Department of Health. Ms. Sinkule earned her master's degree in psychology from George Mason University and her bachelor's degree in psychology from the University of Pittsburgh in Pittsburg, Pennsylvania. She has published research regarding online treatment for individuals with traumatic brain injuries and their caregivers, as well as for individuals with schizophrenia and their families.

Jee Vang is a doctoral candidate at the School of Computational Sciences at George Mason University in Fairfax, Virginia. His research interests are in artificial intelligence and data mining, and his doctoral work focuses on learning causal probabilistic networks. He has worked in software engineering for eight years as a programmer and architect. Mr. Vang earned his master's degree in health services administration from The George Washington University in Washington, DC, and his bachelor's degree in biology from Georgetown University in Washington, DC.